Hypnoanalytic Techniques

Hypnoanalytic Techniques

The Practice of Clinical Hypnosis

Volume II

John G. Watkins, Ph.D.

IRVINGTON PUBLISHERS, INC.
NEW YORK

Irvington Publishers, Inc.,
Executive offices: 522 E. 82nd Street, Suite 1, New York, NY 10028
Customer service and warehouse in care of: Integrated Distribution Services,
195 McGregor St, Manchester, NH 03102, (603) 669-5933

Library of Congress Cataloging-in-Publication Data
(Revised for vol. 2)

Watkins, John G. (John Goodrich), 1913-
        The practice of clinical hypnosis.

        Includes indexes.
        Bibliography: p. v. 1, p. 357-378.
        Contents: v. 1. Hypnotherapeutic techniques—v. 2. Hypnoanalytic
techniques.
        1. Hypnotism—Therapeutic use. I. Title.
[DNLM: 1. Hypnosis—methods. WM 415 W335p]
RC495.W35 1987   615.8'512   87-2597
ISBN 0-8290-1462-4 (v. 1)
ISBN 0-8290-1463-2 (v. 2)

First Printing 1992
1 3 5 7 9 10 8 6 4 2

Printed in the United States of America

Table of Contents

Foreword

This second volume on *The Practice of Clinical Hypnosis* fulfills the promise made in the first volume that appeared in 1987. That volume began with a survey of the history of hypnosis and considered the various approaches to hypnotherapy, most of which had a directive or supporting orientation. This second volume, by its emphasis upon psychoanalytic techniques, gives consideration to an interest revived after a period in which the interest in psychodynamic techniques had cooled. It is to be hoped that through combining hypnosis with some of the practices used in Freudian psychoanalysis the results of time-consuming standard psychoanalysis can be approximated in a shorter period of hypnoanalysis.

This volume is designed to elucidate the use of hypnotherapeutic techniques through giving detailed procedures for adapting such processes as hypnodiagnostic evaluation, the utilization of abreactive techniques, dreams and fantasies, projective techniques, dissociation, transference and counter-transference, and related techniques as rooted in both psychoanalysis and hypnosis.

Each of the chapters is followed by an outline that provides the reader with a convenient review of the topics considered. The data presented and the interpretations are buttressed by an ample list of references to over 350 relevant studies.

The text provides many detailed illustrations of actual interchanges with patients as tape-recorded by the author and his wife, Helen, a fellow-therapist. While some are vignettes to clarify specific examples of the recommended practices, there are also a half dozen fuller case reports showing the interactions in successive sessions, and the ultimate outcomes.

The text will prove useful to all clinicians who are friendly to the use of hypnosis in clinical practice, regardless of their special interest in hypnoanalysis. For those who may be offering instruction in clinical hypnosis, an Instructor's Manual is provided gratis to users of either the first or the second of these volumes.

Because of the author's long experience in the use of hypnotic techniques, his long familiarity with psychoanalysis, his care in recording what goes on between client and therapist, and his interest in relating clinical findings to theoretical interpretations, this book should move forward the acceptance of clinical hypnosis among the healing professions.

Ernest R. Hilgard
Stanford University

Introduction
to Volume II

These two volumes on Clinical Hypnosis aim to provide teaching textbooks for use in introductory and advanced courses in medical schools, psychiatric institutes, graduate schools of psychology, societal workshops and other professional training facilities. They are specifically designed for the needs of the therapist learning the field of treatment by hypnosis and also to serve as reference works.

In *Vol. I Hypnotherapeutic Techniques* the "History" and major "Theories of Hypnosis" were described. These were followed by chapters on "Hypnotic Phenomena," "Suggestibility Tests" and "Induction Techniques." Attention was given to the role of "The Hypnotherapist and the Principles of Hypnotic Induction." Hypnotherapeutic techniques were then described for use in "Surgery, Anesthesiology and the Control of Pain," "Obstetrics and Gynecology," and in "Internal Medicine and General Practice." A section on "Special Conditions," such as smoking, nail biting, stuttering, hiccoughs, alcoholism, drug addiction, weight reduction, insomnia, faulty study habits and applications in the field of sports psychology, was followed by chapters on "Dental Hypnosis" and "Hypnosis with Children." The final chapter in Vol. 1. dealt with "Precautions, Dangers and Contra-Indications" in the use of hypnosis.

The present work, *Vol. 2. Hypnoanalytic Techniques* picks up where Vol. I left off. It covers the more complex hypnotic proceeedures which might be taught in an advanced course. The orientation is eclectic-psychoanalytic.

An Instructor's Manual covering both Volumes I and II is available which presents lecture outlines, practicum exercises, audio-visual instructional aids and test questions designed to assist the clinical instructor. It is available from Irvington Publishers to teachers in the field.

In Chap. 1 of Vol. I we surveyed the history of hypnosis, its significant practitioners and the many changes in the way it was viewed and employed therapeutically. Not only hypnosis, but also the entire field of psychological treatment, has undergone continuous revision. Like the alternating periods of enthusiasm and neglect for hypnosis different approaches in all psychotherapy have changed in popularity over the last seventy years.

At the turn of the century, before Freud's views were known, the more directive or supportive approaches were widely accepted. These included suggestion, reassurance, advice, and manipulation (Alvarez, 1951; Coué, 1922; Déjerine, J. & Glauckler, E, 1913; Dubois, P., 1909; Levine, M., 1942; Thorne, F.C., 1950; (see also Watkins, J.G., 1960, Part II.). The patient came to the doctor, described his symptoms, and was told what to do. The treatment manner was in the traditional medical mode.

As the discoveries of Freud and his associates became more widely known psychoanalysis, or at least a psychoanalytically oriented therapy, became "king." The older directive methods of symptom manipulation were scornfully dismissed by dynamically oriented therapists as superficial and not long-lasting. Although Freud discarded hypnosis various analytically-minded practitioners did make efforts to practice "reconstructive" therapy through an integration of hypnosis and "dynamic" (psychoanalytic) understanding. A British psychiatrist, Hadfield (1940), is generally credited with first coining the term "hypnoanalysis."

As interest in psychoanalytic therapies reached a new high during the period after World War II (1945-1960) a number of publications on hypnoanalysis appeared (Brenman & Gill, 1947; Gill & Brenman, 1959; Lindner, 1944; Schneck, 1954; Watkins, 1949, 1952; Wolberg, 1945,1948). Some books on hypnoanalysis (Schneck, 1965; Meares, 1961) continued to appear during the 1960's, but the prevailing interest in psychotherapy was in behavior therapy, a treatment approach which emphasized symptomatic change in the here and now, and which was not concerned with "unconscious" processes (Franks, 1969). During this period psychoanalysis itself was de-emphasized, and in hypnotherapy there was more interest in applying hypnotic suggestion to a wide variety of disorders (Kroger and Fezler, 1976).

In the late 1970's many behaviorists became again interested in "mental" processes and developed the approach known as "cognitive" therapy (Beck, 1976; Mahoney, M.J., 1977; Meichenbaum, 1977).

Unconscious processes, now termed "covert behavior", (Cautella and Bennett, 1981) were again a topic of respectful "scientific" study.

By the 1980's a renewed interest in psychoanalytic therapies appeared. This was heralded by the development of many new psychoanalytic institutes for the training of psychologists and other non-medical practitioners. A new division (No. 39) of the American Psychological Association was formed to advance the study and practice of psychoanalysis.

Within the field of psychoanalysis itself the earlier attention to "drive theory" (Fenichel, 1945), in which personality functioning and psychopathology was felt to ensue from "Id" drives and their expression through various psychosexual stages of development, was challenged, first, by "Ego Psychology" (Freud, A., 1946; Hartmann, 1958) where attention was focused on the nature of ego defenses rather than on those "drives" which were being defended against. Today there is considerable controversy between the more "classical" theorists and the "object-relation" theorists such as Guntrip (1961), Mahler (1978), Kernberg (1972), Kohut (1978), Winicott (1965) and others.

Object relations analysts emphasize the development of the child from early autism through various stages in relation to the mother figure, to "separation-individuation," whereby the infant acquires an independent "self" structure. The classical hysterical neuroses (around which "drive" theories were first formulated) are seen less commonly today, and the object-relations theorists address themselves increasingly to the treatment of borderline and psychotic conditions. Hypnoanalytic techniques as related to these more recent psychoanalytic theories will be dealt with in Chapter 9, Ego-State Therapy and Chapter 10, Transference and Counter-transference.

This same renewed interest in unconscious processes and the psychodynamic motivations underlying symptoms has sparked a current return of many hypnotherapists back toward the more complex hypnoanalytic techniques which had been described by earlier contributors. Accordingly, it seems it is time now that a new and more up-to-date treatise on hypnoanalytic techniques be launched.

The Field of Hypnoanalysis

It was stated in the Introduction to Volume I (Watkins, 1987) that Volume II would pick up where the initial treatise left off. Those therapists who have acquired the ability to hypnotize and apply suggestive hypnotherapeutic procedures will probably recognize their need to acquire more complex ways of hypnotic intervention, techniques which have been hinted at, but not truly described in Volume I.

Hypnoanalytic techniques are sophisticated procedures, practiced within the hypnotic modality, which are aimed at a more fundamental reconstruction of a patient's personality—as is the goal of psychoanalysis and psychoanalytic therapy. Hypnoanalysis accepts the psychoanalytic principle that neurotic symptoms are generally the consequence of intra-psychic conflict. It aims to reduce or eliminate symptoms by cognitive and emotional restructuring, not merely by suggestion or manipulation. This process is usually accompanied by "insight." Accordingly, hypnoanalysis should be considered a form or variant of psychoanalysis in its broadest sense. Freud (1953a) said that any treatment can be considered psychoanalysis which works by "undoing resistances and interpreting transferences." By these criteria hypnoanalysis is definitely "psychoanalysis" in spite of Freud's rejection of hypnosis, since hypnoanalysts are very much concerned with undoing resistances and interpreting transferences—as will be clear in later chapters.

In actual practice suggestive tactics (especially when applied according to psychodynamic understanding) may also be part of the hypnoanalytic treatment strategy. The therapy becomes "hypnoanalytic" when its suggestive aspects are secondary to the main objective of achieving reconstructive understanding.

Like psychoanalytic practitioners, hypnoanalysts attempt to recover memories, lift repressions, release bound affects and integrate previously unconscious and un-egotized aspects of the personality. They are also concerned with factors of resistance, transference and counter-transference as are psychoanalysts. Like Freud (1953b), hypnoanalysts recognize dreams as a "royal road to the unconscious," and dream interpretation is a major hypnoanalytic technique. Their theoretical views of personality structure and neurotic symptom formation are similar to those of psychoanalysts.

Free association does ultimately un-earth early memories, but many sessions are required to secure the same data which within a shorter time may become apparent through hypnotic hypermnesia or regression. Moreover, in so doing there is little evidence to support Freud's contention that the ego is by-passed, and that consequently personality changes are only temporary. Recent research (Hilgard and Loftus, 1979) has shown that memories under hypnotic regression may be distorted, but Freud found that through "screen memories" the recollections secured by free association could also be distorted. No data seems to be available comparing the validity of hypnotically secured memories versus those elicited through free association.

Dream interpretation has been a valuable psychoanalytic tool, especially in the hands of gifted and intuitive analytic practitioners—such as Wilhelm Stekel (1943c). Hypnoanalysts also employ dream and fantasy analytic procedures (Chap. 6) since the hypnotic modality affords great flexibility in activating, analyzing and interpreting these creations.

The *analysis of transference reactions* is a potent psychoanalytic procedure for achieving reconstructive changes in the basic personality. Such reactions appear during an analysis when the patient projects onto the analyst feelings and attitudes which he/she once experienced toward earlier significant figures (such as a loved mother or a dominating father). As these inappropriate reactions are pointed out to the patient by the analyst's interpretations new insights and growth are achieved. However, many weeks and months often elapse before such responses develop and become manifest in a psychoanalytic relationship. Not only do they develop more rapidly in the hypnoanalytic situation (See Chap. 8), but the patient's regression (Menninger & Holzman, 1973) which brings this about, can be better achieved and "controlled" earlier since hypnosis is, itself, a regression—and one "in the service of the ego" (Gill and Brenman, 1959).

Other techniques like "Hypnodiagnostic Procedures" (Chap. 8) and revitalized "Abreactive Techniques" (Chap. 4) appear to have remedied early criticisms voiced by Freud and Breuer (1953). "Hypnography and Sensory Hypnoplasty (Chap. 5) suggest other ways of deriving information about unconscious processes than by verbalizations alone. Through hypnotically manipulated "Dissociative" (Chap. 9) and "Projective" (Chap. 7) approaches an even greater degree of flexibility is offered the psychoanalytic practitioner. "Ego-State Therapy" (Chap. 10) represents an extension of dissociative techniques that suggest another dimension in psychoanalytic theory—one which to date has been largely neglected. The theoretical origins of this therapeutic technique stem from the writings of Paul Federn (1952) and Edoardo Weiss (1960). However, it approaches (from a somewhat different perspective) concepts concerning the structure and functioning of the self which are found in current "Object Relations" theory (Kohut, 1971; Kernberg, 1972).

It is not necessary to regard hypnoanalytic techniques as competing with the traditional practices of psychoanalysis and psychoanalytic therapy. Rather, they can be viewed as merely extensions and further elaborations of the methods by which Freud and his associates undertook to explore the fascinating inner world of man, one which continually influences our behavior and well-being, but of which we are often so little aware.

Unfortunately, the long time required for a traditional psycho-analysis (three to five times a week for several years) restricts its application to a very limited population. It has been said that what is needed "is a good ten-cent analysis." Hypnoanalysis is not "a ten-cent" psychoanalysis, but it often deals with deep-lying conflicts and achieves genuine personality reorganization in a much shorter period of time, thus making the benefits of psychodynamic thinking and psycho-analytic therapy more widely available.

A chapter on "Forensic Hypnosis" has been added to this volume. Although not concerned with the treatment of patients, this discipline does utilize many of the hypnoanalytic techniques of hypermnesia and regression. It is best practiced by psychological and psychiatric clinicians who have had much experience in treatment and have acquired additional expertise in needs of the courts and the legal profession. For reasons that will be discussed later it is not an appropriate area of practice for police investigators or even psycho-therapists whose training in hypnosis has been at introductory levels. That is why this chapter has been placed in Volume II and not in Volume I.

Finally, since therapy is much more than a collection of techniques, and because its success involves the very "self" of the doctor, we have attempted to place these procedures in a broad and philosophical context. Two practitioners may employ the same "techniques," yet one achieves much better results than the other. In Chapter 12, "Existential Hypnoanalysis and The Therapeutic Self," we will try to integrate these two volumes with the concept that all "techniques" in psycho-logical therapy must be practiced within a constructive interpersonal relationship, and that in the final analysis our success or failure may depend more on *how we be* with a patient than on *what we do* to him.

It is our hope that those skilled psychotherapists and analysts who have had experience in clinical hypnosis will find in this second volume a number of new and exciting therapeutic techniques to add to their practice. Behavioral scientists must continue to explore the inner human condition. Hypnoanalytic techniques offer many so-phisticated ways of accomplishing this, both in the clinic and in the laboratory. Through such approaches perhaps we can improve our understanding of psychological suffering and enhance the meaning of human life.

Chapter 1

Hypnoanalytic Insight Therapy

Suggestive Hypnosis and Hypnoanalysis

Hypnosis has traditionally been viewed as a technique of suggestion, and it does have so many possibilities of directly influencing symptoms that its potential for even greater contribution to the sophisticated "reconstructive" therapies involving insight has not been fully appreciated.

Psychoanalysis and its many variations are based on the assumption that neurotic symptoms are the external manifestations of underlying conflicts, and that by lifting the repression of unconscious factors and achieving "insight" the symptoms will be resolved. In fact, the classical psychoanalyst would probably hold that this is true of all neurotic symptoms, and that unless insight has been achieved into the underlying dynamic structure of a neurosis no permanent cure can be expected. This extreme position is no longer tenable.

As we have seen in Vol. 1. many symptomatic conditions respond favorably to suggestion and similar supportive therapies. However, there are often neurotic symptoms which do not seem to be permanently relinquished unless the unconscious conflicts which are at their root are brought into conscious awareness and reintegrated through that kind of understanding called insight. Hypnosis is prepared to play a role in the therapies which aim at this insight, be they client-centered, cognitive, psychoanalysis, or any of the brief psychoanalytic approaches.

Insight: Intellectual and Experiential

It is important that we clearly indicate what is meant here by this term. Much that passes for "insight" turns out to be only an intellectual understanding limited to the cognitive sphere of personality that has not resulted in a reconstructive alteration. In fact, many analytic therapies go on month after month without significant change even though the patient can verbalize the dynamic constellation which underpins his neurosis. He has achieved only a superficial "insight" which has not truly pervaded his entire personality. Such situations are responsible for the old joke that "after seven years of analysis the patient still bangs his head on the floor, but now he knows why."

Some years ago I interpreted to a depressed patient that he unconsciously hated his father. The evidence from his associations and dreams was quite clear on this point, so unmistakable that he immediately agreed. "You're absolutely right, Doctor. I'm depressed because I hate my father. It's really clear now." However, no change in his symptom occurred until several weeks later when the door of my office burst open. There stood my patient, wild-eyed and with a horror-struck expression shouting, "I really *do* hate my father." That was genuine insight, not his first agreement with my interpretation. His initial understanding had been only cognitive, intellectual, but it had managed during the ensuing weeks to work its way through to an emotional level which mobilized feelings as well. A significant reorganization in his entire perceptual system took place. Now he really understood. He had achieved true insight, and his depression began to clear.

"Insight," as we use it here, means a thorough-going: reorganization of the patient's understanding which is more than verbal or cognitive. It includes an alteration at the emotional level, the perceptual level, the motor level, and even at the tissue level. It is a "gut" comprehension which pervades his whole being in all areas, physiological, psychological and social. It is an alteration in meaning which changes the entire gestalt of his personality. As such it truly resolves inner conflicts and achieves a permanent impact on those dynamic factors which have maintained his symptoms. Defined in this way insight is a significant and profound experience which genuinely influences the patient's entire life style.

Criticisms of the presumed ineffectiveness of "insight" are usually based on a definition of it as simply an intellectual understanding. The techniques to be described here for achieving insight are aimed at this greater and more comprehensive objective even though we recognize that often a superficial cognitive understanding is attained first. In which case it should be viewed as a precursor to a more comprehensive experience that can be translated into permanent changes of feelings and behavior.

Psychoanalytic Criticisms of Hypnosis

Psychoanalysts have usually criticized hypnosis because they assigned to it the role of symptom suppression through suggestion. Even if some insight was achieved they held that this understanding "by-passed the ego" and hence, was not reintegrative. Anna Freud (1946) especially stated this criticism, and it has been repeated and believed by many analysts ever since. It is assumed that when one is hypnotized the ego is simply laid aside, that it is not involved in the uncovering process, and that, accordingly, such material as does emerge cannot be utilized by the patient for genuine change. Any loss of symptoms must be temporary since no change, or at best only a superficial one, has been made in the basic personality. Immediate symptom relief but not permanent cure would thus be expected. The neurotic conflicts, therefore, should reassert themselves, and the symptoms return as soon as the influence of the hypnotist is no long present. This position has been stated positively and repeatedly by the Blancks (1974).

Trance "Depth"

The problem can be viewed in quite a different light if we consider hypnotic depth to be a continuum extending from total, alert awareness, though light hypnoidal relaxation (such as occurs on the analytic couch), into intermediate states, then to deep and somnambulistic regions of consciousness (where hypnoanalytic therapy has generally been practiced). Finally, the deeply hypnotized individual may achieve what Erickson (1952) has termed a "plenary" trance, and perhaps ultimately coma. Hypnosis is then viewed like a dimension of personality, and the question becomes, "Does the most effective therapy occur when the patient is sitting up, wide awake, when relaxed, slightly hypnoidal and reclining on the couch, in an intermediate trance state, or within a profound hypnosis?"

Furthermore, is the therapy best conducted in one area of this continuum, or should there be an alternation back and forth on this dimension, first uncovering repressed material on the deep end of the spectrum, and then bringing it back to the more conscious position for ego-integration?

Viewed in this way hypnoanalytic therapy and psychoanalytic therapy are perceived as similar uncovering and integrating approaches which owe their difference primarily to the position on the hypnotic depth dimension in which they are commonly practiced. Hypnoanalysis is quite capable of employing the traditional analytic techniques of free association, dream interpretation and analysis of the transference, but can do so at different points on this depth-of-consciousness dimension.

However, hypnoanalysts have also developed a number of sophisticated procedures for revealing pre-conscious and unconscious material, isolating and activating defenses, eliciting dynamic patterns of impulse, by-passing or working-through resistances, dealing with transferences, and achieving integrative insight. It would seem, therefore, that practitioners of hypnotherapeutic insight therapy and hypnoanalysis could employ the same therapeutic techniques as do the traditional analysts. However, they have in addition another dimension of operation and a number of unique procedures which can be used to achieve the same result. This might be compared to a military commander who follows the same basic war strategies which have been developed as effective over the years, but who now has available a number of newer weapons and some more recently developed tactics for the achievement of his objectives. He need no longer fight his battles from trenches with primarily the Springfield rifle. It is our position here that, while much of basic analytic *theory*[1] continues to be valid, psychoanalytic *treatment tactics*, which were developed during the pre-World War I period, can be much improved. A reevaluation by psychoanalysts of the hypnotic modality and the greater flexibility of procedure which it offers is past overdue.

A representation of these factors (which were originally mentioned in Vol. 1, Pg. 167) is shown in Figure 1:1. In psychoanalysis the patient is induced to relax on the couch and become preoccupied with inner associations. His field of external perception is restricted and attention focused on his thoughts. But this is precisely what happens when we induce a hypnotic state. The patient is relaxed, his range of external awareness is restricted, and he is induced to experience a world consisting of the hypnotist and his self. Of course, if the therapy is to be primarily suggestive then the focusing is on the words of the hypnotist. However, if it is to be hypnoanalytic then the narrowing of attention is focused on various inner processes.

In the psychoanalytic situation most patients when relaxed on the couch probably develop a hypnoidal or light hypnotic state. Psychoanalysis, therefore, does involve hypnosis, but it is uncontrolled, the patient being left to develop spontaneously whatever state of consciousness he wishes. Had the instruction to lie on the couch, relax and occupy his concentration with inner associations, been continued further we would have termed it a hypnotic induction technique, and many patients would have drifted into a medium or deep trance. The psychoanalyst stops short of this and leaves the patient with a significant degree of ego alertness, but with some ego "relaxation" which Freud (1953a) felt necessary in order that preconscious material and unconscious derivatives could seep through to awareness.

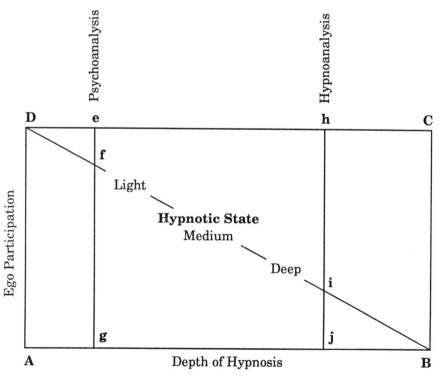

DAB: Conscious Awareness.
DBC: Pre-conscious and Unconscious Material.

Figure 1:1

In figure 1:1 the line on the left (eg) denoting the position of the patient in psychoanalysis shows that most of his ego (fg) is alert, and that only a small amount of behavior and experiential potentials stem from unconscious processes (ef). As one proceeds along the continuum of hypnotic depth from left to right the participation of the ego becomes progressively less, and the emerging of unconscious material increases. In the deep hypnoanalytic position (hj) there is a minimal ego involvement (ij) as more and more underlying unconscious and repressed material (hi) is activated. However, the situation is not at all as it has been traditionally represented in the psychoanalytic literature in which the ego is presumed to have been by-passed in the hypnotic state. Lessened, yes; eliminated, no.

If we regard the activation of unconscious material, and the bringing of it to awareness, as the first part of the analytic process, then a much greater amount is secured in the hypnoanalytic position than in the psychoanalytic one. These data might be compared to the raw material which is provided for fabrication into an article. The finished product is to be the genuine insight which will achieve significant personality change, but it must be fashioned into its final form from the original raw material. Only after so fashioned (worked-through) does it elicit significant personality change. Otherwise, true reintegration does not take place.

In trying to answer the question as to which position on the hypnotic depth continuum would be most effective to combine uncovering with re-integration we might return to our analogy of the factory and the raw material. In the psychoanalytic position (eg) in Figure 1:1 a small amount of raw material (ef) is activated and submitted to a large processing factory (fg). In the deep hypnoanalytic position (hj) a small ego-factory (ij) must confront a huge amount of unconscious raw material (hi). On a theoretical basis it seems reasonable to infer that neither the psychoanalytic position nor the deep hypnoanalytic one would be the most productive area for therapeutic work. Rather, somewhere in-between would represent an optimal balance of these factors.

The greatest promise of therapeutic progress would appear to lie in a psychoanalytic therapy conducted in a medium hypnotic state rather than a deep one. Conn (1959) has emphasized the advantages of working in lighter states of hypnosis. An equally tenable position would hold that we could elicit material during a deep state and then bring it back for submission to a more vigorous ego as represented by the left hand area of the hypnotic-depth dimension. Hypnoanalytic therapy would then consist of a weaving back and forth on this continuum.

In either case it would seem valuable to control this dimension and not leave it entirely to chance. The momentary whims of a patient may impel him to carry through his analysis at a comfortable and convenient intensity level, not one in which he is capable of working. By permitting our "ego-factory" to work at a comfortable level as we submit to it only small amounts of raw material (such as are elicited slowly by free association) our integrating plant works below its capabilities. The uncovering and integration of new material proceeds at a lazy pace, and the analysis takes longer than it needs to. By uncovering unconscious matter at an accelerated tempo we supply our integrating ego with substantial quantities of raw material. And by manipulating the factor of trance depth we provide sufficient participation of our "ego-factory" so as to maximize desired productivity—the most rapid possible achievement of genuine, re-integrating insight.

The process of "working-through," hence, repeated contact between the ego and previously unconscious material, which is such an important element in psychoanalysis, is not dispensed with in hypnoanalytic treatment, but it may be speeded up without the sacrificing of ultimate success. Repetition of material elicited under hypnosis is still essential and will be noted particularly in the effective conduct of hypnotic abreaction (to be described in Chapter 4).

Intermediate Hypnotic "Depth"

As might be expected, material which is elicited and submitted for egotization in the intermediate zone of hypnotic depth may stimulate much anxiety. The confrontation at this point is more severe than at either the psychoanalytic or deep hypnoanalytic ends of the continuum. If I curse my father (unconscious raw material) but he (ego) is not present no confrontation takes place. This would be represented by the extreme right hand position on Figure 1:1. There is no meeting of the incompatible elements. Accordingly, no therapeutic change takes place. It is like trying to teach an unconscious person. If on the other hand my father is present, but I do not express any negative thoughts about him (repression) then also no confrontation takes place. This is like the position at the extreme left hand side of Figure 1:1. The ego is completely present, but it is not in contact with any of its preconscious or unconscious impulses.

However, if I utter an oath against my father while he is present in the room, manifesting my hostility (as is represented by the intermediate zone of the hypnotic depth dimension) then the sparks will fly. A confrontation takes place. If the contact continues, the unpleasant heat (anxiety) which is developed can be dissipated only by a change in the attitudes and acceptances of either or both of us. A new gestalt of understanding and relationship must be forged between us. We can no longer be in conflict with each other, or dissociated from one another. Genuine therapeutic change has been achieved. The process is no different in hypnoanalysis than in psychoanalysis, but a greater flexibility of technique and ego participation has been available to facilitate this objective.

Working in this high-intensity, intermediate zone of consciousness may have some hazards. It is well known that if more material is lifted from repression than the ego can assimilate, and if its defenses are incapable of warding off painful contact with such material, then the individual's usual defenses may be overwhelmed. He flees into a psychotic reaction. I have rarely seen this happen. In most cases the patient's defenses will not permit this to occur. In some way his ego will break off contact with the undigestible repressed material which is now emerging in too great a strength. The patient spontaneously emerges from hypnosis (seeks the extreme left end of the hypnotic depth spectrum) or in a few cases de-cathects his ego temporarily and enters a profound trance state. Although this condition happens infrequently the analyst can minimize any catastrophic reaction by adequate attention to the therapeutic relationship.

The ego strength of the patient is not constant. It is greater at some times than at others. The demands of significant relationships with which it must interact daily can lower it. And the allyship with constructive others in the immediate environment can strengthen it.

Optimal Level of Trance "Depth"

The therapist who practices insight therapy in the intermediate zone of hypnotic depth should be prepared to offer an intensive therapeutic relationship, an allyship involving much "resonance" with his patient (Watkins, 1978). It involves a partial merging of the ego of the therapist with that of the patient, a temporary identification balanced with appropriate objectivity. The patient is reassured and can approach the analytic confrontations with a fuller mobilization of his resources because he perceives that *we* can succeed where *I* alone can not. The analyst who guides his patient through the dark labyrinths of unconscious repressions is like the good parent who takes the child by the hand and goes with him into the dark closet to confront the "boogey man." He has established a therapeutic "withness," a temporary and partial merging of the patient's and therapist's egos. The intensity of the hypnotic relationship enhances such togetherness as therapist and patient make common commitment to the analytic task. This "withness" is not counter-transference, which is a projection of the therapist's needs (often immature) unto the patient.

Interviews under various levels of hypnotic depth may well reveal different facets of impulse and defense. In fact, since hypnosis is also a regression it can sometimes indicate the contents which might have emerged during a classical psychoanalysis. As one proceeds into deeper and deeper levels of hypnotic involvement, content and defenses may be revealed which would be uncovered at much later stages in classical psychoanalysis. Even if the therapeutic plan was to proceed in more traditional analytic ways the pre-scouting value of an overview of the patient's neurosis in depth might aid the psychoanalyst in planning his strategy and facilitate his timing of interpretations. Stekel (1943c) insisted that the first dream in an analysis was like an overview of the entire structure of the neurosis, one whose full meaning only became clear by the end of the analysis. Likewise, a hypnodiagnostic pre-study can often reveal the order in which the various transference reactions might have emerged had the patient free-associated on the psychoanalytic couch. Some analysts may not prefer to use this much control. There has been, of course, even among the older analysts, considerable controversy as to the degree to which the analyst should permit the material to emerge non-directively (Reik, 1948) or evolve according to a plan based on one's theory of personality structure (Reich, 1949).

Hypermnesia and "Working-through"

While hypnotic hypermnesia can facilitate the recovery of memories (experiential although not always veridical), the hypnotic state is also conducive to the activation of feelings and emotions. In hypnotic abreaction strongly repressed affects can be mobilized so that a re-experiencing, not merely a remembering, takes place. Through the hypnotically facilitated release of such bound affect a fuller participation by the patient in genuine insight reactions becomes possible so that newer and constructive meanings can initiate real therapeutic change.

In later chapters specific hypnoanalytic techniques will be described which initiate the lifting of repressions, the activation of transferences, the release of bound affects, and the re-vification of early experiences. One tactic might be noted in comparison with psychoanalytic technique. During psychoanalysis the state of consciousness (equivalent to trance depth) is held constant, or at least is not manipulated by the analyst. The repressions are gradually lifted, and the preconscious and unconscious material submitted to the patient in gradually increasing doses. In hypnoanalysis we may lift a repression, release a great quantity of unconscious, unegotized material and then manipulate the trance depth to submit this larger amount of now unrepressed material to increasing impact with the ego. These are simply two different ways of "working-through." The end result of complete egotization and re-integration may be the same. Only the procedures for its accomplishment have varied.

In summary, our goals and basic strategies in hypnoanalysis do not differ greatly from those in traditional psychoanalysis. The underlying theoretical concepts are similar. However, their employment in conjunction with hypnosis offers the possibility of increased flexibility through altering the dimension of trance depth and the availability of a wider variety of techniques. This often makes it possible to achieve our analytic objectives in a shorter period of time.

Summary

Suggestive hypnotherapy involves primarily the manipulation of symptoms by suggestion. It is a kind of "putting-in." Hypnoanalysis is a "pulling-out." It is the practice of psychoanalysis with the addition of an induced hypnotic state, plus the use of special techniques which hypnosis makes possible. Like psychoanalysis, it attempts to eliminate symptoms indirectly by the lifting of repressions and the achieving of "insight.".

Insight to be effective must be more than intellectual; it must also be experiential involving affective and motor responses as well as cognitive ones.

Psychoanalysts, following Freud's renunciation of hypnosis, have criticized it as being "superficial," "by-passing the ego" and not resulting in permanent character change. These criticisms were only valid in early days when the hypnotic state was induced primarily to potentiate suggestions. They are no longer acceptable. Trance depth is related to the amount of ego participation. In the deeper stages much pre-conscious and unconscious material may be uncovered, but there is less ability to "egotize" this. In the lighter stages there is less material elicited but greater ego participation. The most effective areas for treatment may be in either the light to medium zones of trance depth, or a weaving back and forth between deeper and lighter states.

As in psychoanalysis material lifted from repressions must be "worked-through" to achieve therapeutic benefit.

Chapter 1. Hypnoanalytic Insight Therapy.

Outline

1. The psychoanalytic view of neurotic symptoms as the external manifestations of underlying conflicts.
    a. These conflicts are resolved by the lifting of repressions and the achieving of "insight."
    b. True insight as being also perceptual, affective and motoric, not solely cogitive or intellectual.

2. The psychoanalytic view that hypnosis is merely a technique for symptom suppression through suggestion.
    a. It is presumed to "by-pass" the ego and not result in personality re-integration and permanent symptom relief.

3. Ego participation as related to trance "depth."
    a. Flexibility in uncovering vs. egotization by variation of trance depth.
    b. Hypnosis as a "regression in the service of the ego."
    c. The question of optimal "depth" in therapy.

4. Hypnosis as offering the analytic therapist a wide variety of uncovering and re-integrative procedures.

5. The similarity of psychoanalytic and hypnoanalytic goals but the differences in therapeutic techniques for achieving them.

Footnotes
1. We recognize the more recent developments in ego psychology and object relations theory, such as have been proposed by Hartmann (1958), Kris, (1956), Lowenstein (1951), Mahler (1974), Rappaport (1958), Kohut (1977), Kernberg (1976), and others.

Chapter 2

The Psychodynamics
of Hypnotic
Induction

The more intensely one becomes involved in the study of hypnosis
the more one is drawn to the view that the response of entering an
hypnotic state, deepening and terminating the condition is intimately
related to the inter-personal communications between hypnotist and
subject and to the motivational needs of both. The amateur tends to
think of hypnosis as simply a state entered by the subject in reaction
to certain passes or other cues provided by the hypnotist. Such a
beginner often shows the greatest interest in reading and memorizing
"techniques," completely ignoring that it is the *meaning* of the inter-
personal interaction implied in a so-called "technique" and not the
simple stimulus value of certain words which is of most significance
in determining the kind and extent of the hypnotic response.

Personality Psychodynamics

The psychological sub-science which deals with the complex of
unconscious motivational patterns in the determination of behavior
has been termed "psychodynamics." It considers cause and effect
relationships in psychic life, especially those which are covert. Thus,
the origin of a type of behavior may lie far from the actual response,
so far that neither the subject nor nearby observers suspect its true

cause. Like the music in a popular song of some years ago, "You push the first valve down. The music goes round and around, and it comes out here." Psychodynamics is the study of the "round and around."

Consider a simple, illustrative example. The promiscuous, Don Juan lover has been renowned in literature and opera. At superficial glance he seems to be quite a man. After all, he has possessed many women. One might think that he would be very proud of his masculinity. However, it turns out from the psychodynamic viewpoint that quite the opposite prevails. The Don Juan is very insecure male, doubting his potency, uncertain of his masculinity, and at unconscious levels defending himself against latent feminine or homosexual drives. His seductive behavior is necessary as a constant proof to himself that he really is masculine. Each conquest temporarily allays this inner anxiety but does not last long. He is driven to seek a new affair to quell the small inner voice which whispers that he is really not a man. Only from such a psychodynamic point of view can we understand his behavior, deal with it rationally, and help with an appropriate treatment strategy which will restore to him a sense of confidence that he is truly what he was structurally born to be—a man. Once he has acquired this new understanding, genuine hetero-sexual love becomes possible. A meaningful relationship with a woman replaces his promiscuity.

Similarly, the hypnotic subject reacts in an inter-personal relationship situation to the hypnotist via the communications received during what is called "induction." He or she enters trance, does not enter trance, or does so, but only lightly. Through the study of psychodynamics we are trying to understand the complex of inner and outer motivations which cause the subject to make the response elicited and to learn to control these more effectively with the aim of increasing the likelihood that he/she will react with a hypnotic state deep enough for the effective application of constructive hypnotherapeutic techniques.

Hypnosis as a State of Regression

Various writers (Kline, 1958; Gill and Breman, 1959; Meares, 1961; Copeland, 1986) have emphasized that hypnosis may be viewed both as a state and as a relationship. As a state it has a number of specific characteristics such as lowered criticality, diminished intellectual control, less emotional inhibition, and a return to childish patterns of behavior. This return can be described as a regression (Bellak, 1955).

During sleep, illness, psychosis and psychoneurosis we "regress," hence, return to earlier and simpler patterns of response. Sometimes this regression is forced upon an individual. He/she is confronted with environmental demands which overwhelm the ego, and the person is unable to cope with them. The ego suffers a devastating annihilation. Psychosis results. However in most cases the ego, like the good military commander, knows enough to withdraw from the scene of battle when faced with superior forces. It pulls back, shortens its lines of responsibility, and by conserving its energies within a simpler existence prevents its total destruction. In choosing to do this, such as in normal sleep, the ego rests and awaits the time when with renewed strength and vigor it can venture back to the arena of human struggle. This is called "regression in the service of the ego" (Hartmann, 1958).

Factors Influencing Hypnotic Regression.

When inducing and deepening hypnotic trance we are, accordingly, very much concerned with understanding the factors which will initiate regressive trends in our patient, how these can be stimulated, and how controlled. Actually, all methods of trance induction represent techniques for initiating regression. Gill and Brenman (1959) classify these under two headings: 1. By sensorimotor-ideational deprivation, or, 2. By the stimulation of an archaic (hence, transference) relationship to the hypnotist. Putting it another way, we regress when we do not receive adequate stimulation from the environment, and we regress when we are in intimate personal contact with one who through transference represents an early authoritative figure toward whom we have established immature and primitive patterns of response. The psychodynamic approach to hypnotic induction will, of course, concern itself with both avenues, but it is in the second where it is prepared to make its greatest contribution to our understanding and therapeutic skill.

Let us compare the induction of the regression of sleep with the induction of the regression of hypnosis. In order to sleep we restrict our sensori-motor input. The room is darkened. We lie still. We are made warm by covers and when possible protected from undue skin stimuli by smooth, non-scratch sheets. We do not talk, and we do not want to listen to the sounds of others. In this absence of stimuli the ego withdraws its energies from the sensory organs and nearly eliminates its communication with the outside world.

Conscious thoughts fade and are gradually replaced by those bits of more archaic mental material called dreams in which the logic (or rather psychologic) proceeds according to the rules which govern unconscious or primary-process thinking. The dream becomes like the psychosis, irrational, concretistic, illogical yet still subject to various ego-defensive maneuvers. The ego vacillates between the external world which demands social-reality behavior, and that inner world of primitive drives, which the psychoanalysts call the Id. At this stage the state of regression is not unlike that which exists during deep hypnosis. In fact, there have been many studies comparing ordinary dreaming with hypnotic dreaming (Barber, 1962; Moss, 1967, 1970; Tart, 1964, 1965)

As energies (cathexes) are further withdrawn from the dreamer's ego, mental activity becomes less and less and may finally approach a deep state of coma in which only the continuation of minimal, vital organic functions indicate that the individual is still alive. Erickson (1952) described such a hypnotic state as a "plenary trance," which he induced through prolonged induction procedures in a few subjects. In a doctoral dissertation Sherman (1971) found that profoundly hypnotized individuals reached a stage in which the awareness of "knowledge of individual identity" ceased and the electroencephalogram showed periods of drastic decrease. The pattern of brain energies approached complete cessation, a state that would mark a condition of death.

These various stages also appear in a patient regressed chemically through the anesthetization of his functions on the surgical operating table. And studies on sensory-deprivation (West, 1967) have shown that an individual so deprived experiences hallucinations and similar mental phenomena, even as the sleeper dreams, and the hypnotized subject vivifies or hallucinates inner past or suggested experiences.

In hypnotic induction we facilitate this regression by telling our patient to do such things as stare at a fixed point (restricting sources of visual stimulation), asking that he/she attend to the relaxation in the muscles (lowering motor activities), calling attention to involuntary actions such as eye-closure or hand levitation, hence, demonstrating that increasing parts of the body are becoming de-egotized and are no longer subject to voluntary control. We suggest falling during a standing, body-sway approach (disorienting kinesthetic and equilibratory sense contacts with reality). Or we ask the subject to become preoccupied with a soothing inner fantasy which stresses comfort, rest and peace—again pushing away the outer world. In so doing, the hypnotist tips the balance between cognitive controls and the inner press of more primitive needs. The patient relaxes, closes the eyes and regresses. By relinquishing to a considerable extent direction from conscious mental processes sources outside the ego, suggestions of the hypnotist and unegotized impulses from the unconscious self or related derivatives become more operative. The hypnotized person is not exactly a child, nor psychotic, nor just dreaming, but does demonstrate behavior which is closely related to all of these.

Hypnotic productions often look like the reactions of a dissociated individual, such as are found in multiple personalities. It is not surprising that most multiple personalities have been studied through hypnoanalytic procedures since in the hypnotic state it is so easy to induce the various personalities to appear or disappear. We often forget that the induction procedure is a communication between two parties, and it is the meaning, the essential inner significance of each communicative act, which determines our subject's response, not the fact of administering the technique. To close the eyes means to a subject that one is supposed to rest, to another, to ignore the outer world, to a third, that something is to be "put over" on him without his control, to another, to die, to still another, to pretend or to imagine, etc. Not only may each hypnotic subject interpret the meaning of a suggestion differently, but a single subject may interpret the suggestion one way when given by hypnotist A, who is viewed as a helper, and another way when the same suggestion is administered by hypnotist B, who is regarded as an exploiter. These two different attitudes may have been determined by differences in the real behavior of the two hypnotists, or because inner, personal (transference) attitudes stimulated within the subject by two different people who possess different physical and psychological characteristics.

Special Meanings of the Hypnotic State to the Patient.

Different patients have varied conceptions, both consciously and unconsciously toward hypnosis or its induction. Thus, to relax, either in a chair or on a couch, to relinquish defensive postures, and to give one's self over to the suggestions of another can mean to involve one's self in a state of submission. This same meaning may arise in the patient undergoing relaxation on the psychoanalytic couch. Both submissive needs and fears are stimulated. However, two different patients, both of whom equate being hypnotized to submitting one's self to another, may still react quite differently. To some, this is an enjoyable experience wherein one is no longer held accountable for one's actions or fantasies. One is freed of any guilt. The patient can hold the hypnotist responsible for whatever transpires. Such individuals welcome the hypnotic experience and may sink rapidly into a very deep trance.

However, to another, who has spent his life in struggling for independence, to whom dependence or submission to another constitutes a real threat (one could be taken advantage of), the induction becomes the signal for a "battle of wills." The patient must show the doctor that he/she is resolute and cannot be imposed upon. Unconsciously he must strive to be a Rock of Gibraltar, impregnable in the face of an assault which is perceived as dangerous to the integrity of his ego. The patient is resistant, and either unhypnotizable, or hypnotizable only with great difficulty.

This resistance must be recognized, and either by-passed through appropriate technique and manner, over-powered through superior skill and the mobilization of stronger motivations, or analyzed and "worked-through" to reduce its strength. When one encounters such resistance it is wise to terminate attempts at induction for the present and to inquire of the patient his views about hypnosis, what he has read about it, if he has every seen a demonstration, and what feelings these initiated in him (Stillerman, 1957; Watkins, 1954, 1963).

Occasionally, resistance to induction will arise because of a new fear which had not appeared before. A young woman being treated hypnoanalytically had been trained to respond with a medium-deep trance in about five minutes of suggestions involving eye-fixation, relaxation and the dropping of her arm. At one session she reported late, much disturbed because the newspapers had been carrying the account of a sadistic murder in which a girl had been killed, her body cut into pieces, and strewn about the community.

The patient reacted to the usual trance induction with great anxiety, fidgeting and resistance. Very slowly she involved herself in the hypnotic regression. Toward the end of the induction procedure I had usually lifted her arm by the wrist, suggested that at the count of twelve, when I dropped her hand, she would "fall" into a profoundly deep state. This time as I touched her wrist, she shrieked and shrunk away. No further attempts were made to deepen the trance until she had been asked about her fears. She indicated that today she perceived me as a potential, sadistic murderer, not as a helper. She was frightened. Following the full airing of this feeling under the light trance state she relaxed. A deeper state could be induced, and it proved to be one which was fruitful with the production of much significant material.

On emerging from hypnosis she reported that when coming to my office she had seen a child's shoe lying beside the walk and immediately felt frightened, perceiving it as an amputated foot. Had I failed to sense her changed reaction and proceeded mechanically with the usual suggestions there might have been an overwhelming, traumatic fear response, perhaps even a termination of treatment. By interrupting the induction to inquire into this source of anxiety, not only was it possible to resolve the matter and induce a productive hypnotic state, but also much of value was learned regarding her own psychodynamic needs as they were being projected (transferred) onto the therapist and the hypnoanalytic situation.

We need not be concerned here with the full meaning of her reaction to the sadistic news event and its significance with her neurosis, but rather with its impact on the process of trance induction. What started as a resistance to the hour's work became a valuable source of new understanding and progress. The mechanical application of any induction procedure, however initially effective, may lose much of its efficacy if the therapist is insensitive to the subtle psychodynamic inter-play with can occur within the regressive, hypnotic relationship.

Hypnosis as an Erotic Experience

Some subjects may welcome the hypnotic state as a situation in which one is free to enjoy erotic fantasies. During a regression the later-formed psychic structures tend to be eliminated first, hence, the super-ego (conscience) controls may be lessened, then the ego defenses, leaving immature and erotic impulses more free to gain fantasy expression. This lowering of inhibition is characteristic of both hypnosis and the ingestion of alcohol. As Kline (1958) noted there is a lowering of "criticality."

Sometimes the temptation to enter a trance state becomes so pleasurable that the patient undergoes either spontaneous inductions, or goes into hypnosis at the slightest provocation. This may represent a character trait or the result of much practiced experience in dissociating. However, it can also be a kind of pleasurable seduction, similar to the behavior of schizoid individuals who find indulging in fantasy life more pleasant than real existence. Such a tendency in a hypnotic subject is probably not healthy and may be a contraindication for continued use of hypnosis. In this case the regression is no longer temporary, hence in the "service of the ego," but rather a movement toward a permanent, pathological (perhaps psychotic) state. The patient who is too easily hypnotized demands our careful evaluation and consideration as to what therapeutic procedures are appropriate—and hypnosis may not be one of them.

Sometimes the patient interprets the induction as a prelude to sexual seduction or as itself a symbolic seduction. This can mobilize either wishes or fears, or both. Whether the subject who so perceives it enters the hypnotic state or not depends on the relative balance between the wish to be seduced and the fear of being seduced. Once such a patient has received adequate reassurance of protection from the fear of seduction his/her unconscious erotic wishes may serve as a strong motivating agent facilitating the inductive process.

Fears of Death

The fear of death is universal. Few people are able to master it. Federn (1952) stated that the ego cannot accept or face its own non-existence. Death is equated with the loss of self, stillness, immovability and the end of volition. Accordingly, it is not surprising that some subjects view the induction of hypnosis as dying. After all, we do ask the patient to remain still, to close the eyes and to relinquish volition. If fears of death are mobilized then resistance to hypnosis will increase. Some people are afraid to sleep because they think they may die during sleep. Perhaps this fear was initiated in childhood when they were taught an old bed-time prayer which said: "If I should die before I wake, I pray the Lord my soul to take." Resistance based on this fear does occur, but since most people are not afraid to go to sleep it should not be common.

Hypnosis as a Relationship

Not only the state of hypnosis, but also the *hypnotic relationship* and any interactive communications between doctor and patient have inner and special meanings. In any interpersonal relationship situation, but especially in psychotherapy, the patient perceives "the other" through the eyes of the past. The hypnotherapist is endowed with characteristics, good or bad, which he/she has experienced as inhering in parental and other authoritative figures. Furthermore, this same distortion of perception can occur in the therapist, affecting his evaluation of the patient, his attitude and his choice of therapeutic techniques. We call this phenomena "transference," and in the therapist, "counter-transference." It operates both in the induction process and throughout the treatment. However, because of its importance we will leave its further discussion until Chapter 10.

Fantasies and Induction

Day-dreaming is closely akin to light hypnosis. The schizoid individual constantly revels in such imaginations. But even the normal person often indulges. One of the more sophisticated approaches to hypnotic induction involves the use of fantasy. The patient is asked to imagine a scene and progressively to "live" within it. He/she may then be moved time-wise to secure regression to some earlier age level. The fantasy becomes the experienced reality of the moment—even as a dream in sleep is the "reality" of the moment.

It is always easier to involve one's self in a fantasy experience if this "dream" includes pleasurable stimuli—thus, it lets us enjoy highly satisfying, personal situations. Who among us have not enjoyed day dreams of acquiring success, fame and vanquishing enemies? Especially potent in inducing hypnosis are those fantasied situations which appeal to immature and childhood cravings. For example, skin eroticism has been considered onto-genetically as preceding genital eroticism. Thus, when the hypnotist pictures for the patient the soothing touch of a soft, grassy slope on which he is reclining, or the smooth, velvet sensation about one's body when floating on a cloud, he is invoking tactile, erotic fantasies reminiscent of the maternal touch in earliest childhood. It is not surprising that the patient is encouraged to regress.

A common unconscious fantasy found in psychoanalysis is the desire to return to the womb, to an early, warm, environmentally perfect existence. Rank (1952) held that the process of birth is a violent detachment from that environment which once met all our needs. Accordingly, it represents the greatest trauma of life. We need not agree with his conclusion in order to recognize that when the hypnotist talks about "a soft, warm space with the most beautiful feelings of comfort and peace," he is trying to encourage hypnotic regression though re-vivification of unconscious "somatic memories" of the pre-birth period.

Sometimes the hypnotist suggests that in entering hypnosis the subject will experience great feelings of omnipotence. Thus, the child in the dental chair is asked to close his eyes, to picture a TV screen, and to imagine he is watching "Mighty Mouse"—that little midget who is so successful in over-powering the great cat, dog or other animal representation of parent figures. Or re-living the exploits of "Superman" or "Superwoman" can tap into the child's needs for power. The patient's fantasy wish-life is stimulated to aid in getting a regression into hypnosis wherein sensations from the dental drill are ignored.

In the initiation of such fantasies the pictorial descriptive powers of the hypnotist should be fully utilized. This means vivid description, attention to minute details within the images, the allowance of time for involvement, and the willingness to modify the fantasy as directed by the patient. The more we understand the motivational needs of our patient, the more skillful we become in flexibly adapting our induction techniques to different individuals. In some cases, such as the little dental patient, we may expect that his needs for omnipotence and his desire to best his elders, represent a part of his fantasy life. This is characteristic of almost every child. Often though, we must rely on our knowledge derived from interview contacts with the patient, and the degree of sensitiveness for less obvious communications to which we have conditioned our own "third ear" (Reik, 1948).

The Highly-Resistant Patient.

In spite of the extravagant claims of some practitioners both research and the clinical practice of most hypnotherapists demonstrate that not all patients can be hypnotized. Hypnotic susceptibility may be an inherited and relatively unmodifiable trait (as suggested in Hilgard's early studies (1965). However skill and understanding can certainly increase the number of subjects which are hypnotically responsive.

The general conditions which improve the rate of successful inductions have been discussed in Volume I. Nevertheless, every practitioner will be confronted at times with individuals seeking hypnotherapy who appear to be quite refractory to every approach and to every hypnotist. In fact, some "professional patients" make the rounds of therapists, ostensibly seeking that one clinician who will be successful, but in reality trying to prove that they cannot be hypnotized. They unconsciously perceive hypnosis as a battle of wills and want to demonstrate over and over again that they can defeat every practitioner.

Their initial approach is somewhat as follows: "Doctor, I have been to Doctor A, and he couldn't hypnotize me. Then I went to Doctor B, and he couldn't hypnotize me. Dr. C. tried and failed. But Doctor, I can only be cured by hypnosis. I know *you* can hypnotize me." They then reel off the names of a number of well-known hypnotherapists whom they have consulted. One often notices that they seem more preoccupied with the renown of the doctors whom they claimed failed than with suffering from their reported symptoms—even though they stoutly maintain that their only motivation is to be "cured."

This is commonly a trap designed to ensnare more therapists and enlarge the patient's current collection of scalps. If one accepts the challenge he/she will soon find one's own name added to the list when this patient consults the next practitioner. Perhaps such patients should be rejected at once. And indeed they often mention clinicians who, after hearing their story, refused to accept them. However, narcissism is not a characteristic lacking among those of us who practice hypnotherapy, and it is quite human to wish to succeed where one's respected colleagues have failed. Accordingly, such a patient can usually find more therapists who are willing to try.

Putting cynicism aside one is confronted with a person who apparently has genuine symptoms and who is seeking one's help via a skill that one possesses. We can recognize that under all the passive aggressiveness and needs to dominate there is a struggling human being, unconsciously harboring deep feelings of inferiority, and locked into his neurotic obsession to overcome therapists (who are often parent figures in transference). It is difficult for the sincere practitioner to refuse to at least try.

However, we should do so with a recognition of what is going on and the knowledge that we are being seduced into playing the patient's game. Is there a way by which we might get through his defenses, overcome the resistance, and achieve a successful treatment? Almost every practitioner who has secured some national recognition has been accosted by such individuals, and the more one is known (through publications or reputation) the more likely he or she will be approached. The patient's ego is fed by "knocking-off" big names in the field. He can then brag about their failures to his next victim-therapist.

The following case is illustrative of this situation and suggests some of the many techniques and considerations which may be brought up in trying to deal with such an individual. A man from a distant city in Canada contacted me by phone over several months stating that he wanted a therapist who was a hypnoanalyst and who would treat him by "regression," which he "knew" was the key to his problems. He had seen quite a host of hypnotherapists and psychoanalysts and reeled off a virtual Who's Who in these fields. Moreover, he had read volumes about all the great masters of analytic therapy including Freud, Reich, Reik, Hartmann, Kohut, etc., not to mention practitioners of reality therapy, gestalt therapy, and transactional analysis.

He was a mild, soft-speaking individual, apparently friendly and willing to cooperate. After describing his symptoms (which did not appear to be severe enough to affect his work and normal living activities) he launched into an hour of recounting the failures of all the practitioners whom he had consulted. They were "not competent" and could not hypnotize him. One of them, whom he claimed had hypnotized him, did not have psychoanalytic training, and he needed "hypnoanalysis." Others were too permissive, not authoritarian enough, etc. He talked incessantly, hardly ever stopping. When I asked questions he would interrupt in the middle of them then launch into digressions which did not answer the question. With great difficulty I could find but little information about his early childhood, his parents, his social relationships. There was an obsessive avoiding of anything about his personal life, only a continuous recounting of the failures of his hypnotists. He claimed he could only be treated by an hypnoanalyst of great repute who would do so by an "authoritative" method and then use "regression." Nobody had yet been able to succeed. He was daring me to try and hypnotize him.

In such a case one thinks about what chinks there might be in his defensive armor, what motivations might move him to become involved in hypnosis rather than to seek further reinforcements for his need to dominate. He even complained about the chair he was sitting in. A few seconds after being asked to concentrate (on his watch since he claimed he had once been hypnotized that way by a general practitioner), he would shake his head, break off, and declare that, "It isn't working."

A number of tactical options were possible for the therapist. First, by inquiring about what all the others have done he can avoid doing the same thing. The approach one uses must be different and one for which he is not prepared. It should probably be fairly quick, since if it is slow he will have time to adapt his defenses accordingly. Because of the severity of the resistance one must also consider whether he is defending himself against a possible psychotic break if he should lose control. This could contra-indicate the use of hypnosis. In this case, there were a number of possible indicators in his speech and mannerisms, such as bulging eyes, a rather fixed stare, and slight neologisms. If fear is the primary motivation one's manner will be different than if power needs are the prime underlying force. I judged both were present here, although he loudly denied having any fear of entering hypnosis.

Economic motives were also possible. In which case the fee might be set excessively high to see if he would be willing to invest as much into the treatment, or excessively low to counteract the claim that "all the doctors want of you is your money." One might even try an offer that if the treatment is successful the fee will be substantially reduced. This patient had spent thousands of dollars traveling around to dozens of practitioners, yet he claimed that he could not afford any long-term treatment such as psychoanalysis. It had to be a hypnoanalytic "quickie."

Varying the technique and the therapist's manner seemed to have no differential effect. His response was the same. He would break off from any concentrated attention in a few minutes, shake his head and reiterate his, "It isn't working." Sometimes the "Opposed Hand Levitation" approach (see Vol. I, Chap. 6) is effective. It was not in his case. When I was most authoritative he claimed I was not authoritative enough. Using a "rehearsal method" I had him re-live the experience with the general practitioner. He went into a regression almost immediately, began sobbing and grimacing, but after a minute he spontaneously emerged, smiled and denied the reality of his experience. ("I was only demonstrating to you what I did with Dr. G.").

Sometimes one can appeal to a frightened little boy ego state underlying the passive aggressiveness. Yet here a change to a softer manner met with the same stubborn denial and resistance. Under no circumstance was he will to change.

Finally, when changes of manner, of techniques, more analytic probing for possible sources of conflict and hurt in his life, resonance with sensed underlying needs, and attempts to empathize met with a stone wall, confrontation and direct interpretation of resistance might reach the patient. I pointed out his strong underlying need to sabotage treatment, the satisfactions received from besting each practitioner, the repetitive searching for a kind of therapist—which no one could meet. One must do this in a way in which the maladaptive behavior is interpreted, but the self or person" of the patient is not rejected or scorned. Yet even in this case the fear of entering trance, of losing control, and the need to triumph over the therapist was too great. Only denial and continued resistance appeared. We needed time to establish a sufficiently trusting relationship, but it was not available. He demanded a quick cure, by hypnosis, by regression, and he was not prepared to spend a very long time—just enough to make the attempt fail.

Often resistance is based on transference, possibly the need to defeat a parent figure. My patient would not talk about his parents. Each time a question about them was asked, within five seconds he was no longer discussing his parents but describing in technical jargon some psychoanalytic theory, which he had read. He was willing to talk *about* therapy but not to *experience* it. Repeated questions by me to the effect that, "Let us talk about *you*, your unhappiness and your problems, not what Freud once wrote." were met only with denials and digressions. He was indeed a "Rock of Gibraltar.":

When it became evident that I probably could not help him with any real, underlying problems we decided to terminate our consultations. He did not want to leave, took a long time in going to the door, and even called later in the day to know if I would recommend any other hypnotherapist, obviously to emphasize his "victory". I declined the invitation to burden others of my friends with this case (many of whom he had already contacted) and repeated my firm conviction that he could be helped only when he faced the fact that his need to vanquish therapists was greater than his desire for treatment. I wished him well, and we parted on a friendly note.

No, we are not always successful, even using every bit of technique, skill and relationship we can muster. However, in this case we see a wide variety of approaches applied which had been found to be effective on numerous other occasions. They were reviewed here and this case presented because we often learn more from our failures than our successes—even though it would have been pleasant to have finished this chapter with one of my more brilliant triumphs.

Termination of Hypnosis.

If hypnosis is indeed a regression then its termination means a return to the reality and maturity demands of the present. Just as the physicist must be aware of both centrifugal and centripetal forces, so must the good hypnotherapist consider both the regressive and the progressive needs of the patient. In one sense the termination of each trance is a return to maturity, a re-birth. The regression has truly been "in the service of the ego," not a permanent state. Some patients need reassurance on this point. They fear that maybe they "won't come out of it." The therapist stands on the side of the ego, of reality and mature adjustment. His excursions into the hypnotic regression are limited, purposeful, only for the benefit of the patient, and always to be concluded at some point. The doctor will do well to see that the patient understands this, whether it is communicated directly or by implication.

But in bringing the patient back from the hypnotic state the careful therapist should respect his subject's regressive needs. He must take time and not require that the patient make instant response to the de-hypnotizing suggestions—such as snapping his fingers to terminate trance. The sudden return of ego awareness to the deeply hypnotized patient can in some cases be traumatic. The patient may not be ready to face the world again, not to mention some of the unconscious material about which he was communicating in the hypnotic state. We must protect his ego and not submit it to the sudden battery of external stimuli (or emerging internal material) until it is ready.

The patient sometimes telegraphs his reluctance to leave the comfortable, regressed state to return to unpleasant realities. He stays in hypnosis or may temporarily even go deeper in spite of suggestions to the contrary. The hypnotist must not panic. He merely conveys to the patient an understanding of the patient's enjoyment of the present condition and the wish to remain. He either permits the patient to emerge "when you are ready and at your own speed," or kindly suggests that he may return to this pleasurable state "the next time" when he can re-experience and understand better his present sensations. Under no circumstances should the therapist react as if this was a challenge—which it may so represent. If such a "challenge" continues it may become necessary to understand and interpret its meaning to the patient. However, this is seldom necessary. If told that he will awaken when he is ready, and then left to himself, the patient usually soon becomes alert.

It is important to see that the hypnotic state has been truly terminated and a full state of ego awareness established before releasing the patient to drive home. Accordingly, a few minutes should be permitted at the end of the hypnotic period for interactions in the conscious state.

Psychodynamics is not an exact science. At best we can only aim at increasing our sensitivity in communication and our flexibility in technique. There will be many times when we are at a total loss to understand what is happening within our subject and why he/she seems so completely unresponsive to our induction attempts. But the clinician who consider's the patient's conscious and unconscious motivations, and who pays close attention to his own feelings and relationship with the patient, will improve his "batting average" and develop an increasing effectiveness in the practice of hypnotherapy.

Summary

Psychodynamics deals with unconscious processes, that which transpires between an original stimulus and the final overt behavior or experience. The induction of a hypnotic state is subject to these processes, and the "meaning" which hypnosis has to the patient affects his resistance, the speed with which he enters hypnosis, and its depth. The sophisticated hypnoanalyst will take these factors into account when inducing hypnosis.

Hypnosis has been considered a state of regression, hence, a return to earlier patterns of behavior and thought. It is a regression in the service of the ego, because unlike psychosis, the ego can voluntarily return out of it. There is a significant relationship between the depth of hypnosis and the amount of ego participation, the deeper the state, the less the ego is involved.

Hypnosis has a number of special meanings to subjects, such as an erotic experience,death, an inter-personal relationship, or submission to another. It may be influenced by transference reactions. Individuals may have highly-personalized fantasies when entering or experiencing hypnosis, such as return to the womb or possessing power. If the analyst understands these special meanings he will reduce resistance and be more successful during hypnotic induction.

The termination of hypnosis may also have special psychodynamic meaning to patients.

Chapter 2. Psychodynamics of Hypnotic Induction

Outline

1. Definition of "psychodynamics".
    a. Examples of psychodynamic operation, the "Don Juan."

2. Hypnosis as a state of regression.
   a. Factors influencing hypnotic regression.
      (1) Comparison with sleep.
      (2) Deep or "plenary" trance.
      (3) Variations in hypnotizability related to time, person.
      (4) Encountering resistance.

3. Special meanings of the hypnotic state to the patient.
   a. Submission vs. the need for independence.
   b. Resistance due to fear.

4. Hypnosis as an erotic experience.

5. Fears of death.

6. Hypnosis as a relationship.
   a. Hypnosis and transference.

7. Fantasies and induction.
   a. Return to the womb.
   b. Fantasies of power.

8. The highly-resistant patient.
   a. Techniques for dealing with such cases.

9. Termination of hypnosis.

Chapter 3

Hypnodiagnostic Evaluation

In the practice of psychotherapy, diagnosis should mean more than the attaching of a label to a disease syndrome. Diagnostic techniques enable us to uncover further information about a patient and permit a better understanding. This evaluation may precede the application of treatment techniques, but often it is an on-going process that continually up-dates our comprehension of the condition. Here, we will be concerned with ways of evaluating the patient that involve hypnosis. These include behaviors elicited during the trance state and its induction, and specialized psychological maneuvers designed to explore the experiential world of our patient.

We must assume that every reaction of the patient while in or entering hypnosis has meaning. The sensitive therapist notes these responses and infers their significance in the emerging picture of his functioning and problems. For example, a slight frown appears on the patient's face during an induction. We might wonder if something is troubling him. perhaps we have said or done something which is upsetting, and he is manifesting resistance. If the induction then proceeds very slowly, or is unsuccessful, we may want to ask just what it was that caused this reaction. Or again, a sudden descent into a deep hypnosis during a fantasy of smooth feeling on the skin may indicate skin eroticism. Accordingly, tactile suggestions may be more effective in deepening the state then those which describe lulling sounds. These images may also be related to unconscious conflicts such as are manifested by neurodermatitis or other skin disorders. We try at all times to find out what images, what areas of the body, and what needs are most significant to our patient. Then we couch our inductions, deepenings and therapeutic strategems accordingly.

Affirmative or negative noddings of the head, however slight, can tell us whether we are using effective suggestions or not. Shifts in posture, like leaning forward, sitting back stiffly, tensions, relaxations and sighs can communicate much to the observing clinician. Reactions to alterations in the voice of the hypnotist, when he changes from a strong, forceful manner to a gentle one, may also tell us much about the patient's desires and points of resistance. Sweating, rubbing of the head or wringing of the hands may let us know that some inner conflict has been precipitated, even though nothing other than an induction has been attempted. We may choose to defer further deepening and inquire into the sources of the disturbance.

Variations in trance depth, such as a sudden emerging from hypnosis, or rapid sinking from a rather constant, light state into a deep one often occur as a result of contact with new, conflictful material. Inquiries about the sources and meaning of these reactions can be made directly to the patient without removing the hypnotic state. Or the patient can be de-hypnotized, queried and immediately returned to the trance state.

It is particularly important to observe the manner displayed while under hypnosis. Some patients are relaxed, passive and quiet. They make a response only upon being initiated to do so by the therapist. Others are very active, talking and acting as if they were in the fully conscious condition. Some patients display their resistance by a great slowing in their responses. Others, through rapid associating on many topics, reveal that they are afraid of losing control. The effective hypnotherapist picks up these cues and incorporates them into the inductions. By recognizing the patient's needs and meeting as many of these as possible we lower resistance, intensify the therapeutic relationship and facilitate the treatment process.

The beginner to the field of hypnotherapy often asks upon taking an introductory course,"Just what should I do first with hypnosis?" The best reply is simply, "Do within the hypnotic state whatever you have been accustomed to doing without hypnosis. If you are an analyst have your patients free associate, as they have done before, but hypnotize them first. If you are a client-centered therapist conduct your treatment sessions as you usually do them. Reflect the feelings to the client, but when he/she is in a hypnotic state. If you are a behavior therapist administer the reinforcements or the desensitizations while the patient is hypnotized. The practicing clinician, who has once learned to induce hypnosis can make the transition from psychotherapist to hypnotherapist most easily by continuing the techniques to which he/she has become accustomed but within the hypnotic modality. One of these is the customary intake interview.

Interviewing Under Trance

Perhaps the simplest hypnotic uncovering method is merely to place the patient into hypnosis and take an ordinary case history. The usual questions are asked relating to the patient's symptoms, condition, relationships, job and living situation. This is then followed by an inquiry into childhood, interaction with family members, early illnesses, adjustment in school, sexual experiences, etc. It is like any other intake interview except that the patient is under a state of hypnosis. When doing this the interviewer will usually find a superior recall and greater richness in detail. Memories of events reported in the non-hypnotic state in a sentence or two become expanded into several paragraphs of re-living when elicited under hypnosis. It is as if the bare bones of recollection are, within the hypnotic modality, clothed with many tissues of added detail. Like Reik's "third ear" (1948) one's ability to uncover material further removed from normal awareness seems to be enhanced.

Not only is the flow of memories facilitated, and not only is the amount of recollections substantially increased, but various modifications of questioning technique are possible within hypnosis. For example, one might inquire into the state of mind of a patient at the time that he left his family to enter military service as follows: "You are 18 years old. You have just enlisted in the Service. Your orders have arrived, and you are saying goodbye to your family. You are talking to your father to let him know how you feel about this coming military experience. What are you saying to him?" This is a regression, inducing him to experience the 18-year old period as if it were in the here and now, and reinforcing this regression by asking the questions in the present tense.

Perhaps it is desirable to find information about a patient's relationships with friends when he was a child. One might phrase an inquiry as follows: "You are nine years old and talking to your best friend. What is his name?—"You say, 'Bill'? You're talking to Bill now. What's happening?" The interviewer can even take the role of "Bill" asking the kinds of questions as might a nine-year-old companion and interacting with the regressed patient as boyhood chums would with each other. The patient may reveal to "Bill" many things he would not discuss with parents or with a stranger.

One can frame this interaction psychodramatically such as: "Hey, George, (the patient's name) my Dad says I gotta mow the lawn Saturday. How do you think we can get him to let me off so we can go fishing?" etc. The ensuing conversation between "George" and "Bill" might tell the therapist much about the ways in which the patient as a child interacted with his parents and with other children.

The case-history interview is simply being expanded into a number of different dimensions which are possible because of the focusing effect of hypnosis and its ability to permit role-taking under circumstances that would elicit rejection if attempted in the conscious state. Many individuals have engaged in sexual or aggressive behavior when under the influence of alcohol which they would not have done at other times. The altered state of consciousness provided by the alcohol offers the excuse for a denial of responsibility. So also may people reveal details of their life under hypnosis which they would normally conceal. By telling it under hypnosis they can disclaim responsibility and even deny they said it through actual or claimed hypnotic amnesia subsequently. Hypnosis, like many other psychological defenses, gives us the opportunity both to reveal and to conceal at the same time.

Some of what has been elicited under the hypnotic interview may be material that the patient is not ready to confront and understand consciously. The added knowledge, for the time being, must remain the possession of the therapist's. However, this comprehension can help the clinician plan the therapeutic tactics more effectively, even if the new understanding cannot be shared with the patient immediately.

A college student came to me ostensibly in need of advice concerning her educational and vocational future. For 30 minutes we discussed various possibilities. Almost as an after-thought I hypnotized her. Whereupon she began describing the tangled situation in the girl's dormitory in which she was involved. She had been "recruited" into a small homosexual clique from which she wanted to extricate herself but could not seem to find either the courage or the way to achieve this. Under hypnosis, this whole area was discussed with various possible options which might help her to leave the group without making any enemies. On emerging from hypnosis she manifested an amnesia for the discussion about homosexuality. During the next few sessions each interview was conducted at two levels: first, in the conscious state about educational and vocational matters, and second, under hypnosis and about her relationships with the homosexual group. Some eight sessions later she terminated counseling, having satisfactorily resolved her problem with the homosexual group. She was able to withdraw and form new attachments without antagonizing her former friends. At no time did she discuss the homosexual problem in the conscious state. That entire situation was handled under hypnosis. She thanked me for my help and left, either amnesic of our hypnotic discussions, or without a loss of face by having been confronted with them in the non-hypnotic state. The simple interview, at first diagnostic, and later combined with non-directive counseling, was conducted under hypnosis, but without any complex hypnotherapeutic techniques. There was a kind of unspoken "hypnotic compact" we made, and she would have considered it a breach of confidentiality if I had ever brought up references to the homosexual problem when she was not hypnotized. By preserving her right to dissociative confidentiality under hypnosis I had shown my respect for her needs and facilitated her willingness to reveal the problem and work it through.

In-and Out Technique

Since the data received under hypnosis may differ somewhat from the replies elicited outside of hypnosis a comparison of the two can sometimes reveal areas of conflict. It is reasonable to assume that the material secured under hypnosis may be that which had come under greater defensive needs and hence not verbalized in the fully conscious condition. For example, if a patient describes a family situation under hypnosis and mentions the presence or role of a sister when previously outside of hypnosis he had discussed the same situation but neglected to point out her impact, one might hypotheize that there is something conflictual about this sister, such that it required repression of her in the conscious rendition. As discussed earlier, one of the characteristics of hypnosis is a reduction in criticality, thus permitting previously unacceptable material to be verbalized.

The "in-and-out" technique allows us to interview simultaneously at two different levels, outside of hypnosis and under hypnosis. The patient is hypnotized and given the following post-hypnotic suggestions:

"Whenever I tap my pencil on the table you will go immediately into a deep hypnotic state. When I tap twice you will at once wake up and become very alert."

The patient is then brought our of hypnosis, and the "in-and-out" interview might continue in the following manner:

"Well, I had intended to study for the final exam on Thursday evening. However, a friend of mine came over to discuss a problem with me, and I didn't feel I could cut him off. By the time he left I was too tired to study. I flunked the test, and I felt angry at him for ruining an A in that class."

(Pencil tapped. Patients enters hypnosis).

"Tell me about that time when you said you received a failing grade in an examination."

"Well, I had intended to study for the final exam on Thursday evening. However, a friend of mine came over to discuss a problem with me, and I didn't feel I should cut him off. I was too tired to study by the time he left. I was also angry at him for spoiling my grade in that class. I guess, though, I also felt a little guilty and responsible. I could have told him I had to study and asked him to come over the next day, but somehow I didn't. Maybe a part of me didn't really want to study."

(Pencil tapped twice. Patient emerges from hypnosis.)

"Tell me about that time when you got a failing grade in an examination."

The patient repeats his first description of the situation again omitting the part about feeling responsible and guilty at his failure to postpone the meeting with his friend.

Consciously he blames his friend for the bad grade. Underneath, he recognizes that he was at least partially responsible, but he represses this feeling of personal guilt and fails to take responsibility for the examination, so he reports it only under hypnosis. By using a number of such "in-and-out" maneuvers we become more aware of his defenses and resistances, and can plan our therapeutic strategy accordingly.

Next to its ability to potentiate suggestions, perhaps the most important attribute of hypnosis is the facility with which it permits the crossing of experiential time lines. Within the hypnotic modality memories are more easily stimulated and re-living experiences activated. Unsolved living problems may be re-initiated so that renewed attempts at their solution become feasible with the help of the therapist and with the patient's skills of greater maturity and more recent understandings. Satisfaction of unfulfilled needs and closure of uncompleted gestalts become possible when the memories of these earlier events are re-activated in the here and now.

Of course, this is precisely what psychoanalysis aims to accomplish via transference reactions. However, through the medium of hypnosis we need not always wait until the recall and re-vivification of these earlier events spontaneously arise. Within the intensive hypnotic relationship we can direct and control the regressive process, or at least we can bring it more under control than would be the case in the fully conscious state. Even in psychoanalysis the regressions and transference reactions are expedited because the patient lying on the couch is often in a spontaneously-induced hypnoidal or light hypnotic state. In hypnoanalysis we simple add more therapist control to this factor. Hypnosis does not change either the goals or the conceptualizations of psychoanalytic therapy. It only adds a new dimension to the uncovering and reintegrating processes.

As in psychoanalysis the hypnoanalytic uncovering of earlier behaviors and experiences is not generally on an "either-or" basis. Rather it is more like a continuum in the sense that one can elicit small bits and pieces of yester-year material as verbalized memories and then hopefully move on into genuine re-living experiences involving full emotional as well as intellectual and behavioral responses. We classify such uncovering under two basic headings: hypermnesia and regression.

Hypermnesia and Regression

During hypnosis individuals are often able to remember many situations in far greater detail. For example, under conscious recollection a patient might describe an incident involving a schoolyard fight with a bully, perhaps when he was six or seven years old. The entire incident is related in less than a minute. However, when asked to described the same incident under hypnosis he launches into a vivid picturization of the situation such as the circumstances under which the conflict began, the clothing worn by his opponent, the various blows landed, the outcome, the intervention of friends and teachers, the reactions of parents later at home, etc. What had been told in less than a minute consciously involves perhaps ten or more minutes of descriptive details when recalled under hypnosis.

One must not expect that everything which has been forgotten or repressed will be easily released through hypnosis. The word is "facilitated." Much which lies buried under the amnesias of childhood will continue to remain so even in the deepest hypnotic state

The amount of recall elicited will be a product of many factors, the hypnotizability of the patient, the depth of trance, the relationship with the therapist, and his skill in working in the hypnotic modality. Memories elicited can be factual, but as they are filtered through the perceptual and experiential systems of patients they may have been altered to fit underlying motivations and wishes.

All that has been said about hypermnesia applies equally to regression, and even more so. By regression we mean more than superior memory. Under this term we imply a genuine re-living experience accompanied by emotional, perceptional and behavioral components as they were *presumed* to have occurred at the time they first happened. As we will discuss later this does not necessarily mean the wholistic recapitulation of veridical reality, but rather a re-enactment of the patient's "memory-experience" reality. It is a *subjective* reality; it may or may not be an *objective* reality. However, symptoms are based on the patient's subjective reality; so the material uncovered had therapeutic validity. The patient experiences them as if they were occurring in the here and now. The woman regressed to the age of three actually plays with her dolls. The adult who has recovered from earlier speech defects now stutters. The patient speaks in the first person and present tense, "I'm afraid Billy's going to hit me. Go away, Billy."

Obviously, changes in the physical structure of the individual as a result of having grown up may limit or alter childhood responses. Yet within such changes the truly-regressed individual *appears* to re-vivify and repeat his earlier patterns of behavior and experience.

Regression becomes a more intense and complete form of recall and one which brings into therapeutic focus more of the patient's responding apparatus, affective, perceptual, motoric and experiential. Psychoanalytic "transference" is a kind of regression. Through hypnotic regression we aim at a similar result. Both require much subsequent "working-through, but hypnosis may permit us to arrive at that point sooner.

Many experimental studies on hypermnesia and regression have been published (Ås, 1962; Barber, 1965; Cooper and London, 1973; Dhanens and Lundy, 1975; Huse, 1930; Kleinhauz, Horowitz and Tobin, 1977; Orne, 1979; Udolf, 1983). Our attention here is on hypnoanalytic treatment techniques, so we will not try to review the literature in detail, but rather to present the consensus of research findings to date.

1. When suggestions are given under hypnosis for improved recall

there appears to be a significant increase in memories. Hypnosis alone does not bring any such improvement.

2. The amount and accuracy of recall is related to the kind of material. Meaningful material, such as reports of entire incidents and whole sentences, are better remembered than isolated words or numbers. There is little evidence for hypermnesia in the case of nonsense syllables.

3. Hypnosis seems to facilitate recall of material that is anxiety provoking.

4. Re-vivification of recollections through age regression is generally superior to simple verbalizations as in hypermnesia alone.

5. Age regression is not exact. Material apparently secured from a regression to age eight may include events which happened both earlier or later and may represent the subject's *adult view* of what he was like when he was eight years old.

6. There is apparently a great deal of difference in the material elicited in so-called "age regressions" activated in the experimental laboratory and those which have been observed during psychotherapeutic sessions. Simply telling a person to go to the age of eight is not the same as actually focussing on known eight-year-old events and situations (such as being in an specific 3rd grade class). Many laboratory studies can be criticized on this basis. Regression in an intensive therapeutic relationship with a trusted therapist is not the same as performing in a laboratory with an objective and impersonal investigator. This might account for the conclusions of some researchers that regression is simply "role playing." It may indeed be merely role playing in the laboratory situation. (See Watkins, J., 1989).

7. Both hypermnesia and age regression are susceptible of inaccuracies and confabulations.

These findings do throw considerable doubt on the use of hypermnesia and regression to enhance the testimony of eye-witnesses in courts of law. (See Chapter 11, Forensic Hypnosis). However, research studies provide no justification for discontinuing the procedures in therapy. In fact, they rather support such use.

The evidence indicates that hypermnesia functions best in the recall of meaningful material, and that is precisely the kind of material we wish to secure in hypnoanalysis. Furthermore, material related to anxiety is also best recovered. Anxiety-laden material is often that which is most fruitfully activated, and which we are seeking during analysis. The finding that recall is better under age regression is in line with the conclusion that genuine insight must involve full motor, behavioral, affective and perceptual participation, not merely intellectual verbalizing. The fact that we may often be securing distorted memories does not necessarily contra-indicate the value of obtaining them in therapy. It is common that conflicts have their origins in distorted perceptions and it is in the eliciting of corrective experiences that the therapist achieves the best results. We need not subscribe to an earlier view of learning as the inscribing of experiences on a kind of inner "tape", hypermnesia being then simply the re-activation of this tape. Everything that emerges is of value in the conducting of hypnoanalytic therapy, even though part is confabulated, part is fantasied and only part is objectively veridical. As long as we keep that in mind, we can use hypermnesia and regression. But if these data are incomplete or distorted from whence comes these inaccuracies?

To learn and perhaps later recall an experience we must first record it. This is a matter of perception. Since perception is selective much material may never have been recorded in the first place, and hence cannot be recovered. Furthermore, because of personal dynamic needs our selective perceptions may "choose" to see or hear only certain aspects of an experience. This fact alone limits the material that can be recalled, since we cannot get out what wasn't there in the first place. Items which are cognitively dissonant with already established sets simply don't register.

When the arriving stimuli of dissonant items are so powerful that the individual cannot protect himself by ignoring them, then distortion and other defensive mechanisms may be employed to eliminate or minimize inner conflict. Finally, these same defensive needs may operate to resist their recovery by hypermnesia or regression. The recalled or re-enacted material emerges but with distortions and confabulations. It is precisely such distortions and confabulations which we seek to undo in analytic therapies. Accordingly, we welcome their emergence and availability to change. Horizontal and vertical exploration are hypnoanalytic techniques which enable us to get access to such memories with both their accuracies and their distortions. The question of employing hypnotic hypermnesia in the forensic situation is much different than in psychotherapy. This matter will be discussed in Chapter 11.

Horizontal and Vertical Exploration

Figure 3:1 is a schematic which is useful to conceptualize strategy when employing hypermnesia and regression to uncover forgotten or repressed material. It should be considered only as a useful conceptualization designed for the convenience of the practicing therapist and not as a statement of personality theory. Let the experiential life space of an individual be represented by a solid whose upper surface (ABCD) constitutes the immediate present including all current behaviors, experiences, etc. Let EA be a time dimension running from the moment of conception to the present. Current stimuli impact the ABCD surface and constitute the immediate perceptual experiential and behavioral world. The impacts modify the surface and constitute his "here-and-now." These modifications are recorded and become part of his future memory system. As new stimuli from subsequent moments strike, new surfaces evolve superseding and covering over older ones. The time-line dimension AE lengthens. Data inscribed at earlier periods tends to shrink below the level of awareness. Probably recall suffers first, then recognition as the new experiences retro-actively inhibit the activation of earlier ones.

According to the older, or "recording tape" theories of learning and memory all impacting stimuli would make specific traces, and these would be retained unchanged. Accordingly, to recover them all we would have to do is to regress an individual to the appropriate age level, and we could secure an objective and veridical account of exactly what happened at that time. By regressing him to the six-year-old level (abcd) we could get a true picture of his life and conflicts at that time. Such a view would simplify greatly the job of the analyst, psychoanalytic or hypnoanalytic.

Unfortunately, as we have seen from the previously cited research findings, the situation is much more complex. We can still use our conceptual formulation as in Figure 3:1, but we must consider more carefully just what goes into determining the make-up of the "life-space" solid.

Some of the stimuli involved in the current experience of the here-and-now (plane ABCD) were sufficiently strong as to make specific impacts of which the individual was quite aware. Other stimuli, either because of their lesser magnitude, or because they were in conflict with previous experiences and motivations, made contact, but their impacts were not sufficient to evoke that experience we call consciousness. They were recorded, but being below the perceptual threshold they became part of the person's "covert" or "unconscious" behavioral repertoire—as observed by Hilgard (1986) in his "hidden observer" experiments. Finally, some of the stimuli may never have been recorded at any level, covert or overt. The patient can't remember them, because he never learned them in the first place.

A Schematic Conception of "Life Space"

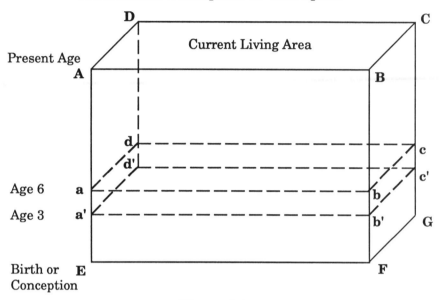

Figure 3:1

The situation is still more complicated by the findings that the impacting stimuli may reach below the surface (ABCD) and modify underlying layers. What happens today may change our memories of what happened yesterday. Furthermore, the process of modifying memory traces is influenced not only by the impacts of immediate stimuli, but it also continues (after experiences have once been inscribed) through the influence of "internal stimuli." These may represent, needs, motivations, traumatic or other previous experiences, attempts to eliminate anxiety and achieve more cognitive consonance, transference experiences with earlier significant figures, etc.

Perceptual psychology (Kubovy and Pomerantz 1981; Hochberg, 1978) notes that we tend to organize experiences into patterns or gestalts. Accordingly, newly received impacts may, by associations, be incorporated into earlier encapsulated patterns. The child regressed to the eighth grade sometimes reports memories or shows some responses appropriate to earlier or later age levels. Experimental studies have often noted that the regressed subject may describe experiences of his earlier period in language more appropriate to an older person. These same findings support the position that communications from individuals regressed to periods earlier than they had learned language may not be merely verbalizing fantasies when they speak in terminology appropriate to a five year old of events which happened before they could have learned such words. Thus, it is common for "hard-nosed" scientists to dismiss as pure fantasy reports by clinicians of the recovery of very early experiences, such as those during the first year of life or birth memories (Cheek and LeCron, 1968). These experiences were presumed to have occurred prior to the acquisition of language. The child at the age of one, may not have learned the word "burn," but he can experience the pain and, at a later age, after having learned the meaning of the word "burn," can attach it to his earlier experience and communicate it to the therapist. The fact, therefore, that recalled and re-enacted data does not necessarily derive from the exact age to which a patient has been regressed in no way negates our use of it in hypnoanalysis. It only calls on us to use greater care and caution in interpreting age levels as we build-up a therapeutic picture of the patient's life experiences. Horizontal and vertical exploration are two techniques for investigating "life space" as conceptualized in Figure 3:1.

Horizontal Exploration involves regressing a patient to some specific age level and then conducting a case-history interview at that age. The technique for regression is to ablate the present and then move the patient in his experience back to the desired age. For example, we might proceed as follows with our patient:

"You are forgetting all about how old you are, what year it is and where you are. You are going back through time and becoming younger and younger. You are 18 years old, 17 years old, 16, 15, 14, 13, 12, 11, 10, 9, 8, 7, 6. You are 6 years old, and you are in school in the first grade. You are sitting at your desk. You can see all your playmates around you and pictures on the wall. Your teacher is standing in front of you. What is her name?"—moving now to surface (abcd), the six-year level.

The steps include: 1. Ablating the present. 2. Moving the patient back step-wise to the earlier age. 3. Rebuilding his experiential world in the regressed age with much vivid description. 4. Testing the adequacy of regression by asking for a specific item (the teacher's name). Once the regression has been secured we then treat the patient as if he were a six-year-old and talk to him accordingly. We explore "horizontally" the surface (abcd) as it was presumed to have been recorded at that time. We try; to secure reports on his relationships with parents and siblings, his reactions to school, his friends, his play and hobbies, his worries, conflicts, etc. In other worlds we are trying to get a picture of his life as it was perceived by him at the age of six. We hope that as much of it as possible will represent actual, objective reality, but we know that it does represent some kind of subjective reality. If he claims that he was mistreated by an older brother and that consequently he feared him, we accept that information (at least at first) on its face value. At some level of his being he feels fear of an older brother and therapeutically that must be dealt with.

Suppose we have already noted that he apparently has a good relationship with this brother at his current age of 21. We wonder what has happened throughout the years? What changes have occurred in his brother-relationship and why? We may choose now to move to *Vertical Exploration.* Keeping to the "brother-relationship" as a common thread we regress him up and down the time line (AE) to find out what happened and when. ("You are no longer six years old. You are becoming younger and younger. Five years old, four years, three years old. Three years old. Do you have a brother? What's he look like? Tell me about him. Do you like him?" We move to (a'b'c'd'), the three year level.

Perhaps we note that his brother was especially jealous of him during his early years because he was his parents' favorite. Later, his brother came to his rescue in a traumatic situation, and he perceived the brother in a new light. He lost his fear, and they became good friends. Through "vertical exploration" we have traced the develop-ment of this brother relationship (as under hypnosis he recalls experiencing it) and can be better prepared to deal with any "un-conscious" blocks which disturb his present interaction with the brother stemming from a transference feeling he held at age six or earlier.

The process reminds one of "mining" his experiential life space by horizontal and vertical shafts. By such procedures we can system-atically explore the three-dimensional living space of our patient throughout his growth and development. Psychoanalysis is more "strip mining" wherein we scrape off the top layer, then the next, etc. Whether we use the psychoanalytic technique of free association or the hypnoanalytic techniques of horizontal and vertical exploration we may still get only a role playing, a partial regression or a more complete regression. Since the latter is what we prefer the question is, "How can we maximize the chances for a true regression? What procedures can we follow to expedite this reaction?"

Simply telling a hypnotized patient to go back to some desired age level may or may not achieve this result. One suspects that some of the research studies which have reported negative results may have used such a simple suggestion—and got only role playing. It is better to remove as much as possible the interferences of the present by ablating current orientation, allowing time for the patient to return to an earlier experiential age, and then describing most vividly some event which took place at that time. It is also important that we use the pr*esent* tense. "You are there. What is happening?", not "What happened when you were six?" In view of the findings regarding hypermnesia for entire incidents as being better than sentences and words the skill of the therapist in attaining significant regressions probably hinge on his first securing a deep state of hypnosis and then on his fluency in picturing a true event in the regressed age. I often use a school scene, assuming we know the patient was in school at that time. Regressed re-living is enhanced when the therapist can visualize himself in the same experiential time frame and co-exist it with the patient. The patient's here-and-now becomes for the moment the therapist's here-and-now. Try to visualize and experience the classroom situation as the patient might have as a child, but without suggesting details. For example, "You're back in the first grade. Look around and tell me what you see. Where's the teacher? What's her name? What does she look like? She's standing in front of the class. What's she saying?" etc. It is important to make the setting as vivid as possible, without suggesting items that may be incorrect. One cannot guarantee that the patient's memory will be objectively correct without some confabulation or fantasying in response to the therapist's "demand" to remember. But the more the patient is non-directively induced to involve himself or herself in the regressed situation the more likely it will be that the hypnotically regressed experience is closer to what really happened.

Indeomotor Finger Signaling

Cheek (1962) has developed a hypnotic form of communication which is partly "dissociative" and partly "projective," but is certainly "hypnodiagnostic." It is an extension of the "interviewing-under-trance" approach but permits the patient to answer questions by finger signally rather than verbally. It was first conceptualized by him and LeCron while observing demonstrations of the Chevreul pendulum

(See Vol. 1, Chap. 4). He has adapted it to the diagnostic understanding and treatment of a wide variety of conditions and has developed it further in a recent treatise (Rossi & Cheek, 1988).

The principle involves informing the patient that his subconscious mind can answer questions without his conscious participation by lifting the first finger if the answer is "yes," the second finger if the answer is "No," and the third finger if the answer is "I don't Know," or "I don't want to tell." In the more recent work (Rossi & Cheek, 1988) the subject (after being told to "let his fingers talk for him") is asked to think "yes-yes-yes" and see "which finger your mind will lift to signal "yes." The same choice is then offered for the "no" response and for a "I am not ready to know consciously yet." In this respect the procedure starts out quite non-directively.

Rossi and Cheek report that, "true unconscious ideodynamic signals are always repetitive and often barely visible." They have extended the motor communication to arm signals and have reported a number o research studies related to ideomotor signaling. The procedure appears to be valuable in getting information past conscious censorship since the subject does not have to formulate a verbal response.

Summary

Diagnosis in the sense of understanding a patient is a continuous process not completed in the initial interviews. Hypnosis can aid in the inquiry by accessing areas of personality not normally available to conscious questioning. Specialized hypnodiagnostic techniques, such as interviewing under trance, "in-and-out," hypermnesia, regression and ideomotor signaling offer the clinician ways of bypassing normal criticality, repressions and other defenses and provide information which can help substantially in planning therapeutic strategy and tactics. The data so gathered is subject to confabulation and pseudomemories. However, regardless of its veridicality it possesses a subjective and experiential reality which is the basic material with which therapist and patient must deal in analytic treatment.

Chapter 3. Hypnodiagnostic Evaluation

Outline

1. Diagnosis as a continuing process of evaluation.

2. Every reaction of the patient is meaningful.
   a. Attention to all changes in patient's posture, gesture and speech nuances as well as verbalizations.

3. Interviewing under trance.
   a. Role-taking during the interview.
   b. Interviewing at multiple levels.
      (1) The "In-and-Out" technique.

4. Hypermnesia and Regression.
   a. Objective reality vs. subjective reality.
   b. Hypnosis facilitates recall of meaningful material.
      (1) Recalled material subject to distortion and confabulation.

5. Horizontal and vertical exploration.

6. The technique of regression.
   a. Ablating the present.
   b. Regressing patient to earlier level.
   c. Reliving patient's experiential world at regressed level.
   d. Testing adequacy of regression.

7. Ideomotor Finger Signaling.

Chapter 4

Abreactive Techniques

Emotional catharsis is a form of release therapy which has been known and practiced for many years. It was from this type of treatment as performed under hypnosis that Freud discovered unconscious processes and proceeded to the development of psychoanalysis. The principle involves the revivification of an emotionally disturbing experience which happened to an individual much earlier, and the release of the affect which has presumably been bound up in the experience. When successful, the result is a great feeling of relief to the patient and often the dramatic disappearance of hysterical or other psychogenic symptoms related to that experience. Freud abandoned the procedure and developed the free association technique of psychoanalysis because he felt that the results of hypnotic abreactions were only temporary. However, Freud felt uncomfortable at having to deal with powerful unbound emotions, and his abandonment of the procedure may have been based more on his personal problems with it (Freud and Breuer, 1953; Kline, 1958).

The abreactive procedure derived from Freud's "Principle of Constancy," in which he argued that an individual seeks to keep stimulation as close to zero as possible. This principle conflicts with the common observation that "people often seek out states of excitement and consider them pleasurable" (Greenberg & Mitchell, 1983, p.26) and also that after periods of sleep organisms arouse themselves to experience increased stimuli. This is one of the reasons psychoanalysts are skeptical of abreactive techniques.

Accordingly, we modify the "principle of constancy" here to suggest that what is sought is not an absence of stimulation but rather an optimal degree of stimulation—and one which alternates over time. Thus, when we have worked (existed) too much or too long we enter sleep where stimulation is greatly lowered. After a period of sleep under-stimulation makes its demands, and we awaken with renewed eagerness for new experience.

Perhaps an analogy is in order. If there is an inadequate amount of heat under the boiler in a steam engine it will not create movement (hence, it is "under-stimulated"). The needs for which the steam engine was constructed (to change heat stimulation into motor behavior) will require that additional heat (stimulation) be applied. In the case of a human individual he will awaken. However, if too much heat is applied to the boiler, and this cannot be translated into overt movement or can be turned into inadequate amounts of movement for its full release, then stress and tension will develop in the mechanism. Likewise, when an organism has received *excessive* stimulation (such as in a trauma), and it has been inadequately released, then the person suffers from tension (anxiety and other symptoms). Abreaction, like a safety value on the steam engine, operates to release the excessive stimulation stemming from the pressure of increased tension. The individual "emotes", and the amount of tension stimulation is lowered to a more comfortable level. A better balance between excessive stimulation and under-stimulation is achieved. The symptoms disappear—at least for the moment. We will discuss later why a single abreaction may be insufficient to bring about a permanent resolution of the symptoms—an observation that Freud made. It is this balance or equilibrium between over-stimulation and under-stimulation which we seek in helping our patient to a more comfortable and meaningful existence.

The human organism often engages in such release procedures spontaneously and naturally (as in sexual orgasm) thus making "abreaction" one of an individual's own self adjustments for the acquiring and maintaining of a desirable equilibrium. Abreactions occur spontaneously to relieve uncomfortable tensions and reduce excessive stimulation as part of normal human self and health maintenance. It is only when the "safety valves" have been unable to open overtly and spontaneously, and release the bound affect, that a psychotherapist (with or without the help of hypnosis) must initiate the procedure and help the patient surmount the blocks which prevent his natural defenses from operating. Abreaction therefore is a therapeutic technique for dealing with tension caused by excessive stimulation which is bound and which has not been released through normal channels of behavior (and experience).

Although Freud ceased his use of hypnotic abreactions Janet (1907) was convinced of the value of emotional discharge and employed the procedure extensively, often inducing crying spells in patients, which he felt needed considerable repetition if the relief from symptoms was to be permanent. Reich (1949), one of Freud's close associates, developed his "Character Analysis," which increasingly emphasized the release of affect that he believed was bound in the patient's "muscular armor." Other workers (Lowen, 1975; Rolf, 1978), using Reich's concept of emotions as being held unexpressed within the muscles, developed approaches to therapy that stressed emotional release through the activation of muscle groups.

In World War I, Simmel in Germany had his soldier patients release rage under hypnosis by attacking and destroying dummies dressed in enemy uniforms. Another active user of hypnotic abreactive therapy at that same time was William Brown (1920). He treated several thousand cases of war neuroses and believed that the cathartic liberation of pent-up feelings brought dissociated segments of the personality back into contact with the ego and resulted in a reintegration of the patient. He deserves credit for recognizing that emotional release must be intensive, continued to exhaustion, repeated, and followed by reassurance and interpretation if symptomatic relief is to be permanent.

In World War II, Grinker and Spiegel (1945) conducted many abreactions with air force personnel who had developed anxiety reactions following bombing raids over enemy territory. They used sodium amytal and sodium pentothal rather than hypnosis to induce an altered state of consciousness and make possible activation of the repressed affect. Also during World War II, J. G. Watkins, at the Army's Welch Convalescent Hospital in Daytona Beach, Florida, employed hypnotic abreactions in treating patients hospitalized after emotional breakdowns during combat on the Italian and French battlefronts. I described these in my book *Hypnotherapy of War Neuroses* (1949).

The traumatic neuroses of war which I encountered during and following World War II are now included within a broader category, called Post-Traumatic Stress Disorders, or PTSD. This category encompasses all syndromes which are caused primarily by exposure to very stressful situations, such as fire, explosions, accidents, loss of loved ones, rape, hijacking, torture, child abuse, etc., as well as war neuroses. The Jews incarcerated in Nazi concentration camps suffered from this disorder.

The symptoms manifested in civilian cases are not unlike those exhibited by the combat soldiers we treated. They include, anxiety, depression, schizoid withdrawal, psychosomatic reactions, phobias, dissociations and psychotic reactions. The egos of these patients have received severe insults from which recovery is difficult and often prolonged, especially when they are not treated in the acute stage. A wide variety of supportive, directive, analytic, humanistic and ego-state approaches may be employed.

Amnesias and multiple personalities (See Chapter 8) usually have severe stress experiences in their backgrounds. The younger the traumas were experienced, the more severe the ego damage, and the more difficult the treatment. Perhaps the good success we had in treating war neuroses was related to the fact that many of these soldiers did not have traumatic childhoods. Their first contact with severe stress came when they entered battle. Until that time they had relatively intact egos. Still one encountered patients who broke under the mild stress of merely being inducted into military service. There are tremendous differences between the ability of various individuals to tolerate stress and not to be damaged, hence, their "ego strength."

Brown and Fromm (1987) have an excellent and most detailed description of PTSD conditions, their etiology and psychodynamics. They also consider in depth treatment strategies from both a behavioral and psychoanalytic viewpoint (including recent object relations theory). They emphasize a conservative treatment approach, seem rather pessimistic about outcomes, and do not recommend abreactions as part of the therapeutic tactics.

As will be discussed more in detail later, our experience seems to be at variance with this position. Although I have treated many more war neuroses, and particularly the acute ones which were seen in an Army hospital, still in the years since the war I have seen a substantial number of civilian neuroses related to severe traumas which occurred both during early childhood and later when the patients were adults. In general, the results with such cases have been fairly good. We believe that abreactive procedures when property conducted, are almost a "sine quo non" for PTSD patients, and we do not believe we could have achieved very significant results without utilizing them. Abreactions, however, to be effective must involve much more than merely releasing affect.

There has been a revival of interest in release therapies using procedures similar to abreactions, for example, behaviorists with their techniques of "flooding" or "implosive therapy" (Stampfl, 1967). From the humanistic stream of therapy comes Janoff's "Primal Scream" (Janov, 1970), an abreactive-like approach that involves regressing patients to the earliest years of their lives and reliving the early pain of parental rejection or other traumas. Perls (1969) and Rose (1976) are other therapists who have emphasized the importance of emotional release over the attainment of cognitive insight.

Many of these more recent workers do not call their procedures "abreactions" but have developed other terminology. However, they insist that emotional re-living and release is essential to good therapy, and in their approaches they employ the procedures described in this chapter to a considerable degree. Some hypnotize their patients; some do not. But when therapists use techniques which emphasize the focusing of attention, concentration and re-experiencing, they may well be inducing trance states indirectly without realizing it.

Freud's self-reported inability to secure a more permanent relief of symptoms through abreaction appears to have resulted from his comparative inexperience with unconscious processes at the time of his early acquaintance with hypnosis and his failure to follow through the emotional release with reassurance, interpretation and reintegration. At any rate, analytic therapists might well profit from a good second look at abreactive procedures.

Criticisms of cathartic therapy come not only from psychoanalysts. Several research studies appear to show that the acting-out of experimentally induced anger in a subject, not only fails to provide true release, but may even increase the subject's angry behavior (see Nichols and Zax, 1977). These authors in a controlled study involving actual patients concluded that there was "definite support for the effectiveness of emotive techniques in stimulating catharsis, and partial support for the effectiveness of catharsis to produce improvement in psychotherapy." However, they reported a number of other experimental studies (Keet, 1948; Berkowitz, 1973) in which induced anger actually increased when presumably it was being released.

The findings can be criticized in that the "anger" in these studies was not *repressed* rage, but rather immediate frustrations experimentally induced in the laboratory. Hence, it was not typical of that which is symptom-causing in patients and cannot be compared with neurotic, long-term, repressed affect stemming from childhood abuse.

Unlike the techniques described here for conducting abreactions these studies did not continue the anger release to the point of physical and emotional exhaustion. Finally, there was no interpretation or egotization of symbolic meanings to achieve reintegration afterwards. Accordingly, these findings cannot be generalized to therapeutically-designed abreactions. (For a more thorough review of studies on catharsis, with and without hypnosis see Nichols and Zax, 1977 and Olsen, 1976.)

From the large number of clinical reports and the few research studies we might conclude that in general:

1. Cathartic therapy involving the release of affect has been shown to be an effective therapeutic procedure in a wide variety of cases.

2. Its best results are secured when it deals with conditions which are acute rather than chronic.

3. It is most effective when treating symptoms that have been precipitated by specific traumatic situations.

4. Abreactions have limited use and may not be effective in treating neuroses that have developed gradually over years and are firmly entrenched through maladaptive behaviors which have had much reinforcement.

Indications for Abreactions.

The first question to be asked when conducting an abreaction is, "Are the conditions favorable for a cathartic procedure?" Abreactions are indicated under the following circumstances:

1. The condition is acute rather than chronic.

2. There are specific symptoms which seem to be related to specific conflicts.

3. The patient has sufficient "ego strength" to undergo a severe emotional buffeting.

4. The therapist is willing and able to co-experience the traumatic event with the patient.

If the symptoms are of recent nature we will think of them as acute. However, that alone is not always important. The fact they appeared rather suddenly may be of greater significance, even though the traumatic incident occurred many years ago. For example, if the patient told us that a certain symptom, such as anxiety, headaches, phobia, depression, etc., first appeared after a very emotionally upsetting experience (or one we would have expected to be upsetting to most people) we have a reasonable basis for inferring some causal relationship. Proximity alone does not determine cause, but it suggests a relationship and is usually worth investigating. Perhaps the patient has said, "When I was seven years old my mother died, and I didn't cry because—. Everybody told me what a brave little boy I was." Or again, we might have heard something like, "I had a war experience. My best buddy was killed when we were fighting together. It was terribly upsetting to me. Right after that I began to have these headaches.," These are the kinds of situations which suggest both acuteness and specificity, and hence are ones more likely to respond to abreactive treatment. They might be regarded as emotionally unfinished business. A situation which would normally precipitate strong emotions has occurred, yet the affect did not appear, at least overtly, to the patient or others. In some way the stimulus which should cause an emotional response (fear, rage, etc.) was presented, but the normally expected response was blocked. Where did the emotional response go? Reich (1949) argued that it was still present, but that the emotion was now frozen or bound in the "character armor," thus creating tension, anxiety and ultimately the neurotic symptoms. The therapist's job is to unbind the frozen affect, release it and achieve closure of the previously unresolved conflict. Since the *normal reaction* was not completed we use an abreaction to re-experience and complete it.

The patient obviously had blocked-off or dissociated the emotion in the first place because he could not handle it, or at least did not feel capable of experiencing it. Now, we are going to confront him with it, so we need to know that he has sufficient "ego strength" to cope with, experience and master that which was previously unmastered. In most therapies we usually have a number of "positives" going for us. Since we have a therapeutic relationship with the patient there is a kind of adding of the therapist's ego-strength to that of the patient's. *We* can endure now what *I*, the patient, could not face alone. With a trusted therapeutic guide in a kind of "withness" the patient is much better able to confront the previous trauma and come out the winner. At the time it occurred he could not deal with it by himself and accordingly had emerged a neurotic loser. It is also likely that if the trauma occurred when he was a child, and as he is now an adult, he, himself, possesses more ego strength.

However, sometimes we may be faced with a patient whose ego is so poorly developed or so conflicted that it is barely able to cope with normal, current frustrations. It is very fragile and might break into an acute psychotic reaction if forced to confront more than it can handle.

In such cases we might wish to study him further, perhaps with the Rorschach, Minnesota Multiphasic Personality or other psychological testing instruments. This situation does not occur often, but when we are not sure that the patient's ego strength plus our therapeutic relationship with him are together still adequate, we may choose to defer the abreaction. We can, of course, work to build up both factors and undertake the abreaction later.

The insecurity of the therapist is an important factor. If we can't take it, then how do we expect the patient to do so. Sometimes the problem is one which you, the therapist, must first solve within yourself. Let us assume that the problem, the patient and the therapist meet the four criteria for favorable conditions, what next?

Inducing the Abreaction

One either starts an abreaction or one does not. There is no half-way. When the decision is made to do it, go into it with all the feeling possible. Don't get part-way into the release of affect and then decide it is too violent. This usually means that the therapist can't take it. Once you open up the patient's bound affect you must continue until it has been fully released. A good surgeon does not open up his patient and then decide that he is not prepared to cope with what he finds there.

Let us assume that through previous sources of information (horizontal, vertical exploration, etc) you know something about the probable trauma, the place where it occurred and the age of the patient at that time. After inducing as deep a trance as possible you then regress him/her to that time and place. (Sometimes it may be desirable to regress the patient to a point in time prior to the traumatic event and gradually work up to it. This may give you an opportunity to evaluate the patient's pre-trauma functioning.)

Next, the scene must be revivified by much description given in the present tense. ("It is June 5th. You are seven years old. Your mother has just died and you are at the funeral. You feel very alone and sad. That feeling is getting stronger and stronger. You want so badly to cry. You are trying to be brave, but you just can't hold back the tears any longer. Let them come. They've needed to come for so long."

Kolb (1988) induced abreactions in Vietnam veterans suffering from post traumatic stress disorder, the more inclusive term now used to include combat neurosis. He employed barbiturates (Sodium

Amytal or Pentothal) rather than hypnosis. To revivify the traumatic situation he played a sound track of combat noises, such as helicopter, rifle, mortar fire and machine gun fire. This served as a strong instigator to elicit regression and a re-living in his patients. Therapists should use every modality possible to build up an experiential return to the traumatic episode.

This scene is vivified until there is a breakthrough, and the feelings begin to flow with nothing to inhibit them. Let the shouts, screams and pounding occur. The more intense the response, the more effective will the abreaction be. Of course, we cannot permit the patient to hurt himself or the therapist. Other than that there should be no restriction on his movements. Don't try to calm him or ask him to "take it easy," or "not to get so upset." We want the patient to be as fully upset as possible.

This experience is continued until the patient is completely exhausted, both physically and psychologically. There are no more tears, and the anger or fear has subsided. Then, and not before, comes the time for reassurance and interpretation. Timing is very important. The therapist has been co-living and co-experiencing the emotional situation. He or she, too, has taken an emotional buffeting. It is time for both to reach a state of calmness and peace. And it is time for the patient to secure an understanding of what it was all about. The therapist must bring meaning through interpretation. But the bound energy which had previously kept this understanding from eogtization has been spent. The resistance is down., Now the interpretations can be accepted and integrated. The interpretations should immediately follow the emotional release. In a short period of time, perhaps a few days, or even a few hours, the defenses will be re-established, and the opportunity for a more permanent resolution of the patient's conflicts will be lost, or at least substantially reduced. Cognitive understanding can more easily follow after the emotional resistance to it has been exhausted.

It is sometimes desirable to repeat the abreaction several times during the same session. Repeat it the next day, a week later, perhaps a month later. The affect is increasingly exhausted until the time comes when the attempt to stimulate it again on the same event arouses no more feeling. It has become a neutral experience, remembered, but no longer capable of causing anxiety or other symptoms. Sometimes a single rendition is sufficient, but be prepared to do repetitions if there is insufficient symptom change after the first.

Some years ago when I was working at the Welch Convalescent

Hospital in Daytona Beach, Florida during World War II a battalion surgeon who had a tremor in his right hand was referred to me. He had diagnosed himself as having a "Parkinson." However, as one of his medical colleagues said, "He didn't know his neurology too well." It wasn't Parkinson but a hysterical tremor.

I noticed whenever he had to salute a commanding officer his hand would shake very violently. He told me that he hated the colonel who was the commanding officer of his hospital detachment. Then he said, "If I could every get that son-of-a-bitch on my operating table, what I wouldn't do to him". This patient was some six foot, three inches in height and weighed over 240 pounds. However, I decided to do an abreaction. So closing the door and putting a table in front of him, I hypnotized him and translated the table into his operating table. A pillow was placed on it, and the hallucination given to him that this was his commanding officer lying there.

"Here he is. What are you going to do with him?" And for the next few minutes he and I committed murder. He was stabbing and cussing "that son-of-a-bitch," ripping with his imaginary scalpel, and I was standing by him shouting, "Give it to him, the son-of-a-bitch. It's what he deserves."

The two of us committed psychological murder over and over. Finally "we" were exhausted. His cussing and screaming stopped, and his body relaxed. Reassurance was given followed by some interpretation about the resemblance of the commanding officer to his own father. He was then brought out of hypnosis. He held his hand up smiling. It was steady, and there was no trace of a tremor.

The Silent Abreaction

The procedures described so far in this chapter have been very intense, sometimes violent, and have encouraged loud verbalization. In many therapist's offices this may not be conveniently done. Professional buildings are not always sound proof. They are build for quiet consultations. Shouting, cursing, and screaming patients simply would not be tolerated. Furthermore, not all therapists are prepared for violent displays of feeling. To better meet the needs of such situations Helen Watkins (1980) has devised a procedure which offers many of the therapeutic advantages of a full abreaction but does not involve the loud noise and violent behavior. She has called it "The Silent Abreaction." It can be more easily initiated than a true behavior abreaction, does not submit the patient to as severe an experience, and yet can be highly effective. It is subject to more limitations than regular abreactions, but is especially useful in dealing with repressed anger.

The technique covers three phases. After the initial hypnotic induction and deepening the therapist describes a scene in which the two of them are walking along a path in the woods. They come to a large boulder which blocks the path. The patient is told that a stout stick is nearby and is asked to pick it up and give the boulder a whack. The suggestion is then made that the boulder "symbolizes" everything that has frustrated the patient, and that it can represent a specific person, a traumatic experience or whatever else is appropriate.

The patient is next induced to start beating on the boulder, hitting it harder and harder until he/she is completely exhausted. The therapist then says, "You can yell and scream and do or say whatever you wish in this place of ours even though you won't be heard in this office. No one will intrude on our scene in the woods." The patient is told to continue this beating until he is exhausted and then to signal this to the therapist by lifting a finger.

The second phase of the technique involves a picturing of the therapist and patient walking up a small rise to a meadow filled with wildflowers. This is accompanied by a vivid description of the sun shining, the breeze gently blowing, and a clump of trees under which the grass is very green. The patient is then told, "Before we can go to the third phase of what we are doing today I need to hear you say something positive about yourself". Many people have been taught not to express anger, and to feel guilty if they do so. Accordingly, this suggestion is aimed at teaching the patient that, "It's all right to get angry." Whatever the patient says is accepted, even if it is a very mild self compliment like, "Sometimes I'm nice to people."

After the positive statement is made the third phase begins. The patient is asked to, "Pay close attention to your toes. You will soon note a warm, glowing, tingly sensation there, and when you notice that feeling signal me by lifting a finger." This sensation is then spread throughout the entire body up the legs into the trunk through the shoulders, arms, neck, etc. Again the patient is asked to signal the therapist by lifting a finger when he becomes increasingly aware of the warm, glowing sensation. At this point the therapist tells the patient that this sensation comes from the patient's own positive feelings about himself, from his inner resources and from faith that he can solve his problems. The therapist then suggests the tingly, warm, slowly sensation will become stronger and asks for a signal of acknowledgement. When the finger signal appears the therapist says, "This additional warm, glowy feeling comes from another well spring. It comes from me as a measure of my belief and faith in you that you will be able to resolve your problem." Coming after the release of anger bound up in the body for so many years, it is a reward for letting go of that anger. The patient is then brought out of hypnosis with the suggestion that the tingling will be gone, but the glow will continue. The silent abreaction can be repeated by the patient at home through self-hypnosis until the anger is gone.

There seems to be no data available comparing the relative effectiveness of a "silent abreaction" with a full-blown one involving overt verbal and motor behavior. From purely a face viewpoint it would seem that a full abreaction which enlists the patient's total expressive behaviors would be better than one which involves only an inner experience. We have had good success with silent abreactions but recommend the more complete catharsis when such is not contraindicated by physical limitations.

The Affect Bridge

Quite frequently the patient shows that his symptoms are related to repressed affect, but we do not know from what time and place in his life they started. We are not informed of any specific traumatic experience which seems relevant. What can be done if we do not know just where to regress the patient? Of course, through horizontal and vertical exploration we may in time locate precipitating incidents, but if we knew just where to go now the treatment might be expedited. In 1958, I tried a novel procedure on a patient for the first time which produced surprisingly effective results. I called it "The Affect Bridge." It was first published in Spanish (Watkins, 1961) and then later in English (Watkins, 1971). Its rationale was as follows.

In psychoanalytic therapy movement from the present to recollections of the past proceeds along chains of associated ideas. The patient says, "I remember when I was 10 years old—, and that reminds me of another time when I—. Memory A leads to memory C because both of them overlap with memory B. Memory B is a "cognitive bridge" which can move us from A to C.

Memory A can lead to memory C, not only because they are both embedded in the common cognition B, but also if they are both related to a common *feeling or affect*. In times of grief we are more likely to remember other situations in which we experienced a similar grief feeling.

Although I have used the procedure frequently over the years that first case provided one of the clearest examples. To illustrate the technique it will be briefly described here. (For those interested in more details see the 1961 or 1971 papers.)

A 35-year old woman was referred for weight reduction following the birth of her child because she had been unable to regain her pre-birth weight. She complained of an obsessive craving for cakes and cookies. At different times this craving would overcome her, and she would rush into the kitchen to satisfy the craving.

During the eighth session she described an incident in which just that had happened. She was in the nursery taking care of her baby when the craving arose, and she satisfied it by gobbling half of an angel food cake. She was placed under hypnosis, regressed to the previous day including the moment when the craving arose, and given suggestions as follows:

"Your craving to eat is becoming more intense. It is becoming so strong that you can think of nothing else. You feel confused. The room is fading. Everything is a great blur. The only thing you can experience is craving. The world is filled with craving, craving, craving, craving."

After the patient had been regressed to (or placed into) the situation which contained the present affect everything except that affect was ablated, and the intensity of the feeling was built-up. The patient's entire experience for the moment was now only a strong mood-state filled with the affect of "craving" and devoid of cognitive content. She was next instructed as follows:

"Now you are becoming younger. You are going back, back, back into the past over a railroad track consisting of craving. Everything is changing except craving. The craving is the same. And you are becoming younger and younger. You are going back to some time in your life when you first felt this same craving. Where are you? What is happening?"

It is important we specify that the patient is to return to a point where he/she felt that *same* craving (or *same* fear, *same* anger, etc. whatever the affect is). All angers may not be psychologically the same, even though they have similar physiological bases. Some "cravings" may well be qualitatively different from other "cravings." We want to activate that specific craving in the here and now which is apparently related (transference) to an earlier incident in which it was originally experienced. If I had not specified the *same* affect the patient might have returned to some other experience, similar, but not the one I was seeking. At this point she replied,

"I am lying in bed. There are slats up and down the bed. I want to suck my thumb, but Mama has tied a cloth on it with bad, black medicine."

The affect of craving when she was in the nursery is the same as the affect of craving she experienced when frustrated by being unable as a child to suck her thumb. Hence, it serves as "the affect bridge" between the two and takes us from the present experience in the nursery to the past one in the crib.

She was next told to "remove the black cloth" and given permission to suck her thumb, which she actually did for some 15 minutes. The "craving" was being satisfied in its original regressed-experiental setting.

Finally, she removed her thumb and said, "I don't want to suck any more I feel so yummy." A new affect has now replaced the craving. It is the feeling of "yumminess." Another affect bridge was run. All experiential content except the affect of "yumminess" was ablated, and she was told to go back to the first time she felt "yummy." Where upon she said nothing, but cupping her hands in front of her mouth she began "nursing."

She was asked, "Do you know where you are," and on receiving an affirmative nod (the ego never fully abdicates, even in deeply regressed hypnosis) I asked if she would be willing to return to the present and bring with her the understanding of what her craving represented, the memories of the crib and the black cloth, plus what the experience of "yumminess" stood for. She agreed, and upon emerging back in the present and fully alert state she broke out into peals of laughter.

"Now I know why I crave cookies and cakes. I don't want to *have* a baby. I want to *be* a baby." During the next 8 weeks she lost 30 pounds, and returned to her original weight. The craving was gone.

Helen Watkins has been using a modification of the affect bridge which she calls, "the somatic bridge." The patient is asked if he/she feels tension in any part of the body. If the reply is "a tightness in the chest," "butterflies in the stomach," or something similar he is asked to concentrate on that part of the body and "go back" to an earlier time when that same sensation was first experienced. Quite often the patient (either with or without a hypnotic induction) will regress to an earlier experience which is then dealt with as in the affect bridge.

Experimental Evidence for the "Affect Bridge."

While many clinicians have reported using the affect bridge successfully, there is also now a substantial body of research findings which support its validity. Bower (1981) has summarized these, including several which he and his associates have carried out at Stanford University. His paper is a significant contribution to learning theory.

Bower, Monteiro and Gilligan (1978) hypnotically induced moods (happy or sad) to create an experimental analog of affect-state-dependent learning. For example, subjects were taught two lists of words, one while happy, the other while sad, and tests for recall given later when the subjects were in the same or the opposite mood. State dependency showed up as better recall of the same-mood list and worse recall of the opposite-mood list. This held when the same was either happy-happy or sad-sad (retention better) and the opposite was happy-sad or sad-happy (retention worse).

In another study they induced a happy or sad mood in their subjects and asked them to describe a series of unrelated incidents of any kind from their pre-high school days. They reported that,"Happy subjects retrieved many more pleasant than unpleasant memories—a 92% bias—whereas sad subjects retrieved slightly more unpleasant than pleasant memories—a 55% bias in the reverse direction." When subjects were asked to describe their childhoods, what they reported, "was enormously dependent on their mood at that time." These findings suggest that I should not have been surprised when my first "affect bridge" patient, while in a state of craving, returned to an earlier incident (the crib) in which she experienced the same craving.

In another study Bower and associates found that when given stories to read, happy readers tended to identify with happy characters and to remember more details about them, while sad subjects tended to identify with sad characters and to remember more about them.

Other investigators, (Teasdale and Fogarty, 1979) found that happy subjects recovered happy memories faster than sad ones, whereas sad subjects recovered sad memories faster than happy ones.

Bower hypothesized an "associative network theory of memory and emotion" to account for these findings. He suggested that an event is represented in memory by a cluster of "descriptive propositions," which are the basic units of thought. These are connected to each other within a semantic-network. The semantic network presumes that each distinct emotion has a specific node or unit in memory which collects together many other aspects of the emotion that are associatively connected to it. The emotional feelings, behaviors related to them and verbal labels assigned to them are connected to the various events in which they occurred throughout different times in one's life.

Accordingly, the common affect provides an associative bridge that permits us to move from one emotional event to another which possesses a similar affect. The theory is extended to account for such phenomena, as "mood-congruity effects," "mood state dependent retention" and dissociation (which will be discussed at greater length in Chapters 8, 9, and 10.)

Bower (1981) concluded with the following statement, "I have described two basic phenomena: first, the mood-contiguity effect, which means that people attend to and learn more about events that match their emotional state, and second, mood-state-dependent retention, which means that people recall an event better if they somehow reinstate during recall the original emotion they experienced during learning."

The Corrective Emotional Experience.

Alexander and French (1946) in a significant attempt to speed-up psychoanalytic treatment stressed the importance of achieving what they called a "corrective emotional experience." By this they meant re-activating an early emotional situation within the analytic transference which had been marked by the patient's inability to cope and to master the situation. By its re-experiencing through transference onto the analyst the patient has a new opportunity to understand it, to perceive its relevance to present-day situations, and to master it. This enables him to respond realistically to current people and similar situations.

To change a situation from a failure to a success it is necessary that it be re-experienced and given a more favorable outcome. That is what psychoanalysts aim to do by way of the transference reaction, and that is also our objective in doing abreactions. When it comes to reactivation, the goals are the same. But as J.G. Watkins (1954) pointed out, hypnotic trance is itself a kind of transference phenomena, at least it provides an altered state of consciousness in which such phenomena can be more easily initiated. Within the trance and the hypnotic relationship we undertake to achieve the same result as advocated by Alexander and French, a "corrective emotional experience" (1946).

If all of the steps for conducting a successful abreaction are carried out we usually do obtain a corrective emotional experience in the patient. However, my wife and colleague, Helen H. Watkins, insists that something is lacking, both in the model of Alexander and French and in the procedures described here for conducting an abreaction. Both models advocate "correction" through re-living, relief of bound affect and new understanding through interpretation, one within the analytic transference and the other within the hypnotic trance. But for true reintegration to take place H. Watkins holds that interpretation is not enough. There must be a re-doing, a corrective action, either in fantasy or in reality, which must be more than a cognitive understanding. The patient *in the regressed state* must make a specific "behavioral" move to change the situation and leave it with a favorable memory, not a failure one.

For example, the patient who has abreactively re-experienced a childhood molestation, and released her fear or anger, must now within the memory images experience herself as pushing back the molester and successfully protecting herself (H. Watkins, 1978). The therapist can help by adding to the patient's "ego strength," thus enabling the sufferer now to master the experience. If the individual has been traumatized by a very fearful experience the therapist (after the releasing abreaction) must in fantasy take "the little girl," hand in hand, back into the feared situation to show her that now she has nothing to fear. Whether or not the patient remembers the corrected version or both versions when she returns to full awareness is not important. What is important is that the corrected version be the one that remains in her "unconscious." It was the original version of what happened (either fantasied or in reality) which was embedded in that covert layer of her personality and which determined her symptoms or present-day maladaptive responses. It must now be the *corrected version* of that event (i.e. the successful coping hypnotically established) which remains in her inner personality structure, so that it, rather than the earlier one, will be the determining agent of her present day behavior and adjustment.

A few years ago when describing the technique for altering pathological memories a psychoanalytic friend of mind remarked, "My God, when you hypnotists start twisting the memories of patients we psychoanalysts will never get them straightened out." And in truth when memories are altered through later influence it may well be that the original version is permanently lost. A number of experimental research studies (Loftus, 1979; Udolf, 1983) have presented data to indicate that once suggested memories have been "frozen" in a subject's mind they may permanently modify or take the place of original veridical recollections. The issue is probably still controversial. However, in psychotherapy with patients we are most concerned with *psychological reality,* not *objective reality.* If a veridical memory causes symptoms and maladaptive behaviors then its replacement by a more benign recollection is in the interests of our patient's welfare. It is what we *think* we have perceived and experienced (conscious or unconscious) that determines our health and adjustment. If a pathological memory can be permanently destroyed and replaced with a health-giving one, then so much the better. We may not always be able to do this. However, the psychological reconstruction of a traumatic emotional experience is a legitimate therapeutic goal. And what may be most important is that the patient take some specific restorative act within his "psyche" to correct the continuous impact on his self-image of a harmful memory.

As an example of this H. Watkins in a published tape (Watkins and Watkins, 1978)[1] recorded an excerpt from an abreactive session in which the patient, regressed to the age of three re-lived a situation in which his mother had locked him in a dark closet (filled with "monsters") because she said he had stolen some cookies. His terror was so great that he had passed-out, and in fact had awakened later in bed regressed in his behavior to a much earlier level. In remembering and re-living the situation he emerges from hypnosis with a severe headache. He cannot cope with the powerful and punitive mother. The therapist says, "I think it's a horrible thing to do to a child. Feel that feeling of resentment and anger. Let it come through, and your headache will stop.—Get in touch with that anger. It's alright to get angry."

But the patient can't do it. He replies, "I can't, damn it. There's something blocking it. There's something that says 'absolutely not'.—Something happened at age two which made me not able to be mad anymore. I just stopped getting mad, the last time I got mad at anybody, really."

The therapist now re-hypnotizes him and regresses him to "that experience that happened to you just before you turned off your anger." He responds with some anger, but not very strongly.

"That's not fair," (hitting the couch). "Mommy. You fooled me."

But with too much fear to continue his anger he starts crying and whimpers "I'm not supposed to be mad."

The sessions continues as follows:

"She hit me with a big belt"

"She hit you with a big belt."

"She told me when I got mad at her she was gonna beat me with the belt."

The therapist now tries to strengthen the child state, so it can cope with Mommy, by suggesting its increase in size.

"You're going to grow up a little bit now. You're gonna get bigger— Can you see Mommy there with the belt?—Now she's gonna hit you with that belt. But you're bigger and bigger, and you can get mad."

This technique doesn't work. The child state still feels too weak to confront Mommy.

"No, I'm just a little tiny kid."

The therapist tries another tactic. This time she strengthens his ego by allying with it.

"Now I want you to pay close attention. I'm not going to let her hit you anymore. I'm going to hold her back, and you can get mad at her. Can you see me holding on to her.—She has a belt in her hand, and I'm not gonna let her hit you. And you can get mad."

The patient, with a therapist-strengthened ego, now takes the necessary action to redress the wrong.

"Can I take the belt and hit her with it?"

Yes. Don't be afraid to. I'm not gonna let her hit you."

The patient laughs and begins to flail his arms, beating the couch hysterically time and time again, at the end of which he spontaneously emerges from hypnosis.

The therapist now interprets: "It's alright; you can be mad now. You don't have to lock yourself into the closet or lock in all your feelings. All those feelings can come out now."

"God damn. You're right, my headache's gone."

The therapist responded with,"I knew if we got the anger out your headache would go away."

The patient can now fully verbalize his rage. "God what a bitch. God what a bitch."

He continues on with a plethora of memories about the mother's mistreatment, and the therapist finally says, "You will remember more and more of all these negative experiences—The energy you have used to repress all this is now available to you for more constructive purposes. The patient looks up with a grin, "How come I feel so tired?"

Laughing the therapist replies, "Well that was a lot of work. You beat the hell out of my couch."

"Poison-Pen Therapy"

Hate abreactions can also be conducted through written catharsis, with or without hypnosis. I have called this "Poison-Pen Therapy" (J.G. Watkins, 1949a).

A very depressed and suicidal woman awoke one night, and spontaneously typed such a letter to her parents. She brought a copy to this therapist. Excerpts from the letter follow:

"Mama and Daddy (in name only), I hope this letter sears your souls and sends you to the everlasting Hell which you so well deserve and which you gave to all your children. You two beasts were so busy fighting all your lives that you did not give your children the slightest love and understanding.—How could you expect to raise children in the hell that you did and get anything but children filled with h*ate, hate, hate*—I was the perfect child—never spanked—wasn't that wonderful? Like hell it was—you held your affection up as the bone I must jump for, and I was always good because I wanted to be loved—not because I wasn't spanked.—I never vomited my food as a small child became I feared the lack of affection it would bring. When I got older I could only retaliate by vomiting.—Truly you are hating people and you will die hated."

The letter was much longer and unfortunately was actually mailed. Even though its writing brought great relief from both depression and the imminent danger of suicide to the patient the therapist should normally suggest this technique only when the patient is requested to bring it in to the treatment, not mail it. One can visualize the reaction of her parents—which might well have created worse reality problems for the patient. The value of such a release comes from expressing the anger at the "parents within the patient," not the old people in reality who would not remember such actions on their own part and simply could not comprehend this message.

Criticisms of Abreactive Techniques

When abreaction is viewed as merely a flooding out of affect, and nothing more, then obviously it may simply be a repetitive acting-out. However, Spiegel (1981), working with Vietnam veterans, demonstrated that hypnotically induced abreactions were very effective when followed by "working-through," the equivalent of the reassurance and re-integration that is stressed here.

Brown and Fromm (1986) have an excellent, scholarly treatise which covers hypnotherapeutic and hypnoanalytic techniques in great detail. In this writer's opinion it is outstanding and a "must" for all serious workers in the field. However, I am in strong disagreement with their views regarding abreaction. They state, "although hypnotic abreaction may be of limited use in certain cases of acute stress symptoms we do not recommend this treatment." Then they advocate a very cautious and conservative approach aimed at avoiding "acting-out" and other "emotional expression."

I and my wife, Helen H. Watkins, have had quite the contrary experience. Starting with the early work with World War II soldiers (Watkins, 1949), followed by over 15 years treating in veterans hospitals and clinics, plus 20 years of private practice, plus many years with dissociated cases (Watkins and Watkins, 1984), we have seen very few of the hazards of which Brown and Fromm warn. In fact, although we, like all other therapists, have had our share of failures, our most outstanding successes were generally the result of profound hypnotic abreactions.

The question may be asked why the disparity between our experience and that of others. We regard dissociated affect, such as is found in traumatic and child abuse cases, as representing a "quantum of pathology" which requires ventilation, expression, release, interpretation and "working-through." One can release this "quantum" violently within a short period, or slowly over an extended time. But this quantity must be released and worked-through one way or another.

A hazard that obviously exists is that the amount of affect released will be too painful to the patient, and his ego will be overwhelmed. In this respect an abreaction is like a "battle" between the "good guys" and the "bad guys." A military principle is that victory goes to him who reaches the conflict area "the firstest with the mostest." In the abreaction it is important that the contact between dissociated "bad" affect and the ego must be stacked with greater strength on the side of the ego.

But the strength or weakness of the ego is not a constant which inheres in that structure. It is measured by the strength of the "therapeutic we-ness," the combined strength of patient and therapist, e.g., "me and my big analytic father (mother, brother)." This "ego-loan" is related to the amount of resonance offered the patient by the therapist. The weaker the patient's ego, the more intense must be the therapist-patient resonance. This strength stems directly from the clinician's "therapeutic self" (to be discussed in Chapter 12) and his commitment to the patient. If the therapist is not willing to submit his own self to the buffeting of a violent co-experience with the patient in the released affect (which may at times involve even fantasy co-murder), then the regressed patient (like a small child) recognizes that his ally, his "therapeutic parent," is not willing to accompany him into the dark closet, "into the jaws of hell." His ego is then not sufficiently strong to prevail in full, unaccompanied contact with the released affect—and the abreaction should not be undertaken.

It has been our experience that even when a most powerful"acting-out" has taken place, the patient seldom emerges from it worse. There has been an emotional release, the resistance is down and the time for reassurance, interpretation and reintegration is at hand. The dire warnings of traditional psychoanalytic theory seldom actually take place. The personality reorganizes, newer ego defenses take place, and the patient moves ahead. We have yet to see a permanent psychosis so tripped off, although transitory psychotic relations may appear—which can have a healing effect if the therapist does not panic.

A young woman with a long-time chronic character disorder involving depression, hostility, constant smoldering anger, and a schizoid manner developed an overwhelming rage in my office. Cursing and screaming she proceeded to throw every book in my professional library on the floor (several hundred), smashed an ashtray, then stormed out shouting, "I never want to see you again as long as I live." Traditional therapy would never tolerate such acting-out, and might even have insisted on hospitalization.

I let her go and wrote her a note saying, "Dear Trude: I shall expect you at our next regular hour. With kind regards, (signed) Jack Watkins." At the next hour she came, profuse with apologies, but beaming all over. Her emotional avalanche had swept away years of depression, repressed anger and narcissistic character traits. She had accomplished more in that one hour than two years of conservative supportive and analytic treatment. With the release of all this bound affect her resistance was greatly lowered. We could now interpret the transferences from her father and her brother—and she could now accept such interpretations.

This was the beginning of an entirely new stage of personality growth for her. Contrary to what might be traditionally predicted, this tremendous progress was not subsequently lost during the many months in which I had contact with her. She resolved a life-long hatred of men, married, and built a new life for herself. Had I panicked, stopped her, rejected her, or returned to a "tip-toeing on eggshells" approach she would never have taken this step forward. "We" had won a decisive battle in her therapeutic struggle.

This was a self-initiated abreaction, but it taught me many things: The healing value of emotional release, the communication of desperation, the revolutions of self in which life-long neurotic patterns of character and behavior can be swept away as the entire governmental structure of the ego is re-organized, the therapeutic opportunity to snatch "victory" from the jaws of chaos and total defeat, the importance of therapist self-control (plus courage), but most of all that intensive relationship and total commitment to one's patient is more important than technique.

This was the first of several similar cases in which great character change followed the abreactive destruction of life-long maladaptive, behavioral patterns. The neurotic who is close to a psychotic break may also be close to a cure.

Abreactive therapy can be dangerous, but it is a very powerful therapeutic technique. Emotional release, and even acting-out, can be turned into a great opportunity in treatment, not merely a liability, if the therapist will take advantage of it. The patient must be protected, either by the restraint of hospitalization or by the restraining hand of the doctor's "therapeutic self." As in any other investments one must evaluate risk vs. possible gain. The first is safer for the moment; but the second is more healing if you can trust yourself and your relationship with the patient.

While certain minimum ego strength in the patient is necessary it appears that the "failures" of abreactions are due more to the limitations in the analyst, rather than to the technique. If you cannot commit your "self" to an intensive co-experiencing in the violent affect, then don't. In other words, if you can't take the heat stay out of the kitchen. Abreactions are not for you, and you should follow a safer release procedure, such as "The Slow Burn", which will not be so threatening, but will take longer. Every therapist must make this judgment for himself or herself.

Kluft (1988) proposed a "slow leak" approach where the patient is instructed to release the anger gradually over a period of time. We completely agree on its value in such cases. However, since it involves some activity on the part of the therapist in controlling it rather than simply "permitting" the patient to regulate its speed, we prefer to call it the "Slow Release" or "Slow Burn" technique.

The Slow Release (or Slow Burn) Procedure.

We must concede that even with the closest resonance of which one is capable, and the utmost of therapeutic commitment, there are times when the abreaction has become so violent or the pain so strong that the patient's ego cannot apparently tolerate its full intensity. He regresses. Even though in the long run the possible gains may outweigh the risks we hesitate to precipitate such a reaction on purpose and prefer to play it more safely, because we (the therapists) are not certain we can bring the patient back to more normal functioning. Sometimes the patient will even inform us that he would prefer to suffer at lesser intensity over a longer time than to involve himself completely in it and "get it over" soon. Patients are often good judges of their ability to tolerate anxiety—although some are "therapeutically lazy" and want only comfort. Ask the patient under hypnosis about his ability to endure these emotional releases. Repressed affect must be released and integrated—either in chunks or in small conservative bits.

In the "Slow Burn" approach we use our relationship to tone down the intensity of the release and encourage the patient to speak it out, work it out, live it out gradually, and extinguish it by being irritated over a longer period rather than violently angry for a short period. The patient may choose to do this. In one case an hypnotically-activated "co-therapist ego state" contracted to desensitize a fear ego state and do the job in "three days," during which the patient would be perceived as hostile by the outside world. He did just that and eliminated a constant source of tension (See H. Watkins, 1978).

We (my colleague Helen Watkins and I) inform our patients that therapy is hard work, that it involves "blood, sweat and tears." To get well they must commit themselves to it—but we agree to make a like commitment ("I will not abandon you."). We also make a point of keeping our commitment, although in some cases it has meant hundreds of hours and many months of free therapy. I remind them after a painful but productive emotional release—as did Frieda Fromm-Reichman (See Greenberg, 1964) "I never promised you a rose garden." They usually feel so much better afterwards, and commonly thank us for having carried them "through therapies" to the other side and co-suffered it with them. It is a time for renewing our "we-ness" relationship.

In cases where the abreaction is being used to relieve the severe suffering which a multiple personality experienced as an abused child we may find that an incomplete resolution of the dissociated rage can precipitate a stage of self-directed anger, perhaps manifested by suicidal attempts or gestures (such as cutting)—from which the patient must be protected. This point will be more specifically described with case illustration in Chapter 8, Dissociation.

Both Comstock (1986) and Kluft (1986) have stressed the almost indispensable necessity for abreactions in the treatment of such patients. However, they have suggested specific ways to mitigate the patient's suffering or reduce its intensity to a tolerable degree. These would be especially indicated if the patient suffered from dangerous cardio-vascular or other physical conditions.

Kluft found this approach valuable in the treatment of elderly patients whose dissociation had existed for a long time and who were not strong enough to face the full fury of their long-repressed rage. In some cases release was so slow that the patient scarcely felt any discomfort, although the reaction continued over an extended period of time.

Kluft also described an approach in which emotional-laden material was brought to awareness in "manageable bits" through a variety of uncovering techniques. The feelings which would be associated with the memories would actually emerge at other times "in solitary moments." He employed "time distortion" occasionally, so that the patient could experience the painful affect as emerging with lesser intensity but over a longer duration. Kluft termed this approach a "fractionated" abreaction.

Although Kluft developed these procedures while treating multiple personalities they appear to be equally applicable for many other conditions. Comstock's suggestions for mitigating the pain of powerful abreactions are also quite useful. They will be discussed further in Chapter 8.

Summary

Abreactive procedures have been neglected in recent years. But the limited and temporary results ascribed to them seem to stem from the incomplete and inconclusive way in which they have so frequently been carried out. Practitioners have released affect, but they have often failed to exhaust it fully and then give the necessary reassurance, interpretation and integration.

They have frequently neglected to repeat the re-living, and have lost confidence in the procedure because miraculous results did not occur after a single rendition. Finally, they have often not been willing to make the necessary commitment to the patient and invest themselves in an intensive, resonant relationship in which they, too, co-experience and co-suffer with the patient. They have misjudged the patient's ego strength and have not presented him with a strong ego-ally.

When applied to specific, known traumatic events that had resulted in repressed affect, inadequate mastery of the precipitating situation and ego damage, and when carried through to completion, abreactions provide valuable therapeutic leverage. They are especially useful in the treatment of Post-Traumatic Stress Disorders. However, they are not without hazard, and require considerable sensitivity, skill, patience and courage on the part of the therapist.

This means that, not only must both the therapist and the patient be strong enough to co-experience them, not only must the affect be prodded to complete exhaustion, and not only must this be followed by reassurance, interpretation and re-integration, but also the entire experience from beginning to end must often be repeated several times if complete release and extinction of the bound affect is to take place. When done properly the ego is better able to cope with stress, and to more clearly establish healthy ego and object representations.

To secure a genuine, emotionally-reconstructed experience reassurance and interpretation may not be enough. The patient must take some positive action to correct the memory of a negative or failure experience and turn it into a successful one.

Abreactions often involve loud shouting and violent emotional behavior—frequently scaring off the timid therapist. It may be unfeasible to carry them out in a therapist's office that is not sound proof and is shared with other professionals. In such cases "silent abreactions" may be helpful. The patient experiences a perceptual release of anger but not a motor or verbal one. Clinical experience indicates that these are effective, but there are not data yet comparing their effectiveness with full-blown abreactions which involve all aspects of the patient's behavioral and experiential abilities.

Even when we are certain that the patient is experiencing transference feelings, inappropriate to the present, and apparently stemming from some early, emotional experience, we are often unable to determine just where and when that incident occurred. An abreaction is indicated, but we need to know just where in the patient's past to initiate it. The "affect bridge" has been developed as a procedure which allows us to return to a previously unknown event in which the patient experienced a feeling state similar to that which he is feeling in the present. This procedure has not only been found to be a very effective therapeutic technique, but it has also had considerable validation from experimental studies on the relation between mood and memory.

"Poison-pen therapy" is a written abreaction which encourages the expression of affect in letters which are not mailed. "Fractionated" abreactions and the "slow leak" ("slow burn") are release approaches that spread the reaction at a lowered intensity over a period of time. They are indicated if the patient's ego is considered to be fragile.

Criticisms of abreactions range from claims that they are ineffective, to encouraging patient "acting-out", to stressing possible hazards to patient or therapist. When the therapist and patient have a close, constructive relationship, and the therapist is "resonating" with the patient, these criticisms do not seem compelling. Abreactions are extremely potent treatment procedures. When carried out skillfully they can often advance therapeutic progress more rapidly.

Chapter 4. Abreactive Techniques

Outline

1. Emotional catharsis, a long practiced release therapy.
    a. Freud's rejection of it.
    b. Controversial research regarding its efficacy.
    c. The corrective emotional experience.

2. Indications for abreactions.
    a. The symptoms are acute.
    b. The patient has sufficient ego strength to endure them.

3. Steps for inducing an abreaction.
    a. Locating the initial traumatic incident.
    b. Regressing patient to this moment.
    c. The therapist co-experiences the abreaction with the patient.
    d. Re-vivifying the experience.
    e. Continuing release to the point of physical and psychological exhaustion.
    f. Interpretation and re-integration.
    g. Repetitions of the abreaction.
    h. Behavioral validation of genuineness of emotional reconstruction.
    i. Hazards and precautions.

4. Indications for Post Traumatic Stress Disorders (including war neuroses).

5. The "silent abreaction."
   a. A perceptual rather than verbal or motoric experience.

6. The "affect bridge."
   a. Relation to cognitive association bridges as employed in psychoanalysis.
   b. Activating the affect in the present.
   c. Ablating all present experience except the pertinent affect.
   d. Regressing the patient back to the earlier experience over their common affect.
   f. The relation of hypnotically activated "affect bridges" to psychoanalytic "transference reactions."
   g. Experimental evidence.
   h. The "somatic bridge."

7. "Poison-pen therapy."

8. Criticisms of abreactive techniques.

9. The slow release or "slow burn" (Kluft's "slow leak").
   a. "Fractionated" abreactions.
   b. Hazards and precautions.

Footnote
1. This tape is currently in the process of being revised and republished.

Chapter 5

Hypnography and Sensory Hypnoplasty

The Use of Art in Hypnoanalytic Technique

This chapter, plus Chapter 6, Dreams and Fantasies, Chapter 7, Projective Hypnoanalysis and Chapter 8, Dissociation, describe a group of procedures which differ yet have much in common. In fact, each pulls on the other, and any one of these chapters could have come first. Each chapter includes techniques which involve fantasy, imaging, projection, subject-object dissociation, and motor communications, both real and hallucinated. The reader may wish to peruse all four chapters at first and then return to each for more intensive study. The order we have chosen here involves a rationale of beginning with the more tangible and concrete approaches, proceeding to the techniques which emphasize projective fantasy, then describing those which center on dissociation and ego splitting. This will lead us more naturally into the complex techniques of hypnoanalytic ego-state therapy in Chapter 9. However, there are good rationales for other orders of presentation.

As a young graduate student I once took a course in the history of modern music during a summer school session. The instructor, composer Edwin Stringham, a distinguished visiting professor from Columbia University, proved to be a most innovative teacher. He wanted to give us an understanding of "impressionism." Accordingly, he not only lectured on its objectives, its history and the lives of its composers, but he also played impressionistic music (Debussy, Ravel, Stravinsky). Still not content, he brought in samples of impressionistic poetry, showed us prints of impressionistic paintings (Degas, Monet,) and photos of impressionistic sculpture. He showered us with "whole brain" learning. He stimulated our imagery as well as our cognition, and we derived a true "insight" into the meaning of that term because he presented it through many modalities, verbal, auditory, visual and kinesthetic.

Recent research (Levy, 1974) in the functioning of the left and right brain hemispheres has demonstrated that they do much more than control the opposite sides of the body. Each has its own, unique mode of thinking, its own *mode* of consciousness. With the left brain we reason logically, express our understandings in verbal terms and are analytical. The right brain presides over such functions as spatial relations, imagery, metaphors and dreaming. In the engineer and the scientist left brain activity is predominant. In the artist and musician it is the right brain which is primarily processing the data. In any given experience one or the other may be dominant, or the two may collaborate, especially when the more intuitive and feeling aspects of our "perceptions" are creatively brought to conscious, verbalized "insight."

A cable of fibers, the corpus callosum, connects the two and apparently provides the exchange of impressions necessary for an individual to integrate these two modes of consciousness. In creative individuals the corpus callosum functions most efficiently. When this connecting link is severed surgically (Sperry, 1973) the individual is in considerable conflict as right-brain information may be verbally mis-labelled by the left brain.

Something of this same nature seems to occur between repressed unconscious processes (which may be more right-brain mediated) and a patient's efforts to acquire conscious, logical, left-brain (e.g. verbal) understanding. The effectiveness of a skillful, sensitive analyst may derive from his creative ability to "tune-in" on the patient's right-brain communications (associations, metaphors, postures, gestures, images and dreams) and communicate them in logical, verbal "interpretations" to the patient's left brain—where they become conscious and controllable. He/she becomes (like my music-history instructor) a transmitter of "whole-brain" learning. He integrates "artistic" understanding with "scientific" understanding, and both are now within the realm of awareness.

The heart of psychotherapy is communication. The patient and the therapist exchange meanings, usually in the form of words. However, communications can take place without words. In our posture, gestures, inflexions, facial expressions, etc. we transmit our meanings to others, perhaps through right-brain activity. In fact, through such indirect communications we often reveal meanings which are unconscious and thus concealed from our own normal awareness.

Artists communicate inner meanings through sculpture, drawing and painting. The later paintings of Van Gogh, by their use of vivid oranges and blacks and by agitated landscapes portrayed so well the storm of depression which was sweeping over the artist—and which led finally to his suicide. The medieval painters in their productions of angels, Madonnas and devils displayed the religious conflicts which pervade that age—and their own selves.

Art productions have been used in psychological projective tests e.g. the House-Tree-Person (Buck, 1948) and the Draw-a-Person test (Machover, 1948). Through these devices the psychologist induces a patient to draw images and fantasies which may portray both the structure of the personality and the inner motivations. Jung (1916) and Rank (1932) analyzed the work of artists in an attempt to understand their psychological processes. Naumburg (1947, 1950, 1953) and Stern (1952) reported the use of drawings and paintings in implementing psychoanalytic therapy (with both neurotics and psychotics). More recently, Grof (1975, 1980, 1985) employed the analysis of art production extensively in his drug-oriented "LSD therapy."

Although art therapy has not been a popular mode of treatment in recent years there are several reports of its practice, such as those by Kramer (1971), Levick (1981) and Wadeson (1980, 1982). The use of art in both diagnosis and treatment has existed for a long time but it has not received the attention it warrants.

Since hypnosis offers an avenue for the creation of dreams and fantasies, as well as a more direct access to unconscious phenomena, most hypnotherapists and hypnoanalysts have relied on communication through words rather than in art productions. Accordingly, the literature in this area is rather meager. Kline (1968) described a procedure which he called "Sensory Hypnoanalysis." This represented an extension of two earlier approaches, "Hypnography" (Meares, 1957) and "Hypnoplasty" (Meares, 1960, Raginsky, 1961, 1962, 1967).

Hypnography

Hypnotized subjects were found by Meares to be more amenable to projective painting than those in the waking state. Initially Meares had his patients draw with a pencil. However, he found that black paint proved more effective than either a pencil or his attempt to use different colors.

He developed a fairly standardized procedure. A "critical depth" of hypnosis was first induced, usually requiring several sessions. Patients would hold the brush very loosely, and suggestions were given, such as: "Here is a paint brush. Here is a paint book. I dip the brush in the paint. Your hand takes the brush. It paints it. Your hand will paint whatever is in your mind." etc.

Some patients had difficulty getting started, a situation which also often occurs when doing automatic or dissociated handwriting (see Chap. 8, Dissociation). The patient was continually urged by repeating such suggestions until painting movements begin. When the brush got dry Meares would say, "The brush is running dry. I take the brush and dip it in the paint." This activity on the part of the therapist was often necessary with very passive patients. Furthermore, when patients were asked to dip the brush themselves they frequently knocked over the paint jar or spilled the paint. For many individuals motor control was inhibited under hypnosis. After the paintings were completed associations to them were elicited before the patient was brought out of hypnosis. Meares also recommended a half hour sleep for the patient after the session before dismissing him.

Paintings under hypnosis often resemble children's productions and initially represent the outline of some object. Prior skill in drawing or painting was not apparently utilized in hypnotic productions. In fact, when the patient was hypnotized his/her normal traits might not show at all. For example, an obsessive-compulsive patient given the normal state to much neatness was very sloppy in his hypnotic productions. This tended to validate the presumed psychodynamic defenses of excessive neatness as opposed to its unconscious opposite (or as Freud hypothesized a regression to anal smearing) and suggests that hypnographic paintings do tap unconscious motivations.

In line with the concrete thinking shown by children and psychotics, paintings of an object tended to refer to a very specific meaning. Thus, the painting of a house did not represent any house but rather a very specific house which was significant in the patient's life. At other times, the object represented a symbol. The "house" might constitute a symbol of a woman, very specific woman, such as the patient's mother—as is commonly found in psychoanalytic dream analysis (See Chap. 6, Dreams and Fantasies). With rare exceptions Meares found that the paintings always represented something which was very important emotionally to the patient. Of considerable interest was his finding that the paintings could not be predicted from a knowledge of the patient's conscious conflicts.

The free associations to the paintings are just as important as the art productions themselves and often are essential if interpretations of their meaning are to be secured. Accordingly, it is best that the association period immediately follow each painting. Suggestions are given such as, "You won't wake up while I talk to you. You talk in a dream. What is this that your hand has painted?" Notice the painting is credited to "your hand," not "you,". Even better might be dissociating the hand further during the painting process by referring to it as "the hand" rather than "your hand."

The process of defense enables us to *express* a covert or unacceptable meaning and *suppress* that meaning from consciousness at the same time. Hypnography affords a modality whereby a patient can *reveal* to the therapist what he has felt the need to *conceal* from himself.

Associations can be elicited which are completely "free." "What do you think about concerning this painting" Or they can be "radial" around specific items in the picture, e.g. "Tell me everything which comes to mind related to this small tree here." The associations are especially essential when the painting refers to traumatic incidents in the patient's life (such as are dealt with in Chapter 4, Abreactions). In fact, such a painting may prove to be the stimulus necessary to induce a regression to the emotion-laden experience and precipitate the abreaction.

Patients sometimes express their underlying meanings by the manner in which it is made rather than by its content, hence, sexual or aggressive motions. The same considerations of gesture, posture, inflexion, facial expressions should be taken into account as one does in any therapy, hypnotic or non-hypnotic.

The more one is experienced in dream interpretation the better use one can make of the hypnographic technique. Meares found that both universal symbols and individual symbols were represented, and that the greatest difficulty in interpretation often lay in the therapist's confusing the two. That is why interpretation should wait the fullest period of associations.

Symbolism in Hypnography*

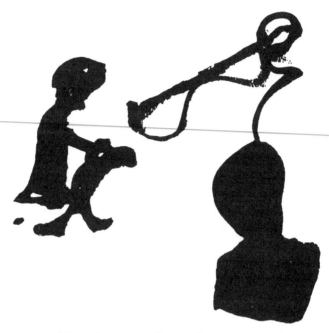

Figure 67. A middleaged patient, who lived with her mother, was suffering from a complete hysterical aphonia. Psychotherapy was virtually impossible on account of her inability to communicate. Attempts to restore her voice with waking suggestion had failed. She was deeply hypnotized, and in a long session, attempts with hypnotic suggestion also failed. When tried with hypnography she produced this painting. The figure on the left represents her mother scolding her as a child. On the right the patient is being struck with the lash of her mother's tongue. Her aphonia was a defence against her speaking rude things in retaliation against her mother. Her voice returned during the session and she has remained well.

* From Meares (1957)

Figure 5:1

When should hypnography be used? Of course, the most logical reason would be when our patient is very taciturn and not given to much verbal expression. Shyness, fear or resistance against revealing self may all be represented in such behavior. This means the therapist should be cautious about revealing to the conscious, alert patient here-to-fore hidden meanings in his art productions. Do so only when he/she is ready to accept such insights. I have found that material revealed under hypnosis will often come spontaneously to mind in the patient two or three weeks later if the therapist will restrain his eagerness to impart this new insight. Common defenses against verbal revelations may not be operative during art communications, and the patient may need a period of protection against an immediate and crude confrontation with them.

Most clinicians will not find hypnography suitable to their manner of treatment. It is somewhat slower than data secured verbally, but it does get at material which often cannot be elicited through words, or at least only with great difficulty. It is a technique which should be in the therapeutic armamentarium of an eclectic hypnoanalyst.

Hypnoplasty is a hypnoanalytic procedure developed by Meares (1960) and Raginsky (1961, 1962, 1967). It involves allowing a hypnotized patient to express inner conflicts through fashioning clay or plasticine models and extends into another artistic modality the same principles found effective for eliciting suppressed or repressed material via painting. However, before describing these techniques it is desirable to spend some time on an intermediate approach developed by Meares which he termed "Plastotherapy." Plastotherapy is simply the use of plastic models by unhypnotized patients as a way of non-verbal communication. Hypnoplasty is merely plastotherapy under hypnosis.

Plastotherapy

The patient was given clay and told, "I want you to model something with this clay. It is fascinating stuff. Feel it."

Occasionally some explanation was necessary such as: "There are many ways in which we can express ourselves. Sometimes we use words. Or we can communicate by gestures, facial expressions or by the way we do things. You can express yourself by modeling. That is why we use this clay. Just let yourself go and make something." I'll be back in a little while." the therapist then leaves the room. Meares felt that the patient was less inhibited when he/she was alone.

In his early work he used Plaster of Paris mixed with asbestos. This slows its hardening and has the advantage that it will form a permanent, hard object which can be studied late at leisure. But Meares discarded this mixture because it was sticky. We also know now about the harmful effects of asbestos. For most therapeutic work ordinary modeling clay or plotters clay, such as are found in toy shops or art shops, is probably best.

A good time to bring in the modeling clay is when the patient seems verbally blocked because of some close-to-conscious conflict.

The change in the therapeutic communication is from verbal (left brain) symbols to plastic (right brain) ones. When confronted with such a projective task there is usually an increase in anxiety since the patient senses that he may lose control of the situation. The therapist's physical absence does not permit the patient to evade by further questions and verbal interaction. Because we are accustomed to using words as defenses this request to communicate through modeling represents an assault on one's personality structure. It by-passes our strongest and most practiced defense mode, the verbal one.

The first productions are either quite innocuous or have a symbolic rather than direct meaning—especially in the non-psychotic patient. However, they should be regarded as having psychodynamic meaning and subject to interpretation. There may be an intensification of affect which can then be used to precipitate abreactions. One can expect much defensive elaboration after the patient is asked to comment or associate to his production. "It's really nothing. Just some object which came to mind. It doesn't have any meaning," etc. However, if one considers the symbolic meanings the modality offers a chance for the therapist to observe more rapidly many of the patient's unconscious conflicts. Modeling (like dreams) is also a "royal road to the unconscious" (Freud, 1953b). The time in analysis required to break down defenses and get at repressed conflicts is shortened.

Since the clay model is an "object," hence, "my" production, but not directly "me," the patient is not immediately confronted with his revelation as in words which he has just uttered. The fact that, unlike a word, the symbol remains in front of his senses requires him to deal with it. He cannot simply dismiss it as with verbal symbols. Emotions of guilt, fear and rage may be immediately stimulated and sudden new insights often occur.

The therapist takes a non-directive role but can come closer to increase relationship impact by sitting beside the patient and cooperate in molding the clay, touching or commenting on the patient's production. Or if desirable the therapist can withdraw and provide distancing, as may be needed by paranoid or otherwise threatened patients. His/her role should be flexible. The patient can be told that, "our fingers make something." This is dissociative behavior similar to hypnosis. The fingers and not one's own self assume responsibility for revealing conflicts. Like the drawings in hypnography the clay models may reveal such conflicts as latent homosexuality, unconscious sadistic impulses, etc.

The patient's associations to his production are extremely important. Theses often become quite specific. For example, a man is not just any person, but may represent the patient's father. A house may be one he lived in as a child. The symbol becomes more concrete in its communication. At first there may be a denial followed by closer approximations of its true meaning as the associations are extended. If the therapist is analytically trained the usual principles employed in free associations during a traditional psychoanalysis (Glover, 1955) can be followed. The only difference is that they start from a tangible clay model and are not completely "free." One can ask the patient simple to "tell me everything that comes to mind in relation to the object." Or one can approach the associations radially. "What comes to your mind in connection with that hole at the top of the model," etc. The symbol may be an abstract concept, a wish, a fear, a significant person in the patient's present or early life. The associations to it generally lead to some significant pre-conscious or unconscious conflict. Meares notes the appearance often of "screen symbols," which like "screen memories" cover up or elaborate the original repressed material into a temporary disguise. They are most likely to appear when the patient's defenses are most threatened, in which case the therapist should be cautious in confronting the patient with too direct an interpretation.

Even though the process may speed up an analysis it cannot completely eliminate the need for "working-through" and experiential time to achieve genuine insights. The therapist should remain relatively passive but can repeat the associations to either the unhypnotized patient or when he is under hypnosis. The associations generally become more concrete and specific under hypnosis. If blockages occur, the patient should be asked to make another model. This often reveals the reason for the blockage. If strong affects break out during the associations the therapist might develop them into a true abreaction employing the principles and safeguards described in Chapter 4.

Plastotherapy should be considered as a projective technique which can serve diagnostically like the Rorschach test but which also can be extended into a therapeutic procedure. Meares book (1960) presents photos of many different models produced by neurotics, psychotics and patients suffering from other conditions. He reported that those molded by psychotics were rather clearly differentiated from those of neurotics.

Plastotherapy is not an integrated system of therapy but rather a tactic within another basic approach, generally psychoanalytic or hypnoanalytic. It has limitations, such as the use of messy materials, the considerable anxiety it often provokes, and the fact that patients will occasionally reject this method of communication. It does reach through defenses more rapidly, can be quite flexible, and affords another modality for the doctor-patient relationship to operate in an analytic treatment situation.

Hypnoplasty

From the use of modeling techniques in the conscious state Meares proceeded to employ these same procedures when the patient was under hypnosis. He believed that a fairly deep degree of hypnosis was essential but conceptualized hypnosis as "a highly dynamic and constantly fluctuating state of mind," rather than a level of trance.

Since active movements of the hands are required, as in hypnography, sleep and relaxation inductions are contraindicated. Meares recommended either the eye-fixation or repetitive movement approaches. Induction was followed by suggestions like the following: "You let yourself go so completely that your body works automatically. Your hands and fingers can do things." The involvement of the fingers was facilitated by such suggestions as, "Your fingers pick up the clay. You do not do it, your hand does it." Perhaps even better would have been, "The hand does it." Notice how "the hand" is dissociated into an object, an "it," not a part of "the me." The patient can be told that he will experience it as "if in a dream" but with the eyes open.

The clay objects fashioned under hypnosis tend to show more primitiveness, be more disorganized, and resemble psychotic productions. Meares noted four different types of symbols: "representational," which is an element of some significant object—but a rather poor likeness. A "conventional" object might be a person with head, two arms, two legs, etc. The "individual" symbol was one peculiar to the individual. It might be quite strange or bizarre. The meanings of these are difficult to determine. The "universal" symbols included the traditional Freudian sexual symbols as well as those representing Jungian archetypes.

In hypnoplasty, plastotherapy is interwoven with the traditional psychoanalytic procedures (such as free association and dream interpretation) but are carried out within a state of hypnosis. Abreactions are initiated, affects are released and interpretations given. Meares believed that analytic therapy proceeds faster in this modality, but he cautioned against initiating too much anxiety during the abreactions.

Example of Hypnoplasty*

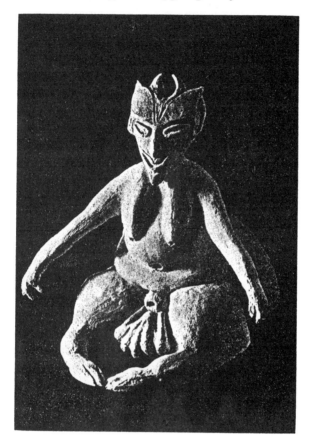

"The Devil"
I don't know why I did it.
It came when I mixed the clay that day.
While I was doing it I was thinking of hermaphrodites.

This is the Devil, who at the same time is her husband. He has the horns and cloven hoofs of the Devil, and a'leering, mask-like face. His male sex organs are shown, but he also has the large breasts of a woman, and huge flabby buttocks.

The patient has recently accused her husband of being sexually abnormal. The truth or otherwise of this is not known. It may be merely a matter of the psychological projection of the patient's own feeling of bisexuality.

* From Meares (1960)

Figure 5:2

Sensory Hypnoplasty

Raginsky (1961, 1962, 1963, 1967) extended Meares' procedures into another dimension, one which provided more stimuli and specific structure. He added variations in color, texture and odor to the plasticine. He reported that these changes stimulated regression to more circumscribed areas of conflict. Thus, patients who were given blood-red plasticine tended to regress to oral levels of development or in women to conflicts about menstruation. When the red plasticine was quite soft sexual fantasies were initiated. Soft brown (stool-like) plasticine brought regression to the anal level and fantasies regarding elimination conflicts. The color white gave patients a "new, clean feel." These were enhanced by the addition of appropriate odors. Raginsky also found that subjects' associations were most revealing. However, unlike Meares he used light trances. It will be recalled that Meares (Vol. I, Hypnotherapeutic Techniques, Chap. 2) had developed the atavistic regression theory of hypnosis, which related the modality to early, primitive levels of function typical of humans as they progressed up the phylogenetic level from anthropoids to humans. Meares, therefore, worked with and emphasized the deeper levels of trance. Ragnisky did not believe deep levels of hypnosis were necessary. Furthermore, because his patients were not so "deeply" hypnotized he had less difficulty in getting them to verbalize their associations.

Psychoanalysis involves restructuring of understanding in the patient based on meaningful interchange of communications between the patient and the analyst. It is anticipated that these "meanings" will be formalized in verbal form, hence, an exchange of words between the two, and that each will come to understanding the "meanings" of these verbal transactions, the analyst's "interpretations" and the patient's "insights."

However, we also know that understandings and meanings can occur within a person which never get verbalized, either to the individual or to others. The personality structure reorganizes around such changed meanings on a covert level. The patient "gets well" without either patient or therapist being able to explain in verbal terms the psychodynamics of that change. We are not referring here to a simple loss of symptoms because of suggestive influences, but rather profound personality reconstruction—which may occur perhaps during such experiences as religious conversions. Most therapists who have worked analytically in depth with patients have seen such examples. The patient improves, manifests a profound change of personality, and there is no reappearance of the symptoms after the suggestive influence and transference relationship with the therapist have been terminated. The patient has apparently "gotten well." We can't explain why, but we accept the "recovery" gratefully.

Since art productions, drawings, paintings, modeling, etc. are often unverbalized, symbolic communications the possibilities for therapeutic changes like the above are ever present. Through free association and/or an analyst's "third ear" sensitivity (Reik, 1948) we can often translate the symbol's meaning into words. But sometimes we cannot interpret its verbal equivalent, even though the creation of the symbol and the reactions of the analyst constituted a genuine interchange of meaning between both at an unconscious level. Sechehaye (1951, 1956) in her "Symbolic Realization" therapy achieved significant results in treating a regressed schizophrenic with such covert exchanges of meanings through non-verbal symbols—as confirmed by the report of her patient (Renee, pseudonym, 1951).

H. Watkins' "Doodle Therapy."

Helen Watkins has experimented substantially with the use of "doodles" as a modality of covert communication especially when her patient has difficulty talking, either overtly or under hypnosis. She frequently inquires whether the patient makes doodles, and if the response is "yes" she encourages him/her to bring in such productions. Sometimes the doodling is done under hypnosis, at other times its meaning is worked out under hypnosis. And at still other times the meaning never becomes verbally conscious to either, but there can be significant symptomatic and personality change subsequently. She reports one case involving doodle communication as follows:

> This woman in her thirties came to me for one appointment. She had previously undergone some 15 years of therapy, mostly traditional psychoanalysis with substantial gain. However, she reported that, "There is still something wrong, something missing, and I don't know what it is." I noticed her writing pad was covered with doodles, and I commented on it. She told me that she was an art therapist and that she draws a lot, showing me samples of her work. I asked about her birth, and she replied that she was adopted. I asked her if her birth mother had tried to abort her, and she replied, "Yes, she told me she was unwed, couldn't keep me, and was embarrassed about her pregnancy." I then said, "I suppose she tried to do

it with a coat hanger?" Startled, she replied, "Why yes, the doctor said I had an injury to my shoulder at birth from the attempt. But how did you know?" I pointed to her doodles. There were coat hangers covering the page.

I then hypnotized her and suggested that she go back to the beginning. She would see a small opening, and she would become small enough to easily pass through this opening into a soft, warm dark room. She lay on the floor of my office, pulled her knees up to her chin, and then scooted herself back into a corner of the room, frightened and huddling into that corner. I told her that she was supposed to live and not die no matter what might be frightening her.

Sometimes later, I described this case to a colleague, who was an obstetrician. She said that when an abortion is attempted the fetus will often try to crawl into the wall of the uterus for safety.

Regardless of how one tries to conceptualize what happened theoretically the fact was that the client reported feeling much better and with a sense of completeness that something was now "right." She felt as if her "analysis" was now finished. Was this what Alexander and French (1946) called "a corrective emotional experience?"

H. Watkins reported another case in which doodles led to the destructive relationship and child abuse which was at the root of a patient's bulimia.

This 20 year old girl was quite depressed at her inability to stop her compulsive binge-purge cycle. Her referring psychologist asked me to use hypnosis to uncover her near-forgotten childhood. She mentioned that she enjoyed doodling, and at my suggestion brought in a page filled with doodles.

In her associations each of them seemed to be connected to a maternal grandmother. At one point I asked her to draw a picture of herself and then under hypnosis to relax in her chair and report whether one arm felt different than the other. My request came because the right arm had been drawn much larger than the left one. She replied that the right hand and arm was larger and much more powerful.

I suggested that it was no longer connected to her, that it was free to move anywhere it wished, and that she could follow it. Whereupon it began to move down the street on which she lived as a child. It proceeded to a house, which she identified as grandmother's, went in the back door to the kitchen, grasped grandmother by the throat and tried to strangle her.

This cued me into a series of abreactions during which she re-experienced many brutal scenes of sexual molestation and cruelty. Grandmother would alternate between starving her and forcing her to eat until she would vomit. The bulimia was resolved, and she ceased the binge-vomit cycle. It was the doodles which cued me into the significant experiences which required abreactions to release wells of repressed anger.

In another case of "doodle therapy" the patient was unable to talk under hypnosis. She would make efforts and then choke. The symptom was a life-long depression. In this case the doodles were brought in by the patient before each session. Their symbolic meaning could only be inferred. However, using the "finger signal" technique described by Cheek (1962) Helen asked questions to find out what age in the patient's life the doodle was supposed to represent. She described the case as follows:

This patient reported to me that she had been depressed since childhood. She hated her critical father and defended her dependent mother. Her parents argued a lot. When I took her down to "a glass paneled room" under hypnosis she saw them "fighting." At the second session she brought in a doodle made with water colors (See Figure 5:3). To me it looked like a womb with a fetus within. However, she had no associations to it but merely said it was just a drawing and had no meaning. I hypnotized her and said, "I am going to count until you reach the doodle you have made at which point the index finger will rise. She could not talk under hypnosis, so I talked to the dissociated hand. When questioned the index finger would rise to signal "yes." The large finger would lift to indicate "no,"

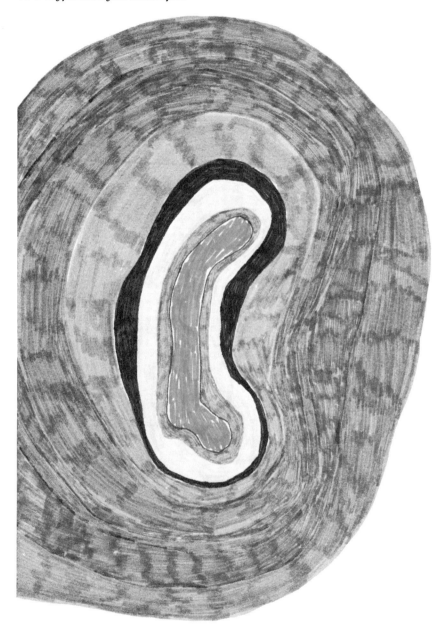

Figure 5:3

and the little finger would respond to communicate "I don't know," then talked to the hand as follows:

"Hand, is this experience prior to birth?"

"Yes." (Index finger lifts.)

"Are you able to take her there?"

"Yes."

"Are you willing to do so now?"

"Yes."

"Let me know when she has undone what she needs to do."

"Yes."

"Any place where she needs to go?"

"Yes."

"Uterus?"

"No.

"1st year?"

"Yes"

"Are you able to take her there?"

"Yes."

"Would you be willing to do so right now?"

"Yes."

"Let me know when she has done what she needs to do."

"Yes."

"Is it important that she recall at the conscious level what she has just experienced?"

"No."

Each session the therapy continued as she brought in more doodles and responded with finger signals as to what she (the patient) should do and where in her life space she should go. No meanings were ever verbalized. Her conscious experience was that she was in a dark place. Sometimes she felt fear or teared but nothing else. However, at the third session she brought a drawing which resembled a sperm (see Figure 5:4). In the second session after that she brought one which resembled the union of sperm and egg (see Figure 5:5). When it was asked, the finger signal reported that this represented "conception." Two weeks later Figure 5:6 was brought in. It resembled a fertilized ovum, but no associations could be elicited in either the hypnotic or the conscious state. However, following this "fertilized ovum" doodle a profound change came over the patient. Her depression lifted, her eyes brightened and her face released. Her grades in college improved, and she complained no more. Her feelings of inferiority

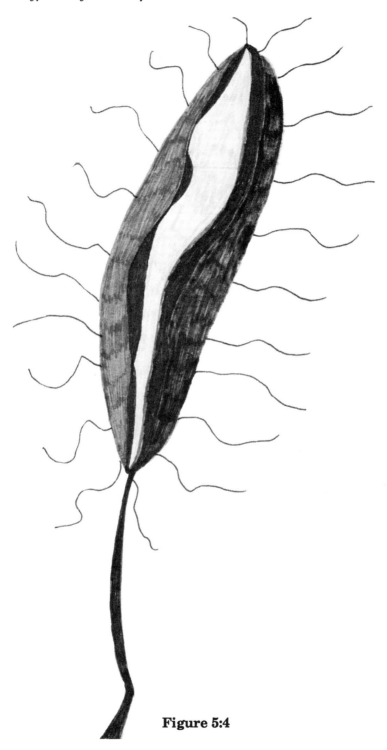

Figure 5:4

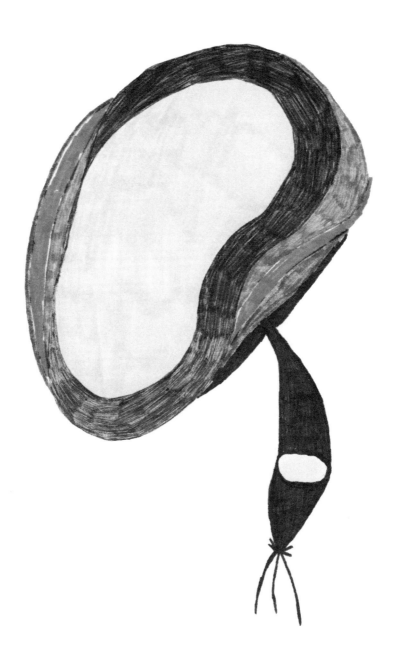

Figure 5:5

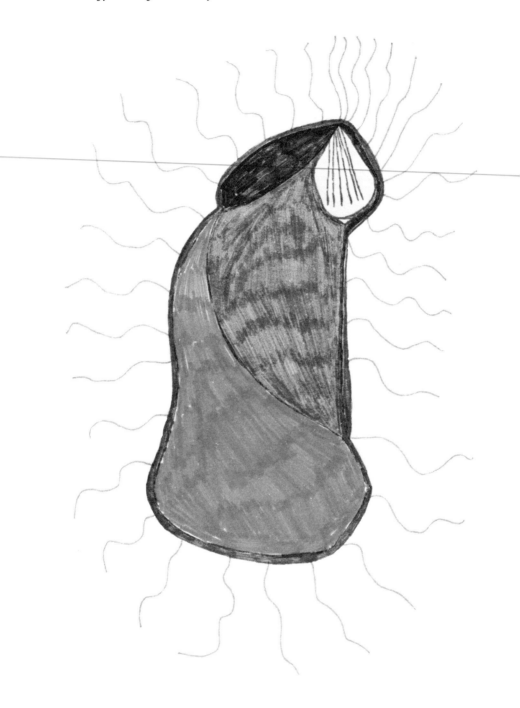

Figure 5:6

seemed to disappear, and her relationship with her boyfriend greatly improved. Therapy was discontinued, but when she returned for a single session five months later all of her gains had continued.

What had happened? What communications were exchanged through the doodles and my reactions to them? One can, of course, speculate that the doodles transmitted the symbols of a new birth, a new chance, a new sexual relationship with her boy friend, a fantasy of mother and father getting together, and many other hypotheses. But these would be only speculation. I only know that through these doodles somehow constructive therapy took place, that it was not simply suggestion, and that it endured beyond the time during which a positive transference reaction could be expected to hold. At some unconscious level my patient had achieved a "covert insight" through her symbolic communications to me and to herself, and she had resolved some inner conflict. I decided to let well enough alone and rejoice with her at the change.

Summary

Non-verbal communication through art productions can provide meaningful therapeutic interaction. Drawings, paintings, "doodles," and plastic modeling are useful media for implementing this. Associations are most essential to get at the underlying meanings of the symbol creations. These may be elicited in either the conscious state or under hypnosis. At times the use of such symbolic productions can help the therapist when the patient is unable (or unwilling) to communicate verbally.

At other times these symbols can help a patient to resolve inner problems by re-arranging meanings covertly in such a way that neither the therapist nor the patient knows their true meaning in words. The patient knows them unconsciously and resolves his/her inner conflicts. Recovery takes place, but we have not explained it psychodynamically. It has made an inner sense to the patient who has achieved a kind of "unconscious insight."

Meares had his patients sketch images with black paint with instructions only to let the hand make whatever it wished and without conscious attention. He called this procedure "Hypnography," and reported that it tapped covert processes which could not be consciously expressed.

Plastotherapy" is a form of treatment in which the patient expresses himself through modeling with clay or similar material. Meares combined this with hypnosis to develop an approach he named "Hypnoplasty."

The procedure was extended further by Raginsky using colored plasticine. He called it "Sensory Hypnoplasty." By varying both color land texture of the modeling material he offered the patient other dimensions in which to express conscious and unconscious motivations. Kline (1968) combined Hypnography and Hypnoplasty into an approach which he termed "Sensory Hypnoanalysis."

H. Watkins has developed an approach ("Doodle Therapy") in which "doodles," apparent random scribbles produced by patients without conscious attention, are analyzed to determine covert meanings. Sometimes they lead to areas needing therapeutic abreactions.

The potentialities of art productions as a modality in hypnoanalysis have not been fully realized.

Chapter 5. Hypnography and Sensory Hypnoplasty

Outline

1. Art as a modality of communication in psychotherapy.

2. Left brain vs. right brain activity.
   a. Images, dreams and "art" as right brain functions.

3. Hypnography, the use of painting under hypnosis, as a modality for "unconscious" communication in psychotherapy.
   a. Productions initially child-like and similar to dreams.
   b. Unrelated to painting experience.

4. Plastotherapy, the use of modeling clay in psychotherapy as a means of communication.

5. Meares' Hypnoplasty, the modeling of sculptured miniatures under hypnosis.
   a. The utilization of plasticine to offer different colors and textures for expression (Raginsky's "Sensory Hypnoplasty").

6. Kline's combination of Hypnography and Sensory Hypnoplasty (Sensory Hypnoanalysis).

7. H. Watkins' "Doodle Therapy," the analysis of meanings in "doodles" which are drawn without conscious attention/
   a. "Doodles" to determine areas needing abreactions.

6. "Covert" or unconscious insight.

Chapter 6

Dreams and Fantasies

A "reality" experience is supposed to be a response to perception of stimuli originating outside an individual. Science makes much of the need to "test reality" by "objective" observations. Yet the kind of reality with which psychotherapists deal is often internal and subjective. When our patient says he "hurts" we cannot directly feel it, experience it and verify it. We are reduced to accepting his report supplemented by our observation of his overt behavior. Because we, too, have experienced pain we may "understand" his feelings, and perhaps through resonance (Watkins, 1978) replicate within our own self a facsimile of that experience. For the moment then we may be able to "suffer" in a similar way, qualitatively if not to the same degree.

But dreams and fantasies, like our patient's pain experience, render scientific study more difficult. Some systems of therapy, such as behavior modification and those which stress "inter-personal" relationships, try to achieve scientific goals by objective observation only. They do so at the expense of overlooking a vast body of "reality" which is internal, subjective, yet to the patient just as real.

These experiences, unlike normal perceptions, are initiated by stimuli which lie within the patient, and are not directly visible and controllable by the therapist. Beahrs (1986) has dealt significantly with this dilemma. He notes that uncertainty, or the principle of indeterminacy which Heisenberg (1958) formulated for physics, must also apply in psychotherapy. We observe, understand, diagnosis and intervene constructively into intangible processes within another individual but with uncertainty and relatively little verified technology. Yet to the astute clinician the study of dreams and fantasies, not only permits insights into the patient's inner processes, but also opens a modality for constructive change. This is because it is the patient's inner and experiential reality, his unique perception of events, rather than the external events themselves which often cause his symptoms. This principle is well-recognized by cognitive therapists (Beck, 1976; Meichenbaum, 1977) as well as by psychoanalysts.

The good clinician, therefore, must learn to "feel his way around" in the patient's inner reality. It is like a blind man groping in the dark and relying on other modes of perception to discern the nature of a world in which he is trying to bring some new control. Freud (1953b) called dreams "the royal road to the unconscious." In this chapter we will try to indicate how the hypnoanalyst can use them diagnostically and therapeutically.

Images, Fantasies, Dreams and Hallucinations

Right hemisphere brain processes govern images, fantasies, dreams and hallucinations. These phenomena have certain attributes in common. On the one hand they originate primarily from internal stimuli, and on the other hand they are generally experienced by the individual as if they were visual. They differ in that images can be produced consciously and represent circumscribed bits of experience. Fantasies are often consciously initiated also but may display longer, more story-type productions. They have more "body" and organization than simple images. Images and fantasies are "subjective" experiences. The person senses them as being self-created, a part of his self.

Imaging under hypnosis has been extensively studied. J. Hilgard (1979) found that hypnotizability is highly correlated with the ability for vivid imagination. Råmonth (1985a, 1985b) studied "absorption," the capacity for total attention in an imaginative activity or an object of experience. Crawford (1982) and Spanos and McPeake (1975) found this "absorption" also highly correlated with hypnotizability. When absorption is high the images become the reality of the subject, and outside stimuli are ignored. Images may be suggested by the hypnotist or created spontaneously by the subject. They become a powerful means of communication from unconscious or preconscious processes within a patient and can be a most valuable tool in hypnoanalysis.

Dreams and hallucinations are subjective phenomena but experienced by the individual as "object."[1] He senses them as something which is happening to him, not something he is doing. Perhaps the only difference between dreams and hallucinations is that the first occur during sleep and the second happen while presumably the person is awake. However, at the time they are experienced the individual "sees" them as he would perceive an external object whose image is focused on his retina. Images and fantasies generally occur during "normal" states of consciousness or in hypnogogic reveries which may be compared to a very light state of hypnosis.

Dreams and hallucinations on the other hand appear during some altered state of consciousness, such as sleep, deep hypnosis or psychosis. They are unconsciously motivated. "Imaging" and "fantasying" are used by different writers to describe the same class of phenomena. From the psychoanalytic point of view images and fantasies represent "pre-conscious" experiences. Dreams and hallucinations manifest more "unconscious" and "concrete" mental activity. Hallucinations have often been considered as dreams in the awake state.

Both dreams and hallucinations tend to express meanings less directly, employ more symbolism, and require greater effort to interpret their meaning—manifesting what Freud termed "primary process" thinking. Yet all four represent right hemisphere activity primarily and require different approaches in dealing with them than do conscious, verbal communications.

Free association, the verbalizing of consciously controlled thoughts has been a basic method in psychoanalysis. Fantasy might be considered as a form of free association using images instead of words. The patient withdraws attention from the external world, is passive, and allows a series of visual images to pass through consciousness. He usually describes them in words only after the experience and not during it since the ego activity required for verbalizing (left brain activity) interferes with the right brain imaging.

If we think of trance depth as lying on a continuum from hypnoidal, through light, medium, deep to somnambulism (See Chap. 1, Figure 1:1) then images and fantasies would occur during lighter states of consciousness, while dreams and hallucinations are experienced more in the deeper states of hypnosis. This is in line with the experiences of hypnotists that a fairly deep degree of trance is required to suggest hallucinations. We might also hypothesize that the lighter the trance in which a visual-perceptual experience occurs the more the production will be guided by secondary (conscious or pre-conscious) processes, and, hence, the easier it will be to interpret its meaning. On the other hand, fantasies or "dreams" reported during or following deep trance states are much more likely to contain primary, concrete thinking and require the sophisticated methods of dream interpretation developed by psychoanalysts.

There are a number of studies (Barber, 1962; Moss, 1967, 1970; Tart, 1964, 1965) comparing "hypnotic dreams" with "sleep dreams." There has been controversy between different contributors, some holding that hypnotic dreams and sleep dreams are similar, others concluding that they are very different from one another. However, many of the studies did not control the factor of *trance depth*. Walker (1984) reviewed many studies and concluded that hypnotic "dreams" were more like directed fantasy than nocturnal dreams. However, she also challenged the concept of "trance" itself. The problem seems to reside in the extent to which the images and fantasies reported under hypnosis have been subjected to the psychodynamic distortion which psychoanalysts find in the manifest content of nocturnal dreams. Hilgard and Nowlis (1972) reported that some 63% of 172 subjects indicated that their hypnotic dreams were like real, night dreams. Hilgard (1986) concluded that hypnotic dreams lay somewhere between night dreams and Thematic Apperception Test stories.

We take the position here that imagery experienced as "visual" simply constitute different points on a continuum, from images, through fantasies, and dreams to true, overt hallucinations and represent a diminishing level of ego control but without clear dividing boundaries between them. Our problem as therapists will be to decide at what level we will make our interpretation. However, even as the "manifest" level of interpretation has been found to achieve significant meaning in true dreams, the psychoanalytic and symbolic level of translation has been shown to be of value in such "ego-creations" as stories on the Thematic Apperception Test (Murray, 1943). Let us start with a few findings on the dreaming process itself.

The Physiological Basis of Dreaming

Dement and Kleitman (1957) reported data showing that dreaming tended to be associated with rapid eye-movements (REM) and occurred during light or Stage I sleep. It was first thought that the movements of the eyes represented their focusing visually on different aspects of the dream image (Dement and Kleitman, 1974). Later findings have not confirmed this. During a typical night of sleep REM periods will alternate with Non-REM periods. More REM activity is observed the longer one sleeps. It has been discovered that mental activity occurs during both, but true "dreams" tend to appear during the REM period. During non-REM periods thinking is more related to the day's activities and does not manifest the symbolic and regressive nature of true dreams (Vogel, Foulkes and Trosman, 1969; Foulkes, 1969).

The Psychoanalytic Theory of Dreams

From a study of his own dreams Freud (1953b) formulated a theory of their formation. He believed that the dream was the guardian of sleep. An inner conflict arises between "instincts" and the "ego" or "super-ego." The tension and anxiety it creates as repressed material tries to force its way into consciousness can be alleviated or dissipated through a kind of acting-out of the conflict in fantasy form, hence, the dream. However, since the material has been repressed below the level of consciousness, because of its incompatibility with the conscience (super-ego) and self-view (ego) of the individual, it can emerge only if in disguised form. The original material he termed the "latent" content of the dream; the form in which it emerges is the "manifest" content. We remember and are consciously aware only of the manifest content.

The manifest dream was made up of the "day's residues," by which Freud meant the dreamer's experiences during the day prior to the dream. Pötzl (see Shevrin and Luborsky, 1974) presented subjects with very brief glimpses of material via a tachistoscope. Material from the scene which was not noticed consciously at the time appeared in their dreams later indicating that pre-conscious impressions can be incorporated into manifest dream content. This inclusion of subliminal material into manifest dreams was also verified by Fisher (1974).

The "dream work", through such processes as symbolism, condensation, displacement and substitution, presents us with this manifest version of the original which is more acceptable than the latent meaning. The dream thus protects sleep by concealing the latent meaning and revealing it indirectly only thorough the altered, manifest version. The amount of defensive change which is involved in the dream work of disguising its latent meaning is related to the anxiety attached to that meaning and to the motivational drive to express it. Accordingly, if a certain meaning is very threatening to the conscience or self-image of a person we can expect much difference between the manifest dream and its latent meaning. On the other hand, if there is a strong drive to express this underlying meaning the degree of disguise may be less, but the patient will be under greater conflict. The task of the analyst was to assist the patient in deciphering and interpreting the original meaning, thus revealing another piece of "the unconscious." Dream interpretation became another basic analytic technique along with free association.

Alfred Adler (1963) considered dreams as a problem-solving activity and not necessarily related to Freud's "instinctual" demands. They could represent normal, everyday problems. Dreams also employ symbolic language, not only to solve problems, but also to rehearse solutions and prepare for translation of these solutions into more adaptive, overt behaviors. They can be inegrative in nature and facilitate the process of differentiating self from object representations (Baker, 1981).

Moss (1961) determined experimentally that dream symbols constitute a language of "the sleeping mind," even if latent anxiety is not involved. This tends to vindicate the position that dreaming is a right-brain activity which uses images rather than words to communicate. Baker also noted that dream images in the adult may stand for "transitional objects" (like dolls, teddy bears and security blankets) which took the place of mothers or other original objects in the child's life that were lost or had to be relinquished. In the dream, mental symbols take the place of the more tangible symbols to which the child was originally attached.

The Interpretations of Dreams

Many different systems of dream interpretation have been devised. The literature on the study of dreams is voluminous extending from the earliest civilizations to modern experimental studies. For those who wish a general acquaintance with the literature on dreaming the following constitute a representative sample ranging from the anecdotal and theoretical to the more recent research studies: Gutheil (1970), Hall (1953), Mahoney (1976), Rossi (1972), Rycroft (1979), Ullman and Zimmerman (1979), Wolman (1979), Woods (1974), Woods and Greenhouse, (1974).

Means et al (1986)suggested a systematic four-step procedure: 1. Collection and examination of dream images; 2. Clarification of the affectual and kinesthetic components; 3. Revification of the dream elements and their associated affect, and 4. Integration of the "dream meaning" with the dreamers past and present life experiences.

Most of the early psychoanalytic writers (Federn, see Weiss, 1960;

Freud, 1953b; Erich Fromm, 1951; Jung, 1958; Stekel, 1943c) have devoted considerable attention to the study of dreams. Stekel advocated an "intuitive" approach to dream analysis. French and Erika Fromm (1986) have emphasized the activity of the ego and the problem solving objectives of dreams. They believe that the dream analyst must employ both intuition and "scientific" (e.g. objective) exploration to arrive at correct interpretations.

There is general agreement among the writers that dreams have personal meanings to the dreamer and that they represent communications from covert mental processes which can often be interpreted to bring about increased understanding and insight. We will make no attempt here to review that great area, but will concentrate on *techniques* for interpreting dreams, inducing them, and therapeutically manipulating them as part of hypnoanalytic therapy.

Steps in Dream Interpretation

Even as too much activity by the analyst will mobilize more resistance, too much passivity allows the patient to proceed at such a "comfortable" rate as to prolong the treatment unnecessarily. An appropriate balance is desirable. It will be shown later in this chapter that dream interpretation in hypnoanalysis is an even more active mode than in psychoanalysis but does not necessarily result in the classically-predicted harm. Accordingly, our position here is that we can generally apply more active techniques in working with dreams than the conventional and conservative approaches have recommended. The following represents a general outline of techniques employed by this clinician for exploring a dream p*rior* to using hypnosis.

A. Eliciting and recording the dream report.
    1. Some therapists ask the patient to write down their dreams. Others believe that the dream which is forgotten before the therapy session should be allowed to remain in oblivion unless the patient's defenses permit it to be recalled spontaneously.
        a. If it seems desirable for the patient to write down a dream he might be helped with the following suggestions.
            (1) "Keep a pencil and pad by the bed. Write down the dream when you first awaken. Dreams tend to fade the longer we wait after waking up. The most significant parts of a dream will be the first forgotten."

(2) "When you first awaken do not jump immediately out of bed. Relax into a half-sleep state and revive the dreams of the night, reviewing them through mentally. Afterwards, write them down at once."

b. If the patient comes with his dreams unwritten the therapist may either listen to their oral presentation and analyze accordingly or write the dream down him/herself for detailed consideration.

(1) It is desirable for the more inexperienced therapist to have dreams written out either by the patient or by himself.

c. It is sometimes warranted to ask the patient to report his dreams twice, noting any changes in the record.

B. Interpreting the dream.

1. Initial questions to be asked by the therapist.

a. "When did you dream this?"

b. "Have you dreamed it before?" (Repetitive dreams are most significant.)

c. "What happened during the day preceding the dream?"

d. "What thoughts were on your mind when you went to sleep?"

e. "With what problems were you concerned during the preceding day?"

f. "What seems to be the main problem in your life at the present time?"

g. "Were you the hero (heroine) or victim in this dream?"

h. "Did you become involved actively in the dream, or were you a passive observer?"

i. "What do you think this dream might mean?"

j. "What are your associations to the dream? Just let your thoughts go and tell me everything that comes to mind whether it seems important, relevant or not."

2. After the patient has exhausted the unguided, general associations, then move to more specific points "radially."

a. "What about the large trunk which appeared in the dream?"

b. "Can you describe it in more detail?"

c. "Tell me everything that comes to mind in relation to the trunk."

d. "What do you remember in regards to trunks?"

e. "What is a trunk?"

f. "What's a trunk for?"

g. "If I had come from a foreign country with little knowledge of the English language and asked you what the word "trunk" meant what would you tell me?"

h. Ask for both the general and specific characteristics about each item in the dream. Hence, "You saw a 'bear' in the dream. What kind of bear?"

   (1) "Just what was the bear doing?"

   (2) "How do you feel about bears?

   (3) "Would you say that a bear was weak? Strong? Masculine? Feminine? Passive? Aggressive? Cruel? Cuddly?," etc.

Since dreams use para-logic, symbols tend to be equated with their true meanings over a bridge in which the symbol and that which it represents have some part or element in common. Research has shown (Kline, P., 1972) that Freud was not entirely wrong when he reported that long objects, like poles and swords, were penis symbols, and that openings and containers, such as boxes and house were feminine symbols. They commonly are, but it would be an error for a therapist to generalize that all such objects do. Each person has uniquely individual meanings which often emerge through associations.

The therapist with a sensitive "intuition" may often divine the meaning of dream symbols in some patients without securing associations. Some people almost naturally seem to have an intuitive ability to sense unconscious communications and translate dream symbols. Reik (1948) called this "the third ear." Children often have it better than adults, indicating that our stress on objectivity, "scientific" validity, and logical argument during schooling (left-brain activities) has taught us to inhibit the sensitive and intuitive right-brain thought processes. In other words as we grow up this intuitive ability (which is the mark of a good therapist or analyst) tends to get lost. However, this therapeutic sensitivity is amendable to re-training.

Stekel, although scorned as superficial and not "scientific" by many of his colleagues, was nevertheless recognized as a sensitive master of dream interpretation. In addition to his two volumes on dream interpretation (1943c) he published a series of case studies on such topics as *Sadism and Masochism* (1939a), *Impotence in the Male* (1939b), *Sexual Aberrations* (1940), *Frigidity in Women* (1943a),

Peculiarities of Behavior (1943b), and *Compulsion and Doubt* (1949). In the two-volume work in each of these areas Stekel described many cases which he had analyzed plus innumerable dreams.

He held that the first dream in an analysis constituted a kind of overview of the entire neurosis, and that by the end of the analysis the patient would understand its full meaning and the dynamic structure of his neurosis. Even though such a claim has not been experimentally substantiated we can learn much by studying his approach to dream analysis.

At the beginning of each case Stekel would describe the background and history of the patient, plus the presenting complaints. He would then report the patient's first dream followed by his direct and intuitive interpretation of it. He continued this pattern throughout each case by presenting the development of the analysis, several of the patient's dreams, and followed with his intuitive interpretations (which a reader must confess appear both brilliant and logical, if not subject to scientific verification). Stekel seemed able to react sensitively to the symbols and subtle unconscious communications in the dreams of his patients and thus fathom their meanings. In fact, he often bragged how, through his "direct" and intuitive analysis, he could shorten the time of treatment and achieve therapeutic results more rapidly than his colleagues, who were bound by the slow, free-association approach.

I had previously noted that, through intensive study and resonance with the analytic intuition of Theodore Reik (1948, 1956, 1957), one could sharpen one's sensitivity at picking-up covert communications in the associations of one's patients. Accordingly, I decided to study Stekel's recognized skills in dream interpretation similarly.

I would read his description of the background of each case and then the patient's dream. At this point, I would lay his book down and write out my own direct, "intuitive" interpretation of the dream. Next, I would compare my interpretation point by point with his, noting identities, similarities and differences. I would then take another of the dreams he reported from the same case (or from some of the 1200 others which he published) and do the same. It was an exercise in programed learning.

After practicing this exercise through several hundred dreams I found that my interpretations began approaching his more and more. Often they would be almost identical. This, of course, does not prove that either his or mine were correct. It does show, however, that I was learning to respond to the same cues to which he reacted and in a similar way. I was incorporating his approach to dream interpretation. Subsequently, I noticed that my abilities to "intuit" dream and projective fantasy meanings in my patients was greatly improved—to their benefit. This was a kind of unconscious training for me and an extension of the skills acquired in my own analysis. Therapists can develop their analytic skills from reading, observing and modelling other skilled practitioners. Young analysts do it all the time in their "training" analyses.

Dreaming and Hypnosis

The addition of hypnosis to the technique of dream interpretation does not diminish the value of the original psychoanalytic procedures. Free and radial associations continue to be desirable approaches, but nothing can substitute for the analyst's knowledge of symbol formation and intuitive sensitivity. However, hypnosis adds another dimension which permits us to initiate, intervene and control dream activity. Let us consider first how the hypnotic modality allows us more leverage in the analysis of dreams which are normally created by the sleeping patient.

Dreaming tends to occur in Stage I sleep, which is the lightest. This makes sense as we think of a progressive continuum in levels of consciousness from wide-awake alertness at one end to deep, almost coma-like states at the other. Cognitive activities do not suddenly disappear. They gradually diminish. And as the degree of awareness and mentation lessens certain functions decrease faster than others. Thus in classical psychoanalytic terms the "super-ego" is the first casualty. As its vigilant function diminishes, the dream material which emerges is less subject to conscience and "parental" controls. Individuals dream vividly about activities which in the normal awake state would be taboo to them. Extra-marital escapades and similar activities, which the person's "super-ego" inhibits and prevents from being carried out in real life, begin to appear. Very primitive impulses may become manifest. (When the super-ego's away the id will play.)

It has been said that "ontogeny recapitulates phylogeny," that is, the individual in his development from the fertilized egg to the mature adult repeats the evolutionary history of the species *homo sapiens*. Socialized control as represented internally in the super-ego has come late in man's development. Accordingly, since sleep, like hypnosis, is a "regression in the service of the ego" (Gill and Brenman, 1959) we should expect the most recently formed psychological structures and processes to be the first to succumb as the regressive state begins to take over, and more primitive ones appear. For example, in deep sleep we often assume a curled, fetal position under the covers.

During Stage I. sleep there is much bodily movement, tossing and turning and also eye-movements which have been found to correlate with dreaming activity. As the sleep progresses to Stages II, III and IV both physical and mental activity becomes less. After the super-ego is inhibited there is progressively less "ego" activity, and dreams are more likely to reflect primitive motivations and processes. As the fantasies reach into this area they are more likely to be forgotten when the dreamer awakens. This is partly because they occurred at a deeper level of consciousness, and partly because, being more primitive, they are likely to differ, not only from the subject's accepted (super-ego) norms, but also from his self (ego) perceptions. Thus the ego would be the next to go, with the most primitive (id) processes, those which governed in earlier ontogenic and phylogenetic human development, being the last to manifest themselves before complete coma takes over.

Something of this same order occurs during alcoholic intoxication. The drunk first loses social inhibitions, makes crude sexual passes, and/or is aggressively hostile. With the ingestion of more liquor he becomes passive and loses both mental and physical coordination. Finally, he "passes-out" and enters a coma-like state of stupor in which all semblance of consciousness and normal behavior disappears.

As sleep becomes deeper dreams take on a more concrete nature reflecting primitive and earlier-developing brain processes with less higher-level cerebral activity. This is also true with hypnosis when it is deepened from hypnoidal and lighter levels, through medium, to profound somnambulistic trance—and finally to that coma-like condition which Erickson (1952) termed a "plenary" trance.

It is generally accepted that most people dream, even when a patient reports no dreams. This may result because the dreams required repressing, hence, forgetting, or because they were dreamed in such a deep state that they are no longer subject to recall, or to both factors. Hypnosis may permit us to go back and recover these dreams, even as it can often help to break through amnesias.

With the patient hypnotized as deeply as possible we instruct him to go back, recover and re-dream any dreams he had the previous night. Often we will find dreams now reported, and we have new material with which to work. This is more likely to occur during the initial stages of an analytic treatment.

Frequently we encounter a dream which is consciously reported in only the briefest form. A patient once brought in the following: "I dreamt last night that I was almost struck by a car."

He was hypnotized and told, "Go back to your dream of last night when you were almost struck by a car. It is happening again just as it did then."

The patient stated, "I am standing with a friend at the corner of Arthur and Beckworth. A red convertible driven by a blonde woman comes barrelling around the corner and almost hits me. I jump back, fall down and skin my knee. My friend says, Why doesn't that bitch look where she's going?'"

Notice the amplification with increased details. The working-through of meanings related to a "red convertible," "the blonde," "the friend," and his remark open up new vistas to this patient's treatment.

Not only does hypnosis increase the opportunities to bring greater dream recall, but we can also use it to suggestively create dreams, either by initiating dream process, or by inducing dreams about specific topics. Under hypnosis the patient can be given the suggestion that he will have dreams tonight, or that he will dream about his relationship with his mother.

For example, I once suggested to a hypnotized patient that she would dream about the treatment and her therapist. At our next session she presented me the following:

"I dreamed I was sitting on the lawn listening to a fatuous young man orating from a stump. He seemed to be very pleased with the sound of his own voice." I not only was alerted to her negative transference toward me, but I got the message to shut up and listen more. As I behaved better, her therapy improved.

In another case I asked under hypnosis for a prognosis dream. The next session the patient reported: "I dreamed that I went back to my old home town. It was terribly run down. The streets had been neglected, the trees were dieing, and nobody seemed to be in charge. Then I had another dream. It seems that I went back again to the town two years later, and there was much improvement. Somebody had cleaned up most of the garbage and planted some new vegetation. I had the feeling that finally they had voted-in a mayor who was going to do something." Needless to say I felt much better about the future course of the therapy.

These dreams, of course, are quite transparent and need little working-through to secure meaning. Yet still it is amazing to a therapist who asks the patient directly, "What do you think this dream means" to get an "I don't know" answer. If dreams are used frequently in therapy patients become more skillful in interpreting them. They also get more sophisticated in creating dreams which are difficult to analyze. As they become more educated, so also do their defenses. This suggests that the therapist should not exclusively use dreams as a *modus operandi*, but should alternate them with other analytic procedures.

The question can be raised as to whether some patients may not be intelligent enough to decipher the dreams they report in therapy, especially if their intellectual abilities are quite modest. Psychoanalysts have raised this same question in regards to the screening of acceptable candidates for analysis. Some have proposed that patients should be at least above average in intelligence if they were to understand their neuroses. However, an individual's neurosis has been compounded from his own cognitive abilities. Consequently, its simplicity or complexity must reflect the intellectual abilities of its creator, smart person—smart neurosis, dumb person—dumb neurosis, and a person is always bright enough to understand his or her own particular neurosis. Unfortunately, some people's neuroses are too smart for their analysts, and thus their defenses are never penetrated in the treatment. Fromm and Kahn (1990) have demonstrated that, after learning self hypnosis, many patients are quite capable of inducing and interpreting their own hypnotic images and dreams.

Analyzing Dreams under Hypnosis

All of the techniques used in psychoanalysis for interpreting dreams can be employed in hypnoanalysis. Just hypnotize the patient and apply them. Thus, since a subject is often able to tell the meaning of a dream directly, especially when its latent meaning is little disguised, simply ask the hypnotized patient what he/she thinks is the dream's meaning. Next, apply free and radial associations of the elements of the dreams, but this time with the patient under hypnosis. Any or all of the questions suggested in the outline presented on pages can be applied under hypnosis.

The therapist should consider how deeply the patient is in trance when evaluating to what degree the manifest material has been distorted from its latent meaning. There are many dissociative and projective techniques which can also be employed to elicit the meaning of symbolic dream representations, but discussion of them will be deferred to Chapters 7, 8 and 9 where they can be illustrated in detail.

Finally, it is possible to intervene in dreams or at least into the reliving of them. This approach without the use of hypnosis, which they call "active imagination," has been practiced by Jungian analysts for many years (see Gerhard Adler, 1948).

Let us suppose that the patient describes a dream as follows:

"I was walking down the street of a strange town when I noticed a tall, dark man wearing a long cloak approaching me. I felt much fear and woke up."

The analyst might approach the interpretation as follows: "Close your eyes and visualize the dream.[2] You are walking down the street in this strange town, and you are seeing a tall, dark man approaching you. You are frightened and want to escape. However, I will walk with you, so you need not be afraid." (Strengthening patient's ego by relationship.) "Walk up to him and look at his face. Who does he look like? Have you ever seen him before? Where?" etc. Continue questioning to establish who or what "the man" represents.

Now try, "Ask him who he is." Say, "What is your name?'".

The above incident represents the way a Jungian analyst might practice "active imagination."

The same active intervention can be applied with the patient under a light or deep hypnotic state. Let us not think of hypnosis as being a completely different treatment modality from psychoanalysis, but rather that at times it can provide greater leverage, flexibility and an altered state of consciousness in which to apply the analytic procedures one might use without it. Freud rejected hypnosis, probably because he was afraid of the powerful reactions which it could evoke (Kline, 1958). He then wrote down his rejection as a kind of dictum for other analysts, which many of them have followed quite religiously. Otherwise, they might well today be integrating hypnotic procedures with their regular psychoanalytic techniques. The published words of great innovators (right or wrong) carry enormous weight with their followers.

In Chapter 7, Projective Techniques, these fantasy and dream-intervention techniques will be illustrated at length. However, for the present the working-through of a particular dream might be of interest.

A patient presented the following dream:

"I was walking down a city street when I saw a large colonial mansion which was on fire. I was trying to put out the fire but not succeeding very well."

The patient was hypnotized, told to return to that dream, and when he could see the burning house to lift the index finger of his left hand. The finger lifts.

"Now, while you are watching the burning house, time is going to reverse until you see the house just before it begins to burn. Let your finger lift when you can see it that way." The finger lifts.

"Describe the house."

"It's white and has two large pillars, one on each side of the door."

"Go up to the door. Let the finger lift when you get there."

The finger lifts.

"Fine, open the door and go in."

"The door is locked. I can't open it." (Resistance)

"Perhaps if you looked around you might find a key which would open it." Patient squirms in chair and moves head about.

"I don't see any key." (More resistance).

"There's a door mat there. Have you looked under it."

"Yes, there does seem to be a key there." Resistance is lessened, partly because we are now only trying to find a key (concrete thinking) and are not keeping in the foreground of consciousness the goal of opening the door. We now ask the patient to apply the key to the door lock. Notice the symbolic communication of "finding the key."

The patient begrudgingly, "Well, it's hard to turn it."

"Keep trying."

"Yes, I've opened it now."

"Go in. What do you see."

"Just a long hallway."

"Go down the hall until you come to a door that is slightly open." (We make it "slightly" so as not to challenge the patient's defenses too directly. He can still resist going into that room.)

"What's in the room?"

"Nothing."

"Keep looking. Maybe there is some furniture there."

"There's a rocking chair in the center of the room."

"What does rocking chair remind you of?"

"My mother had a rocking chair. She used to hold me and rock me in it before putting me to bed."

Associations have now led us, through resistance, from "burning house" to "mother." We will not pursue the inquiry further except to note that eventually he was able to see his mother rocking in the chair.

While we do not accept Freud's belief as to the universality of the Oedipus Complex in all male neuroses, nevertheless, it does occur at times, and this happened to be the time. His sexual impotence did represent his sexual tie to his mother, and his passivity covered up his "burning" desire for her. In classical psychoanalytic symbolism houses often represent women, who represent the first "house" in which we live. Mothers are large compared to children, hence "a mansion." They are not sexual (the house is white), and like all women they have an entrance between two pillars (legs). Once we got through the initial resistance the meaning of the dream became clear, but the patient was not yet ready for its complete interpretation. Direct confrontation at this point with his erotic feelings for his mother might well have scared him away from treatment. Although more working-through was required, the therapist has secured from the dream the direction the treatment must take. We had applied the Jungian "active imagination" method and intervened in the dream under hypnosis to decipher it.

Hypnotic Dreams

The patient can be asked under hypnosis to "dream" about some general or specific problem while in the trance state and to report it immediately afterward. There is controversy as to whether such "dreams" are the same as those which occur in nocturnal sleep. Some therapists prefer to use the term "to image" instead of "to dream" in describing the phenomena—and in their instructions to the patient. Since to most people "dreaming" has a special connotation different from simply "imaging" it is probably better to use the word "dream" in our suggestions. However, we do recognize that a "dream" reported by a lightly-hypnotized patient has more the character of a conscious day-dream than that of a true nocturnal dream. Wright (1987) noted that the hypnotic dream more closely resembles nocturnal dreams which are reported several days afterward (hence, subject to more defensive amnesia) than to those described immediately after awakening. The deeper the trance state, the more likely it is that the production will manifest the defensive elaborations which separate an overt dream report from its latent meaning. However, Moss (1970) through the use of Osgood's "semantic differential" (1964) has shown experimentally that the symbols elicited in hypnotic dreams, although differing from those in nocturnal dreams, nevertheless have real meaning and relate to significant conflicts within the dreamer, both overt and covert ones.

Sacerdote (1967) used hypnosis to induce a sequence of dreams about a specific therapeutic problem. Each one would build on the previous one. Through a set of successive approximations the true essence of the problems was approached. We know that hypnosis is not the same as sleep. However, Sacerdote felt that hypnotic dreaming was more productive if hypnosis was induced by using the word "sleep," since most people expect to "dream" when they are asleep. Gill and Menninger (1947) used a similar approach by suggesting that patients dream a second dream to help explain a first one which was not clearly explicable.

Hypnotic dreams can be combined with many other hypnotherapeutic techniques. Schneck (1974) reported he found that hypnotically-induced nightmares were the equivalent of normal nocturnal nightmares. Thus, Regardie (1950) traced the development of conflicts by studying hypnotic dreams under age regression. Since hypnotized subjects are closer to their own unconscious it is not surprising that they may be better able than conscious individuals to decipher the meanings of dreams other than their own. Erickson and Kubie (1941) described how one subject was able to interpret the automatic writings of another. One wonders whether the analyst who is able to relax into a hypnoidal or light hypnotic state might find his intuitive sensitivity to dream communications enhanced. An experimental study testing this hypothesis would be welcome.

Both dreams and psychotic hallucinations present us with concrete ideation. It has been suggested that dreams represent a psychosis experienced in sleep, or that psychosis is a dream when we are awake. Since hypnosis is a modality for intervening in dreams it is not surprising that some therapists have employed it to intervene in the mental processes of psychotics.

When Scagnelli (1977) was confronted with a schizophrenic patient who was most fearful of losing ego control, both to the therapist without and to the fantasies within, she first taught him autohypnosis, e.g. how to control his own states of consciousness. She then developed with him a procedure by which he could manage and "control" his hallucinated "monsters" and other frightening phantasmagoria through hypnotic dreaming. As he practiced this "creator control" technique he began to master his psychotic indeation and learned to distinguish subject from object representations. Fourteen months later he had re-integrated and formed a stable self-identity. He had learned not to be frightened and helpless at his own unconscious. His former hallucinations had changed into normal dreaming— which he could control. This technique shows great promise in working with psychotics.

Summary

Images, fantasies, dreams and hallucinations are visual creations which may communicate preconscious and unconscious processes. Dreams and hallucinations, although subjectively created are experienced as if they were external "objects." The techniques used by psychoanalysts for deciphering dreams can be employed with added leverage in hypnotized patients. A wide variety of hypnotic techniques are available for initiating dreams, interpreting them and intervening in them for both diagnostic and therapeutic purposes. Hypnotic dreams differ from sleep dreams, being closer to conscious fantasies but may approach the concrete thinking in sleep dreams during deeper states of hypnosis. Dreams tend to occur during Stage I. (REM) sleep. However, the eye movements have not yet been shown to represent scanning of an internal "visual field." The psychoanalytic theory of dreams holds that through "dream work" the original latent dream is transformed into the manifest dream experienced by the dreamer.

Dream interpretation can be by associations or done "intuitively." Under hypnosis, dreams may be reported which consciously are not remembered. They may be hypnotically suggested, and may then be interpreted. Sometimes dreams may be initiated which suggest prognosis for the treatment. "Active Imagination," a Jungian approach, can be applied under hypnosis. It involves the analyst's direct intervention into the dream process. Dreams may be suggested to help psychotics establish more stable object representations.

The study of dreams in conjunction with the hypnotic modality offers the analyst increased access to unconscious processes.

Chapter 6. Dreams and Fantasies

Outline

1. Images, fantasies, dreams and hallucinations.
   a. Images and fantasies, conscious and preconscious productions.
   b. Dreams and hallucinations stemming from unconscious processes.
   c. Images, fantasies, dreams and hallucinations related hypnotically to increasingly deeper levels of trance.

2. Hypnotic dreams similar but less regressive than sleep dreams.

3. The physiological basis of dreaming.
   a. Dreams occur primarily during Stage I. (REM) sleep.

4. The psychoanalytic theory of dreams.

5. The interpretation of dreams.
   a. Association
   b. Intuitive.
   c. Steps in dream interpretation.

6. Dreaming and hypnosis.
   a. Memory of dreams under hypnosis.
   b. Hypnotically suggesting dreams.
   c. Analyzing dreams under hypnosis.
   d. Suggestion of prognosis dreams.

7. Hypnotic dreams.

Footnotes
1. In Chapter 9 the two-energy theory of Paul Federn (1952), will be presented. It provides a rationale for explaining how subject and object experiences are changed from one to another.

2. We shall not argue the point here as to whether or not the analyst has unwittingly induced a hypnotic trance by involving the patient in a fantasy.

Chapter 7

Projective Hypnoanalysis

"You can't trust anybody these days." While there is some truth to the assertion that many are not trustworthy the claim that nobody is, reveals more about the honesty of the speaker than the situation. Projection is a common psychological defense whereby an individual imputes to some one or thing in the outside world aspects of his own self. The very honest person tends to be more trusting of others—often to his own detriment. An individual loaded with repressed hatred may present a smiling face but insists that he is the victim of somebody else's vendetta. It is a common defense to protect the integrity of one's personality when it is filled with disparate elements. In severe cases projection develops into a psychotic paranoid reaction. The unique way that one perceives the world can tell much about one's own personality since different people perceive it so differently.

Projective Techniques

This tendency of humans to externalize or "project" their own motivations, attitudes and feelings onto their perceptions has been capitalized by a set of psychological diagnostic devices called "projective techniques." In the hands of a skilled diagnostician they can disclose facets of a patient's functioning of which he or she is quite unaware. They offer a modality for revealing that which has been concealed. Some of these, like the Rorschach Ink-Blot Test, can disclose such structural aspects of an individual's personality as the nature of his defenses, the impending possibility of a psychotic breakdown, the degree to which the patient can control emotions, the extent of inner fantasy and his compulsiveness or other traits. Some projective tests, such as the TAT (Murray, 1943) or the MAPS (Schneidman, 1947), can probe inner psychodynamic processes and reveal attitudes towards parents, toward self, or even the current state of the transference relationship with the therapist.

The Rorschach test (Rorschach, 1949) composed of ten cards on which are ink blots is the most widely studied of the procedures. Ink blots (like clouds) are vague unstructured stimuli. They offer the opportunity for different people to see them in very different ways. In the TAT, pictures are shown to the subject who is then asked to make up stories about them. The principle behind all these projective techniques is to present the subject with vague unstructured stimuli who is then encourage to structure them according to his own unique personality needs.

These tests, accordingly, employ an entirely different concept from "objective" personality tests. In objective tests each item is rendered as specific and succinct as possible so that the possibility of the subject misinterpreting it will be minimized. In the projective tests we intentionally make the stimulus vague so that our patient can "misinterpret" it in his own individual way. Both approaches can yield data on personality functioning. However, projective techniques tend to tap the more pre-conscious and unconscious aspects of personality. Hence, they are more valuable in psychoanalytic or hypnoanalytic therapy.

This writer coined the term "projective hypnoanalysis" in an effort to pull together the three approaches which are most significant for gaining access to unconscious processes: psychoanalysis, hypnosis and projective techniques. At that time (Watkins, 1952), I hoped by combining all three into an integrated therapeutic methodology to develop a powerful therapeutic approach which might be superior to any of the three alone. Unfortunately, while it did combine several powerful probing techniques it did not give the attention to transference and relationship factors which I now find so important (Watkins, 1978). However, technique plus relationship is better than either alone, and so this chapter is devoted primarily to a good case example condensed from my earlier book (Watkins, 1949).

Many writers, both before and after its original publication, have described approaches combining projective, dissociative and fantasy procedures (Erickson, 1967; Brenman and Gill, 1947; Kline, 1967; Wolberg, 1945; Schneck, 1965). Spontaneous drama, hypnotically induced, has been tried (Moreno, 1946; Moreno and Enneis, 1950; Shaw, 1978). Even behavioral cognitive researchers (Cautella and Bennett, 1981; Meichenbaum, 1977) have re-discovered the value of projective covert fantasies in facilitating behavior changes—although they have formulated them under behavioral theory concepts. The approach here has been described and practiced by others under many different terminologies, such as "guided fantasy," "active imagination," "imaging," etc.

Projective hypnoanalysis combines the procedures described in the chapters on abreaction, hypnography, hypnoplasty, dreams and fantasies, plus dissociated handwriting and "ego states" (which will be described later). However, this is a good place to illustrate the integrated procedure. Up to this point "techniques" have been most emphasized. In subsequent chapters we will give more attention to relationship and transference factors.

The following case was originally published (Watkins, 1949) as a good example of projective hypnoanalytic techniques. However, since it is no longer in print it is reproduced here (with theoretical and therapist notes) in greatly shortened form. The following are excerpts from the more significant sessions.

The Hypnoanalytic Treatment of an Entrenched Phobia

Patient "X" was a young lieutenant in the army who suffered from a constant feeling that somebody was out to "get" him. He experienced this as a fear of the dark which had been continuous for three years prior to the beginning of treatment. He was seen for sixty-five sessions spread over a period of ten months. No claim is made that Patient X was "fully analyzed." The treatment, however, did represent an exploration in considerable depth, an insightful resolution of his symptom, and a substantial growth in his personal maturity.

This case was the first example of interaction by internal ego states which this therapist had seen. It initiated the beginning of an extended study of dissociated entities which developed some thirty years later into the formulation of the theory and techniques of "Ego-State Therapy" (See Chapter 9). The patient will be referred to as Patient X.

Session of October 26th

Early in the treatment the Thematic Apperception Test was given in the hope that it might offer clues to the psychodynamics which underlay this fear symptom. The patient's responses to two of the cards are presented here to be compared with responses offered to the same cards by two distinct "ego states" within the patient which emerged later in the treatment. From the patient's alternating behavior styles he was obviously a borderline multiple personality, although I did not so recognize it at that time.

TAT Picture No. 11
(Weird prehistoric scene)
"We have had a earthly disturbance—earthquakes and land-slides. Can't make out this object in the extreme front. The object in the left is blended into the backgrounds. It could be an animal. I can see webbed feet. It could be a delusion. These are animals here. They are round. It may even be prehistoric times. It may be years ago. It looks like dinosaurs. I can't see much else in this picture."

TAT Picture No. 12M.
(Young man reclining on couch asleep; Older man leaning over him with hands in front of young man's face.)
"Well, we have here a boy. He is a young man. He is lying on his couch. He is the son of this man, the old man, and he has just come back home and has laid down to rest. He has slept too long, and his father is trying to wake him. The boy hasn't seen his father for many years, and this is his first trip away from his job. He wanted to come home to tell his father that he was going to get married and invite his father to go with him back home. The older man had lived in that community for years and years. He finally decided that the boy should go home alone, and at a later date return to pay a visit to his father—which he does. He gets married and has a little boy and is very happy. The father gets old and dies. The young man lives happily ever after."

(Therapist note: In TAT Picture No. 11 the patient reacts with anxiety and confusion, wishes it away (It could be a delusion."), and is obviously upset by the long necked dinosaur-like animal resembling a penis in the foreground.

To Picture No. 12M the patient portrays the reconciliation of a long-absent son with his father, his decision to embark on a hetero-sexual commitment, "marriage," and the father's willingness to accept his independence and maturity. He then predicts his own future as a happy adult.)

Under hypnosis two underlying entities were revealed, George, a rather psychopathic ego state, and Melvin, a weak but high super-egoed personality. George was strong, rough, promiscuous and little concerned with the needs of others. Melvin, on the other hand, was high principled but ineffective. Melvin and George were hypnotically activated and given the TAT test cards separately. Their personality differences are quite noticeable from their responses to the same two cards as previously given to the conscious patient.

Session of December 4th

TAT Picture No. 11
(Responses by "Melvin".)

"These are prehistoric times. There is a giant lizard at the left. Right over here are some animals. Naturally, the giant lizard is trying to get at them. He isn't able to get the animals, however, because they run out over the road, and they escaped."

(Responses by "George"—in a very angry voice.)

"There's nothing in this picture. What do you want to show me something like this for? It is ridiculous. Any one who would draw pictures like this must have his head in the fog. What the hell! This looks like a lizard. It's a stupid picture. I can't see anything about it." And the George personality threw the picture down.

(Therapist note: Melvin perceives a threat by the lizard who is "naturally trying to get at" the smaller animals. They escape by running away. George sees no threat but rejects the entire picture.)

TAT Picture No. 12M.
(Response by "Melvin")

"This is a sickly boy. He has been supporting his father and working very hard. He comes home at night. The old man doesn't like it because he has to work so hard. He is sickly too. One day the boy flops on a couch. The old man walks over to him and tries to soothe him. He wants to help the boy along. This is an intelligent boy, but he's working at a job that he's not fitted for; so the old man gets dressed and goes to the factory to talk to the foreman. He then gives the boy the right kind of job. The boy is very happy and successful and gets promotions and raises in pay."

(Responses by "George")

"This is a club house. The boy is traveling across the country. He has a few hundred dollars sewed in his shirt, but he doesn't want to spend it. The damn fool ought to know not to keep it there. The old man sees the boy and figures he might keep it on him because he looks good. He goes over and takes the money out of the shirt. The old man beats it. The boy wakes up and is broke. He goes to the police, but the police don't believe his story. They won't back him up. Instead they throw him for three days in jail as a vagrant. He wants to get back at the police, but he can't do it, and when finally they take him off to the city limits he goes away beaten and broken. He want to do to others what they did unto him."

(Therapist note: To Melvin, father-figures are kindly, helpful and solve his problems. To George they are menacing. To Melvin, stories have happy endings; to George they end tragically. To Melvin, heroes are hard-working, honorable people supporting a loving father; to George, they are bums or hoboes with a bitter, cynical view toward life. In the conscious response of Patient X to this card the hero reconciles with the father (but not too closely) then becomes mature, marries and builds a happy life. In the hypnotically activated Melvin ego state there is a caring father and a sickly, martyr son who doesn't leave the parental home—neurotic solution. In the hypnotically activated George ego state the solution is psychopathic. The hero is the victim of uncaring fathers, first the old thief, then the cruel police. He then becomes cynical and uncaring toward others.

Much of X's past career had been like George, but obviously Melvin, the super-ego part of his personality, who wishes by hard work to gain the approval (and be dependant upon) a loving father, has been condemning his way of life. And so there is inner conflict.

Mr. Y and his Knife.

Various projective hypnoanalytic techniques were next used to study the interactions between the main personality and its ego states.

Session of January 14th

George, Melvin and X Hold a Conference.

X reported a reappearance of fear at night. He knew he was not asleep, but he could not open his eyes. They kept sticking together. He had been unable to sleep the entire night. He experienced several dreams but could not recall any of them. He was hypnotized after considerable resistance. Under trance he could easily recall the dreams which he could not remember in the conscious state.

"Would you tell me what it was you dreamed last night?"
"I dreamed I was talking to a man who was eating "peaches."
"Peaches—what about peaches?"
"Wheelbarrow—the man was eating peaches out of a wheel-
    barrow, and he had eaten all of them."

Therapist note: Patient X's real name is closely associated with peaches. A "man" is orally destroying him. Wheel-barrow?

Patient X refused to associate but immediately launched into a description of another dream (resistance).

"There was a big black bird flying through the air. I tried to
    catch the bird, but I couldn't."
"Who did this bird represent?"
"He was Mr. Y—some kind of enveloping power."

(Therapist note: He used the term "Mr. Y" to represent his phobia and hence, "the man" who would stab him in the dark with a knife.)

A Conversation with The Hands

Since no other associations could be secured we tried the "disso-ciated hand" technique (See Chap 8, pg....). It involves hypnotically anesthetizing and paralyzing the writing hand, which is then asked questions. Since "the hand" is no longer under the patient's conscious control it is "free" to reveal "secrets" or otherwise by-pass ego defenses and super-ego inhibitions.

In this instance both hands were dissociated within a deep trance and connected to the underlying ego states as follows:

"Your right hand is losing all sense of feeling and movement. It is no longer under your control. Now it is under the control of George—the George personality. It will write whatever George wants to say."

This was accompanied by rubbing the hand and suggestions hallucinating the hand away from the wrist. The same suggestions were then related with the left hand.

"Your left hand is now no long under your control. It will write only for Melvin."

"In a moment I shall wake you up. You and I will continue our discussion, but you will not have control over either of your hands. George will write with the right hand, and Melvin will write with the left hand. They will make their own comments independently of you or of each other."

The patient was then seated at a desk, pencils placed in each hand, and sheets of paper conveniently arranged. He was then awakened. He seemed a bit surprised and stared in a puzzled manner at the two hands over which he had no control.

The George Hand: WHERE IS X? (The entire patient.)

W: X can speak with his mouth. You are not in trance now. You're wide awake. You and I can talk as usual. Only your hands are not under your control. The two hands will write for George and for Melvin. Do you think maybe George might be able to interpret some of your dreams further?

The George Hand: THE MAN IS EATING ALL THE GOOD THINGS THAT BELONG TO "X". (Note previous dream of a "man" eating "peaches out of a wheelbarrow.)

W: What about the man in the dream?

The George Hand: THE MAN IS (The hand filled in a small place with black pencil lines and then continued writing.) DARKNESS, BLACK, BLACK. (Resistance even by a "dissociated hand.")

The Melvin Hand: (This hand drew a picture of a peach and labeled it. Then it wrote.) WHY DOES "X" FEAR?

The George Hand: BECAUSE HE IS AFRAID OF HIMSELF. (The threat is from within.)

The Melvin Hand: DOESN'T HE HAVE WHAT EVERYBODY ELSE HAS?

The George Hand: "X" IS A NORMAL, SENSIBLE MAN WITH NATURAL INCLINATIONS FOR THE PROPER METHODS OF LIFE. FRUSTRATION AND INFERIORITY COMPLEX WILL NOT HELP HIM.

W: Do you notice the significance of the dream choosing peaches to symbolize your various abilities and possibilities? It's associated to your name, isn't it? What relation do you think all this has with your feelings of guilt?

X: The numbness is going away out of the Melvin hand. I thing it's gone entirely now. It feels perfect normal. (X lifted his hand, opening and closing the fingers.)

W: Is the George hand still numb?

X: Yes, it is.

While this was going on the George Hand, apparently still dissociated, started "doodling" on the top of the sheet of paper. The Hand first made an 8 and two zeros, then a picture of a house, an odd pattern, some circular scribbling, picture of a funny old man, and a circle (see Figure 7:1).

W: I think maybe George might tell us more about the guilt feelings. (Therapist pushing.)

The George Hand: IF A MAN DOESN'T TAKE ADVANTAGE OF OPPORTUNITIES GIVEN HIM HE DESERVES NOTHING. LET THOSE WHO FEEL GUILT SWIM IN THAT GUILT. WHAT DIF-FERENCE DOES IT MAKE AS LONG AS HE GETS WHAT HE GOES AFTER? KILL OR BE KILLED—MELVIN WOULD SAY THAT WAS WRONG. HE'S NUTS! IT'S JUST A PHRASE LIKE EAT OR BE EATEN. THE STRONGEST SURVIVE. YES, OF COURSE—WHY CAN'T YOU SEE THAT YOURSELF. CAN'T YOU UNDER-STAND. WHY GO ON WITH THIS NONSENSE? YES. (Both X and W [therapist] stared at the hand in astonishment.)

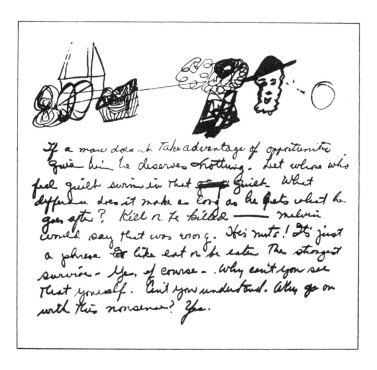

Figure 7:1

W: Is George angry?

The George Hand: YES.

The George Hand was then re-associated by merely rubbing it until feeling and movement were restored. After "The Hand" had been connected again to X, the therapist and Patient X began discussing news events of the day. "X, look what your hand is doing."

X glanced over and remarked, "What about it?"

"Doesn't it seem a bit odd that it is making all that doodling on the paper? Does that mean anything? Can you think of anything in associating to those figures?"

X tried but could not associate in any way to them.

The patient was now placed back on the cot, and a deep trance induced. "You will open your eyes while staying asleep and look at these funny pictures that you drew. What do they make you think of?"

Patient X opened his eyes and gazed at them. "Nothing—I can't think of anything."

"Tonight you will have another dream. This will indicate still further the nature of your guilt feelings."

"I think it's a good idea. I don't want to forget the dream. I'm going to take paper and pencil to bed with me."

"Do you think you could associate any more ideas in connection with the two dreams you told me? What about the bird—you said something about an enveloping power?"

Mr. Y Loses his Knife

"I don't see anything about the bird now. I remember something, though, that happened the other day. I was out walking in the dark, and suddenly I had the feeling that Mr. Y was there, but Mr. Y no longer had his knife."

The therapist repeated this in a non-directive manner. "Mr. Y has lost his knife?"

At this moment the patient became very excited. With raised pitch and a voice filled with emotion he repeated, "Mr Y has lost his knife. Why didn't you tell me this before? Mr. Y has lost his knife."

The therapist asked, "Why has Mr. Y lost his knife?"

Suddenly X sat up on the cot with his eyes wide open, emerging instantly from a deep trance.

"I've got the most wonderful feeling, the most wonderful feeling I've had for a long time. *Mr. Y has lost his knife.* Now I can handle that guy. I feel as if a great weight has been lifted from my shoulders. I'd like to find a dark place right now. I what to try it out. I'm sure I'm not going to have any more fears." The therapist tried to quiet his enthusiasm. "Better not be too optimistic. You've had feelings something like this before."

"Never like this before. This is important. Mr. Y has lost his knife."

"Do you think perhaps this means that part of your fear is gone? Maybe it represents a partial gain in insight because you now realize that guilt feelings are at the basis of your fear. Recognition of this point may have reduced the fear symbolically by causing Mr. Y to lose his knife—thus making him a less fearsome creature."

"Yes, maybe that's true. Maybe that's what caused it. I only know that I'm happy—that I'm not afraid. I can handle that guy. This is the most important thing that has happened in the whole analysis. *Mr. Y has lost his knife.*"

(Therapist note: Has Patient X now lost his "castration fears?" And if so, why? He has accepted for the first time that his external fear is related to an unconscious sense of guilt, repressed into "Melvin" and denied by "George" with psychopathic-like behavior.)

Following this moment the treatment proceeded much more rapidly.

Sessions of Jan. 16th, 17th and 21st.

Dreams of Fear and Frustration.

A number of dreams were now hypnotically initiated to try and learn more about Mr. Y. X was hypnotized and the trance state deepened.

"I'm going to count up to ten. When I do you will dream again about Mr. Y. One, two three,...ten."

Patient X began to twitch all over. He started with anxiety. He exhibited tremors, and his breathing came in a labored manner. This continued for a minute. He would relax; then it began again and would disappear once more after a minute or two. Finally, he began to talk.

"I was standing in a big place or field—like a desert. In front of me were a dozen different lanes or roads. I wanted to go on one of them and get some drinking water because I was getting right thirsty. I started down the one on the extreme left and had gone about ten paces when suddenly a fierce animal appeared in front of me. He had bared his teeth and grimaced at me. I turn back. Then I tried each one of the roads, and each time there was the animal, and he showed his fangs and wouldn't let me through; so I came back and lay down on the ground. I was very, very thirsty, but I didn't really care. I couldn't go on. That was all."

"I think maybe you can add more to this dream. Do you want to go back and finish it? You can describe it as it is happening."

"I'm very thirsty, but there is a little girl coming toward me. She's taking me by the hand. She is taking me out of the woods, but I can't stop her. Nothing can stop her; but there is no animal, and we come to a light spring, and I kneel down to drink. I look in, and I see the face of the animal. I look again, and only the little girl looks down. The animal is gone. I drink, and the little girl is gone now, but I don't care because I can go on by myself, and the water is so very, very good."

(Therapist note: Is he to be rescued from Mr. Y by a little girl, e.g. accepting femininity and immaturity? Is this the only solution to his problem? Or is the little girl a symbol of his own femininity, his "animal?")

"What does the little girl make you think of?"

"She is the helping hand."

"What do you mean by the helping hand?" (X had previously referred to his Mother as "the guiding hand.")

"It's you and others. Some one to guide me. She's just a little baby. What a little girl should do, I should be able to do. She needs to be led herself." (Is dependency the problem?)

"Can you think of anything else about her?"

"No, she just means the helping hand—oh I see a beautiful horse, a beautiful animal. He's that black horse again, isn't he?" (Referring to a previous dream.)

"Yes, he is. All right, you're going to catch him and ride him. He is coal black. There is nobody on him." (Therapist trying to see if X can "master" and control Mr. Y by hypnotic suggestion).

"I don't think I can catch him. I'm trying to catch him. I've got hold of his nose, but he keeps moving away and in a circle—running away. Now he's gone. I would just rather watch a horse like that. I knew I shouldn't try to ride that horse. He was very beautiful." Patient X turned his head reproachfully toward the therapist, "You said to ride him."

"I'm going to count up to ten once more, and then you'll have another dream regarding Mr. Y one, two, three,...then."

After X had dreamed for five minutes, he began to relate the following: "I was at a party, a Halloween party. Everybody was there. I knew them even though they had their faces covered with masks. A girl came up to me and took me by the hand. She was in a mask, and she said, 'Follow me,' and then led me downstairs off into a little wood. Then she said, 'Do you know who I am?' And I said, 'I don't' know.' She said, 'Don't you want to find out?' Then she said, 'Catch me.' And she ran into the woods. She was quick, and I couldn't catch her. I heard her laughing and laughing. I wanted to catch her. I wanted to stop her, but I couldn't catch her. You were driving me on to catch her. Something tells me I can't catch her. I wish that I could. I could hold her hand. She's playing tag with me."

"Are you afraid of her?"

"No, she isn't sinister, but she makes me very nervous and excited by her actions. I wasn't afraid of her. I could leave her alone if I wanted to. I didn't even have to follow her down. She is only toying with me now—because you are here to help me."

Patient X was now awakened from trance. He could add nothing more to his description of the dreams.

During the following session further work was done with "dissociated handwriting," and several other projective techniques were tried including a "tautophone" or "verbal summator" procedure* (See Shakow and Rosenzweig, 1949; Skinner, 1939; Trussell, 1939.)

---

* In the original "tautophone test" subjects were played garbled sounds and asked what "the voices" were saying. Will Patient X "hear" unconscious communications in "the voices?"

After the patient had been hypnotized, and his right hand dissociated, he was asked to listen to a tape, which was played backwards, and tell me what the voices were saying. He showed resistance, would not write at first, and insisted that he heard only jumbled material. The dissociated hand displayed a lot of negativism, making wavy motions up and down. It then started to write.

The Hand: I DO—(I don't know.)

W: Of course you know.

The Hand: JUMBLE, JUMBLE. (See Figure 7:2)

W: That's right. But what do these jumble voices say? They say something.

The Hand: THE HAND CAN'T TELL. "X" WILL TELL.

(Therapist note: The tautophone procedure does not in itself produce the "voices" hoped for, but it does stimulate another round of significant material to emerge.)

X: (speaking) It sounded pretty badly jumbled, but I do have a dream which the voice has made me think of. There is a horse. It is the same horse again, and he has a beautiful saddle and bridle. Everybody

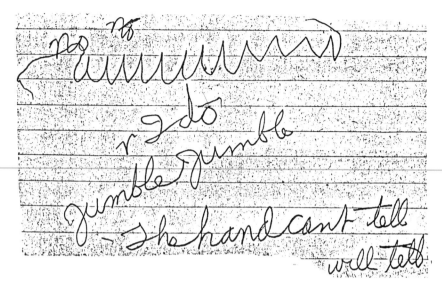

Figure 7:2

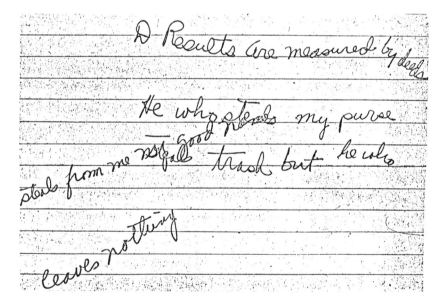

Figure 7:3

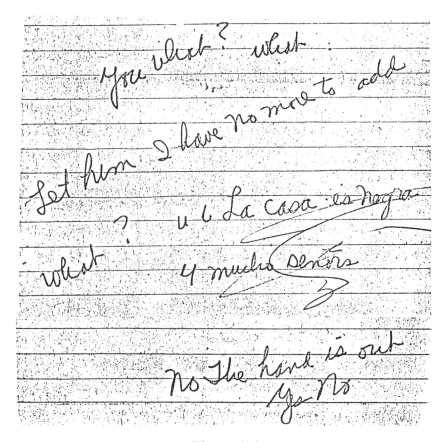

Figure 7:4

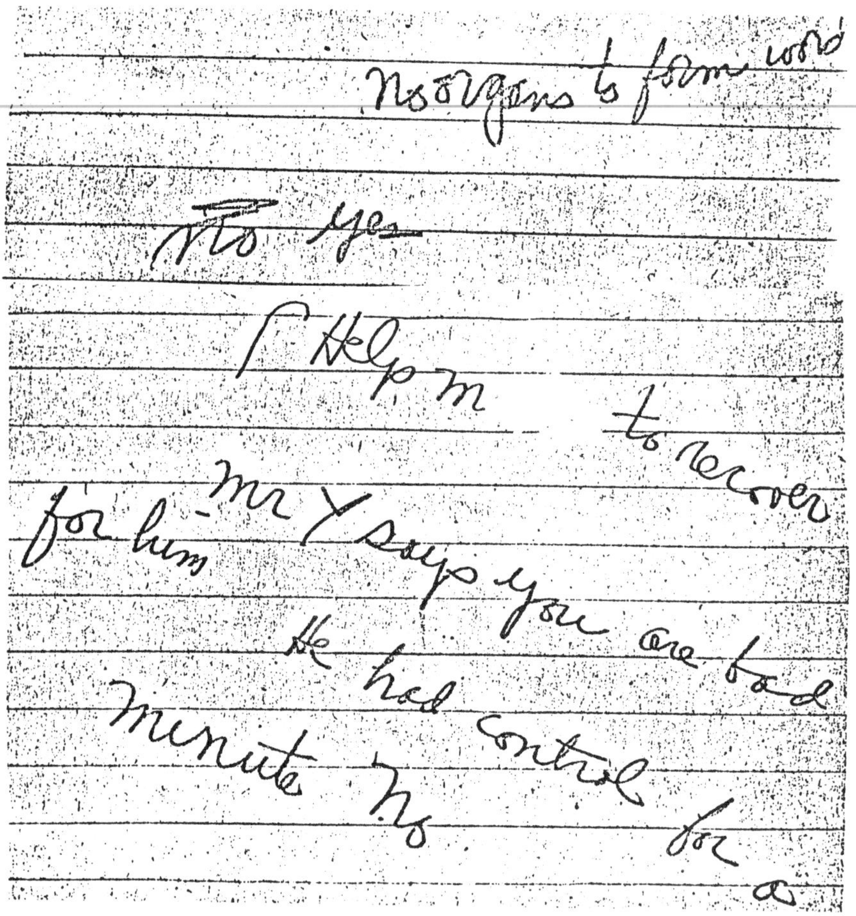
No organs to form word
No yes
I Help him to recover
for him
Mr X says you are bad
He had control for a minute
No

Figure 7:5

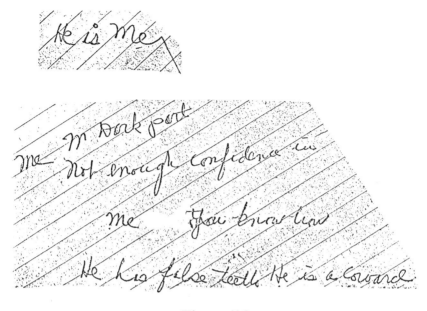

Figure 7:6

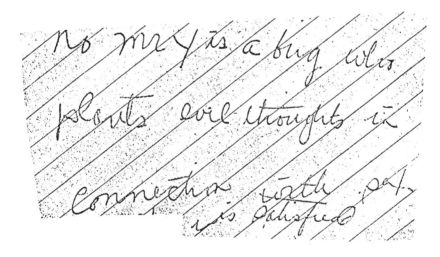

Figure 7:7

is trying to get on it, and the horse wouldn't let anybody get on. He just stood there. I got one foot upon the saddle, but I couldn't get up. The reason I couldn't get up was because I had roots in the ground.

W: Do you think maybe The Hand could explain better your inability to mount the horse?

X: What do you want to let The Hand write for? I don't want The Hand to write. Why can't I say it myself?

(Apparently X is afraid that The Hand will reveal something he doesn't want to become aware of. Hostile remarks like this continued for some time. Finally The Hand began to write.)

The Hand: RESULTS ARE MEASURED BY DEEDS.

W: How do you mean that?

The Hand: HE WHO STEALS MY PURSE STEALS TRASH BUT HE WHO STEALS FROM ME MY GOOD NAME LEAVES NOTHING. (See Figure 7:3.)

W: Who has stolen X's good name?

The Hand: YOU—WHAT? WHAT?

X: (Covering his head with his hands) I'm not going to talk any more.

The Hand: LET HIM. I HAVE NO MORE TO ADD. (See Figure 7:4.)

W: What do you mean by "let him?"

The Hand: LA CASA ES NEGRA Y MUCHO SENORS (The house is black and many men.)

At this point The Hand became quite rebellious and refused to write for some time. Eventually it was induced to hold the pencil again.

W: (pushing) I think The Hand can reveal more.

The Hand: NO. THE HAND IS OUT.

W: You mean the feeling has returned to the hand?

The Hand: YES NO

W: What do you mean by that?

The Hand: NO ORGANS TO FORM WORDS.

W: Do you mean that The Hand is incapable of further writing?

(The Hand first wrote "NO" and then "YES," finally scratching it out. Then the patient became very angry. He started pouting like a small boy. He threw the pencil away. He threw "The Hand" away. The therapist put the pencil some six times back in the fingers of The Hand before The Hand would grip and continue writing.)

The Hand: I HELP "X" TO RECOVER. MR Y SAYS YOU ARE BAD FOR HIM. (A feeling of relief and a loss of tension seemed to come over the patient.

Then he continued writing.)

The Hand: HE HAD CONTROL FOR A MINUTE. (See Figure 7:5.)

(Therapist note: Here is a brief change of executive ego state.)

W: Can you tell me more about Mr. Y?

The Hand: HE IS ME. MY DARK PAST.

W: Can you explain more about this?

The Hand: NOT ENOUGH CONFIDENCE IN ME, "X". (See Figure 7:6.)

W: What do you mean by this? (The patient once more became irritable, but The Hand finally started scribbling again.)

The Hand: YOU KNOW HOW. HE HAS FALSE TEETH. HE IS A COWARD.

W: Does that mean that Mr. Y represents that part of you which is cowardly?

The Hand: YES.

W: In what way are you cowardly? What are ;you afraid of?

The Hand: NO MAN BUT VARIOUS DAILY ENCOUNTERS.

W: Do you think that the fear of Mr. Y has anything to do with your wife or marital difficulties?

(At this point Patient X became very anxious and tense. The Hand did not want to write. It threw the pencil away a number of times. Finally, the patient was induced to hold the pencil again, but The Hand would not write.)

W: I am going to count up to five when I say "five" you will have to write. One, two, three, four, five.

The Hand: NO. MR Y IS A BUG WHO PLANTS EVIL THOUGHTS IN CONNECTION WITH SEX. After a pause it continued writing, X IS SATISFIED. (See Figure 7:7.)

At this point feeling and movement began to return to The Hand, whereupon it was re-associated to the body. The session was continued verbally.

"You can discuss matters now without using your hand. The Hand wrote something about sex. What does this mean?"

"This means desires for other women." Then he added concerning Mr. Y, "He's the guy that put the bug where it shouldn't be—X is afraid of losing his potency."

"Why?"

"Well, look at the life I've lived—continuous sex relations with women. Don't you think it would take away some from my strength—from my ability?"

(Therapist note: In psychoanalytic theory Don Juans have latent homosexual impulses which they repress and deny by having affairs with many women.)

X was asked why he had two weeks of resistance.

He replied, "You know, Mr. Y was cornered. We were so close to his home. He was flanked on all sides. If he went forward, he ran into you. If he went to the right, he ran into you. If he went to the left, he ran into you; so he didn't have any place to go except to come back on me, and that is what made me all excited, anxious and tense. He's right over the crest of the next hill. He hasn't got much ammunition left. I'm going to get hold of him and drag him out."

At this point X, still under hypnosis, began to ramble about many apparently inconsequential matters. He discussed the recent fire department handling of the auditorium fire. Then he commented about Mr. Byrnes's talk on the English loan. For about fifteen minutes he continued in this manner.

(Therapist note: Sometimes when one eases up on pressure very revealing material will emerge.)

He seemed childlike at this time, so I suggested, "Let's play a new game."

Patient X picked it up instantly. "That's a good idea. It'll break the monotony."

"When I count up to thirteen there will suddenly pop into your mind the number of days it will take until we finally uncover the last of Mr. Y and get him out of his lair."

Patient X smiled, "Make it fourteen."

"All right. One, two, there,—thirteen, fourteen."

Instantly X remarked, "Twenty-one." While the therapist was counting X was making a number of rather odd-looking passes with his hands in the air. He seemed much interested at the number which had emerged.

"That's a lot of fun. Let's play that game again."

"All right. I'm going to count up to eleven, and some important word about what will happen to Mr. Y will emerge—only the word will be scrambled form. One, two, three...eleven."

Patient X started reeling off the following letters:

"R-E-M-B-A-E-C-O-G-Y. I know what the word is. It's 'remember.' I'm going to remember something which is significant and will have something to do with Mr. Y." X awakened from trance.

The therapist opened his appointment book, which had a page for each day, and started slowing counting pages: "One, two, three,—. At first X didn't understand. Then he opened his eyes in amazement and smiled. Finally, when number twenty-one was reached the therapist drew a large circle around March 7th.

"So that's the day we're going to beat Mr. Y. I remember now. I told you it would be twenty-one days, didn't I?"

After some ten minutes the session ended, and Patient X started to leave the treatment office. When he reached the door he turned around and looked back. "By the way, how are you coming with your book?"

"Oh I get to do a little work on it from time to time."

"How many chapters are in it?"

"There'll be thirty-three" (the number planned at that time).

"I though you said there were twenty-one."

The therapist laughed. "There aren't twenty-one chapters in *my* book. There are twenty-one chapters in *your* book—and remember, the last one is twenty-one. Isn't that right?"

Patient X laughingly agreed.

Session of Feb. 28th. A Turkey and an Eagle.

During the sessions a variety of association and projective procedures were employed. They illustrate how psychoanalytic and hypnoanalytic techniques can be used together.

X was placed in a light hypnoidal trance after considerable resistance.

"I'm going to count up to nine and something will pop up in your mind that is significant. One, two, three,...nine."

"Barnyard fowl."

"What do you mean 'barnyard fowl'?"

"Well, this means chickens, pigs, hogs, etc." He was unable to associate further, but after some time he said, "There was a turkey which got the idea in my mind—relatively large turkey."

"What about the turkey?"

"Well, the turkey has got big feathers like a peacock or somebody who is strutting."

"Who is it that struts?"

"Well, that's myself. I put on a big front."

"Now, X, I want you to make the fingertips of you two hands touch each other. That's fine. Now each one of those fingers represents a root of Mr. Y. Pretty soon you're going to have a tingling feeling at the tips of one of those pairs of fingers."

X lay quietly on the cot. After a while he said, "It's in the third finger."

"All right. Remove all the fingers except the third fingers. Keep the tips to them together. Now right between those two finger tips a word is going to form. It will have raised letters on it, like the kind the blind feel. This word will slowly emerge, and you're going to be able to spell it out."

Patient X started spelling,

"P-R-O-A-N-T-I-R-A-N S-U-B-S-T-A-N-C-H-I-I-O-N-I-S-T."

Greatly surprised the therapist inquired, "Do you think you could spell it again?" (correct spelling, Proantiransubstantionalist)

Patient X spelled it again exactly the same way—even with the double "i"—then he added, "I read it years ago. Proantiransubstanchiionist.. It was way back in the Civil War, and it was about a man who had a certain kind of social standing. They gave that name to him. He was a man that had a pro and con against certain elements. He had two different kinds of standing at the same time."

(Therapist note: Perhaps like bi-sexual?)

"What do you think the word means?"

"It means absolutely nothing—maybe it might apply to me, because it goes two ways at the same time."

"You can concentrate real hard on those two fingers. Let's see if another word doesn't begin to squeeze in between them."

In a minute X spelled out the word "A-L-L-E-V-I-A-T-E," and then added, "You know what 'alleviate' means? It means to alleviate my symptoms."

"Right between your two fingers will run a ticker tape. It will have raised words on it. You will be able to spell the words."

Patient X began spelling, "H-O-M-O-B-I-O-L-O-G-I-C-A-L-H-O-M-O." He then spelled "P-R-E-S-S-I-V-E." "There's no word 'pressive'."

"Maybe you mean 'oppressive'?"

X became very playful. "I'm a radio station—tick, tick, tick." Then he started spelling some more. "P-R-O-C-L-I-V-I-T-E. Proclivity? What does that mean?"

"I'm going to count up to seven. When I say 'seven' an idea telling you what 'proclivity' means will pop into your mind. one, two, three...seven."

"Of all things in the world. Proclivity is you—Proclivity Watkins. You have a proclivity for pulling things out of me." Then he added, "Do I have to hold these fingers together any more? You know I can't open my eyes. I've been trying to."

Another projective technique was tried.

"In front of you there is a great fire. You can see it. It is a great picture in fire."

Patient X immediately seized on this unstructured stimulus and started fashioning a concept with it. "Yes, I see this fire very, very clear. It stands out like the wings of a bird—an eagle. The eagle is getting larger and larger. He is just standing there like a statue. What does the eagle mean?"

"I'm going to count up to five, and when I say 'five' an association will come to your mind which will tell you something about what the eagle means. One, two, three, four, five."

"Huh, when you said 'five' the bird disappeared."

"Let's try another angle. Answer yes or no quickly. Now regarding this bird, is it—you?"

"No."

"Is it—Melvin?"

"No."

"Is it—George?"

"No."

"Is it—Mr. Y?"

"No."

"Is it—me?"

"No."

"This time I'm going to count up to seven, and when I say 'seven' a scrambled word will come to your mind."

Patient X started spelling, "H-E-R-A-E-T-C," then added, "but I can't interpret it."

"All right. I'm going to count to seven once more. This time you will be able to spell the word in a little better form. One, two, three...seven."

"I knew you were going to analyze it. I told you so. Well here goes. C-H-E-R-T-E-A."

"Does it mean 'cheater?'"

"No. It means 'teacher.'"

"Tell me what the word teacher brings to mind."

"Well the teacher struck me—Miss Jordon was her name. The boy in front of me turned around and whispered something. She came over and slapped me because he was a pet of hers. I then threw a bottle of ink all over her—all over her white blouse. She took me up immediately to the principal, and the principal, after finding out what was wrong, censured her instead of me."

"Yes, but I don't see what all this has to do with 'eagle.'"

"Don't you see? An eagle is a leader—a teacher. You know, I'm going to be a teacher. I want to be an eagle that can fly and not have a broken leg. That means I need education and support because my own wings, my own education, are broken."

"What about that long word, proantiransubstanchiionist?*

* Correct spelling "proantiransubstantiationalist" is an obscure term from the Civil War period referring to an individual holding conflicting views of reality and commitment, hence, one of divided loyalties.

"What's that got to do with it?"

"Don't you see that it is a big long word? That is the front that I have to have. I always put up a big *impressive* front. (The reader will recall that X had spelled out the word 'pressive.') That's the kind of a guy I am."

He further integrated these concepts by pointing out that he wanted to be an eagle—a leader, but he felt he was more of a turkey, a show-off.

A War for Survival

During the next week a tremendous period of resistance began. As the last of the twenty-one days began to pass, and the significant date of March 7th approached, Patient X became more tense, more nervous. His fears at night became stronger. Following the session of February 28th he did not report for some time. He conjured one excuse and rationalization after another not to come in. It was obvious that a terrific battle was going on within him. He, himself, had set the date of March 7th for the final uncovering, yet down deep inside Mr. Y was waging a tremendous conflict to remain hidden in his unconscious stronghold.

On March 6th Patient X came to the office, looking wan, tired, and haggard. His eyes showed the lack of sleep. He was nervous, tense and jittery, and his face was covered with the deepest depression.

"We've been on the wrong track. I know there's no use of us going any further. We're never going to find the solution to my problem. I'm just going to have to live with it, I guess, for the rest of my life." Mr. Y was obviously pleading to have the treatment called off at this point.

The Masquerade is Ended.

For two weeks a decisive battle had been going on within Patient X. His nights were spent in helplessly tossing around the bed. The few moments of sleep were filled with vague forms of fear—dreams, fantasies. Headaches appeared often. At times tremors shook his body. Like poison he had avoided the therapist. March 7th was approaching, and Mr. Y, cornered, was fighting like a wild beast.

Session of March 7th

Patient X opened the door. He came in and sat down. For a few moments he did not say anything. The expression on his face was a mixture of anguished apprehension and stoical fortitude. After a while he spoke.

"There are dreams I meant to tell you about, but I can't think of them."

X was placed on the cot, and suggestions to induce hypnosis were started. In view of his state of agitation, the therapist had felt severe misgivings as to the possibility of actually inducing a trance at this time. These were not groundless. Indeed, after the session was finished Patient X himself said, "When I came in I didn't think you'd be able to hypnotize me today."

However, after a period of fifteen minutes the patient's right hand slowly rose into the air and touched his head, the pre-arranged signal which had been used in each hypnotic session to indicate to the therapist and to the patient himself that a deep degree of trance had finally been reached.

"X, you are in a cave, a dark cave." (Symbolic of "the unconscious"). "There are steps leading down the cave, not into darkness, but into a light which is ahead. You are going to go out into this very bright light." The therapist counted steps.

The patient began to describe his dream. "It is all shining. There is a big, open, hollow tunnel. Light is in one section—there is nothing in the tunnel. There is only an old tunnel," X growled belligerently. "You got me to come down here."

We try more projective techniques.

"Maybe there are some pictures on the walls of this tunnel. Look around and see."

"Yes, it has markings. Someone chiseled them on the stone. I am trying to see what they say. These markings were written years and years ago." (It happened a long time ago in my life). "Oh, the light is going out." (Resistance.)

"You're very strong now, much stronger than you used to be. You can put the light on again, You can *will* the light on. I am going to count up to ten, and as I do, you will be able to will the light back on. One, two, three,...ten."

Patient X smiled. "Yes, the light is back on again. Let me turn it on and off again. I want to see if it will work. I wonder if I could make colored lights too." (Perhaps meaning, 'can I have control of this situation?')

A few moments elapsed while X "turned the light on and off again." After his smile indicated satisfaction, he was prodded again to describe what he saw.

"It is so light now the wall is turning all white. There are nurses and doctors around me. I see myself as a boy. It is at Saint A—'s Hospital. I had my tonsils taken out; there's nothing to it, but across from me is a boy who's blind. I wonder where he is now. My mother just brought me ice cream. This throat feeling is hard to go down, but it does in time." X cleared his throat and began to speak in a hoarse, whispering voice describing his feelings.

(Therapist note: Much symbolic communication going on here. He is reminded of a childhood surgery because he is faced now with "psychological surgery" on an immature self. "The boy" has been blind—psychologically. He is now about to see, but it is painful to speak about what he is to reveal. He has oral pain. His throat hurts.)

It was suggested to him that he look once more at the message on the wall, but he ignored this and continued, "I see myself being taken out of the hospital. I sit around the house. The boy friends come in to see me now. Naturally, they think I'm brave—the only time I've been in the hospital for an operation."

(The session today, like the tonsil operation in his childhood, calls for "bravery." He must face an unpleasant insight.)

"How old are you?"

"Ten years old."

"I'm going to count up to ten, and something will come to your mind that is very important—very, very important. One, two, three, four,—,.

"You don't have to make it jell. I see now." (X is ready.)

"There's a bully. His name was George S—. Huh! Did I every tell you about him before? He was much older. I used to go out to the railroad yards and jump to the same trestle. I was the only one who was brave enough to do it. If I missed, there would be no telling where I would have fallen to. This boy said he wanted to come up there with him, and I went up, and we were in box car. He took his peter out. He wanted me to do something—to kiss him Then he said, 'Do it, or I'll beat you up,' and he rushed at me. It was a railroad car filled with sawdust, and I got terribly mad and beat him and beat him—kicked him until he cried and hollered, and then I came to my senses, and I left. He got out, 'cause I saw him later. I whipped him terribly. He was much bigger than I was. How could I do it? There was some kind of a revulsion in me—something terrible. I felt a lot better afterwards. Imagine me beating George. It would be like beating Joe Louis today. I was still afraid of him, though—even afterwards."

Here was the missing link, the handle on the last door, the fear of Mr. Y with his knife. the great emphasis on athletic prowess, manhood and leadership, the explanation of his many sexual affairs with women, the enormous rage and super-human strength in beating this older boy—and now finally, the tremendous blinding fear of this childhood incident, which had been so repressed and forgotten. They all added up to what Patient X was afraid to face within himself, the existence of which his whole life had been one constant striving to deny. Almost instantly innumerable pieces of jug-saw puzzle fitted together, and the pattern they made was *latent homosexuality*.

In the days when this case was treated homosexuality did not have the acceptance it has today. Homosexuals were treated with the utmost derision. Being called one was a most powerful insult, and boys were taught that being one was about the most terrible thing which could happen to them. To be known as one was to be a social pariah, avoided by all "decent" people. Furthermore, to be a homosexual meant in the popular view to be castrated, to be a woman.

These attitudes were strongly held in both the times and the culture where X was raised. No wonder that he fought so hard (with "revulsion") against the older and stronger homosexual seducer. But though he won the fight with George S. he did not realize that the invitation to homosexual pleasures had attracted him and left him with unconscious desires which required all the resistance and defenses he could mobilize, not just to avoid carrying them out, but merely to avoid recognizing that he might want to. His remark that although he had beaten George S. he was "still afraid" of him meant he was "afraid" of his own impulses.

Insight to be helpful must reach down deep within the patient himself. Could this understanding be initiated into X without creating a panic? Could this concept, obviously so terrible to X as to have warped his whole life, be integrated into his understanding? The session continued.

"This older boy—you said you felt fear toward him."

"Yes, it was intense."

"What kind of feeling was it?"

"I never knew what it meant—it just came from within. Since that time I've thought a lot about that boy. I wanted to tell you about him, but somehow I forgot to."

"Did you ever have any other experiences involving homosexuals?"

"I've seen so many men approach me. I can tell them when I first see them. I know them right and left. I know what they eat, drink and sleep. I've had enough of them as friends, but my relations with them have always been platonic. I can spot them a million miles away."

X mused a bit to himself. "How do you think I can tell them? My brother is the same way. Isn't it funny that I can spot them? Doesn't affect me, though. Don't get angry at them any more. I just believe they are sort of sick. I knew a girl, and she was a lesbian—a very good friend of mine; only she got angry at me when I started to go with a girl she had a crush on. We had *that kind* of a relation. I wouldn't let a man do that to me—but a woman, yes. I got to enjoy it quite a lot" (oral sex).

The therapist further explained that there was a certain amount of homosexuality in latent form in all of us—that there was nothing wrong about having an F (female) component—that it does not take the form of actual homosexual relations in most cases, but that many persons are afraid to face it in themselves. At one point, when the discussion centered about homosexual relations, Patient X remarked, "I wonder what it would feel like to do it."

The discussion now returned to the waves of anger which overcome many men on being approached by a homosexual—the great desire they have to strike or injure the homosexual.

X remarked, "You know, that's me." Then he began to smile all over.

His attention was next called to the fact that overt or actual expression of homosexual tendencies was regarded by the old Greek society as an accepted form of sexual expression. He was told that all he needed to do was to frankly recognize that he, like many other men in the world, had this F component within him, and that once he recognized it and ceased fighting it, he would no longer fear it.

Then the therapist asked, "How did this manifest itself in you?"

X replied, "You know, Mr. Y—Mr. Y with his big knife, the knife is like a penis."

At this point the tenseness began to disappear in his body. He remarked, "The darkness has faded away. Everything is becoming light."

"By the way, X, do you know what day today is?"

"Oh yes, it's March 7th, isn't it? That's the day you said Mr. Y would be uncovered."

"I didn't say it. You said it. Now, I'm going to describe a dream to you and you can finish the dream. You see yourself out in a field, and there is a big black horse in this field."

Immediately X said, "Like a flash I'm on top of that horse. I'm galloping off—I'm galloping off. I can ride it—I can handle it." (I can handle my impulses.)

The therapist continued, "Now I want you to see another dream. You are at a masquerade. Everyone has on masks. You know them all except one young woman. She runs downstairs with a mask on. You chase after, and she says, 'If you want to see who I am, catch me first.' Now go ahead and finish the dream"

Patient X jumped. He writhed—he fidgeted—he wrinkled his face. Finally he replied, "I've caught her. I'm removing the mask. Huh—that's me. I'm the woman." (The F component finally unmasked.)

Once more the therapist suggested a dream. You're on a desert again. There are many roads leading out in all directions. You are very thirsty. What happens?"

"I am walking down the road. There is no wolf any more. He is gone. Now all the many roads merge into one, and there is a clear straight road. Everything is fine. There are roses around it."

"You can walk down this road. Tell me what you see. Is there a house?"

"Yes. Only now the house has changed. It has been painted white. Now it has solid, brick foundations under it. It is well built. It is now changed from the shaky foundations to solid ones."

"You know what the house means, don't you?"

"Yes, it means me."

"That's right. And now you'll no longer fear the old traces of homosexuality because you understand them. You don't have to repress them any longer. You realize you can have an F component within you, like many others, only you're not afraid of it any more."

"You have nothing more to hide from yourself. Mr. Y is gone. Melvin and George are gone now too. They merged into one person. That's you. They will not need to fight each other any more."

(Therapist note: Dissociation, although not overt to the point of creating true multiple personalities, did separate X into at least two covert ego states which alternated in governing his feelings and behavior. Was the psychopathic "George" personality an introject of George S.—hence, an identification with the aggressor?)

"I am going to count up to five, and when I do you will wake up. You will feel good, and you will remember distinctly everything we have discussed. One, two, three, four, five."

Patient X opened his eyes and smiled. "Isn't it fun. I don't feel wild exhilaration. I just feel a calm sense of satisfaction—a feeling of relief as if a burden has gone."

The material was now re-discussed with him in the conscious state, and it was planned to go over his entire treatment with him, word for word. Then his chart could be closed, and he could be discharged to civilian life.

(Therapist note: In Chapter 1 of this volume the meaning of true "insight" was discussed. It is not always easy to know whether the patient has achieved it or only an "intellectual insight," often to impress the therapist during a period of positive transference. One of the ways to test it is to feed back to the patient neurotic, uncompleted dreams which have arisen during the course of his analysis. It will be recalled that I tried earlier to get the patient to "ride the black horse," and to "catch the masked girl." He could not do it then. Now, after recalling the traumatic seduction incident with George S., and after securing some meaning into it all, he can ride the horse. He can also catch and unmask the teasing girl—which he recognized as his own self. When closure can be brought to such neurotic dreams we have more support for the belief that the "insight" is genuine and that true progress has been accomplished.)

One more Battle

Moses and Aaron once looked over a hill and saw the Promised Land of Canaan, but it was only a glimpse. The Children of Israel wandered in the wilderness for years before they were permitted to enjoy that promised land. Sometimes insight is like that. The cause is unearthed—the patient sees—he understands. It looks all to clear. Then the fog of resistance closes down—the clouds congeal—the light is obscured. The explanations are rejected. Mr. Y still had one round of ammunition.

Beginning that night, March 7th, all the anxieties and fears returned to Patient X—returned in the most acute form he had ever experienced. For four nights he went through a virtual hell. He spent his nights again rising and tossing, and his days gritting his teeth, striving to swallow the anxiety. That which his whole life had been trying to deny had now finally emerged to the surface. He had been made to look directly into the mirror at himself, and what he saw was not pleasing.

It was March 11th before he again reported in to see the therapist and describe the tortures through which he had been going. The therapist gave him some reassurance and once more pointed out the necessity of understanding and accepting, not rejecting. Patient X was now involved in that stage which psychoanalysts have termed "working-through." He left slightly reassured, but the death agonies of Mr. Y continued for seven more days.

Finally, On March 18th his anxieties had subsided somewhat, and he returned. Reassurance was again given, plus further discussion as to the meaning behind the material uncovered. He left feeling much better.

The next day, March 19th, the hour was spent in an exhaustive review of the entire treatment. Line by line, word by word, event by event, the material was discussed, placing the pieces in the pattern where they made sense as interpreted in the light of the uncovered key—the latent homosexual component which X had been desperately trying to conceal from himself for many years.*

* So many items now made sense. You may recall the session of February 28th when the patient's dissociated hand wrote, "H-O-M-O-B-I-O-L-G-I-C-A-L-H-O-M-O," and the delving up of the word, "P-R-O-A-N-T-I-R-A-N-S-U-B-S-T-A-N-C-H-I-I-O-N-I-S-T", an unusual Civil War term meaning a person with two different kinds of social standing, standing in his unconscious for heterosexual and homosexual. Another time he dreamed of being chased from behind by a car with "a big nickel-plated engine" (A male genital symbol). His ability to "know" homosexuals "right and left," plus "what they eat, drink, and sleep" attests to his underlying resonance with them. There were many more such items which arose but which we have not mentioned in this brief account of the treatment.

By March 26th he reported sleeping well for five days. Except for a slight uneasiness he felt little disturbed. There were no more nightmares. He was not awakened at night, and concerning his fear of the dark he said, "I just forgot it."

Obviously no "complete analysis" had been accomplished. Certain strata of his unconscious mind had been penetrated. The existence of latent homosexual impulses were revealed and the fear of his own feminine component with considerable "castration anxiety." He apparently derived insight into these and mastered his fears. His chief symptom (fear of the dark) disappeared.

We might ask such questions as why these homosexual fears first originated? What were the childhood fantasies that occurred in his sexual development? How did his Melvin and George ego states split off—and so many other questions. But we had reached a point where the treatment could be stabilized. It was time now for X to go home, to leave the military environment and return to civilian life. There was time for only one more meeting.

Session of March 28th

"You know I had a dream recently. I saw a baby. It was dying. It did die. Its heart protruded making the skin extend. I saw it suffering, and then it was dead." (Is the "baby" his own neurotic immaturity?)

He was next taken back to the field and shown the black horse again. He said, "It is very wild. It is running away from me. He comes back—he runs away—he comes back—he circles me—he stops. I get in the saddle. Now I'm on top of him. He is a wild animal—he throws me off. I'm getting on again. He jumps over fences and throws me off again. I get on again. We are running down the road. He takes off into the air. I can ride him. And now he disappears. He is just a flash in the distance." (I can master my neurosis?)

"You will have a dream now which will indicate your future. Will you be riding the horse in the future?"

X sat quietly for five minutes, twiddling with his fingers. When asked, "Have you finished your dream?" He replied, "Yes, first I saw an Army barracks like we have here. Suddenly one of them began to change into a house, a nice house. It had a small fence around it. Outside the house was a horse. I started to go to the field, playing polo. I can't imagine why—riding him."

The therapist reassured, "You can ride *your* horse."

"All right. You are now at a masquerade ball. There is a girl there who has a mask on."

"She probably needs to keep her face covered because her face is horrible—my face." Then he laughed, "That's good joke."

"Who is this girl?"

Immediately X replied, "I don't want to chase her. I know who she is."

"Are you afraid of her?"

"No, of course not. I'm not afraid of her."

He then began to rub his eyes. "I'm getting awake."

"What happened to George and Melvin?"

"Oh," replied the patient, "they have taken long trips—gone away, and they are not coming back. Poor Melvin." He mused a moment. "If they had combined their best traits in one person—what a person."

"Maybe they have."

"I want to get back to civilian life and start driving—the old push—the old force, like I used to have. If I were cleaning streets, I'd have the cleanest streets in the block. Mr. Y will be just a bad memory." Patient X opened his eyes and smiled.

Just before leaving the hospital X was given a Rorschach analysis. It was not secured under optimum conditions, hence, the total number of responses was low. However, the results were indicative of normal personality functioning, with little evidence of neurotic maladjustment. Ego strength was good and regard for reality high. His intellectual approach to problems was along more general and obvious lines. Mild anxiety and depressive features were noted. Although he exhibited sensitivity to emotional stimuli from his environment, his capacity for emotional identification with others was still not fully mature and stabilized. The general Rorschach pattern was that of a reasonably normal personality without severe psychopathology.

Chapter 7. Projective Hypnoanalysis

Outline

1. The mechanism of projection.

2. Psychological projective techniques.
    a. Rorschach Ink Blot Test.
    b. Thematic Apprception Test (TAT).
    c. Tautophone (Verbal Summator).
3. Jungian "Active Imagination."

4. Dissociated handwriting.

5. Dream interpretation.

6. Symbolic communication.

7. Projective forecast of conflict resolution.

8. Evidences for the validity of apparent "insight."
    a. Resolution of neurotic dreams following "insight."

Chapter 8

Dissociation

In Vol. 1. Hypnotherapeutic Techniques, Chapter 2. Theories of Hypnosis listed dissociation as among the more prominent theories of hypnosis. Janet (1907) used this term in referring to hypnotic phenomena, and later Hilgard (1986) developed a "neo-dissociative" theory of hypnosis. After all, the hypnotized subject exhibits dissociation in many ways. During induction the subject is focused on the voice of the hypnotists and his own inner processes to the exclusion of other stimuli from without. Hypnoanesthesia (see Vol. 1. Chapter 9) involves the dissociation of pain perception from an injured tissue. In an hypnotically-induced compulsion a behavior is dissociated from normal, conscious volition. And in hypnotic hallucinations inner experience is dissociated from reality perception.

Accordingly, hypnosis may be considered as, itself, a form of dissociative behavior and also as a modality for creating, manipulating and terminating dissociations. Not only are there numerous dissociative procedures which can be utilized within hypnosis in diagnosing and treating may disorders, but the modality is almost a *"sine quo non"* in the treatment of amnesias and multiple personalities. We will first consider those hypnotic techniques which can be used throughout hypnoanalysis, and then ways in which they can be employed in dealing with "natural" dissociations, such as amnesias and multiple personalities that have spontaneously appeared without the patient being hypnotized.

Dissociated Diagnostic Techniques

The presence of dissociation can be inferred from interviews, observation of behavior, case histgory, reports of "time out" by the patient or by the Perceptual Alteration Scale (Sanders, 1986). It is usually initiated by some early inner conflict or trauma.

Inner conflict within the neurotic disorders is caused by the impact of two contradictory elements on each other. Thus, a sexual desire for a friend's wife or husband may be in conflict with a conscience need to be regarded as a moral person. Anxiety and other symptoms can result. The sexual drive may be repressed, and the subject is unaware of it.

In such conditions psychoanalysis tries to receive communications which reveal to the analyst the unconscious motivations when they are still beyond awareness to the patient. The psychoanalytic techniques of free association, dream analysis and transference are employed to "wrest" from the unconscious of the patient the "secret" impulses which underly this conflict.

How does one get a patient to "reveal" such unconscious secrets while at the same time permitting him to "conceal" them from his own awareness. The anxiety arises because the two elements of the conflict are both "on stage" at the same time. The patient mentioned above may be partially aware of a sexual attraction to his friend's wife, but be unwilling to let such a recognition reach full comprehension. He cannot verbalize the conflict because to do so would be telling himself as well as his analyst its true nature. If we could but devise a way whereby his "unconscious" self could inform us of the hidden desire while his "conscious ego" is still kept in the dark about it, then we would have pre-knowledge of the conflict and could plan our therapeutic strategy accordingly. Of course, we recognize that the information so derived may have to be withheld from the patient until a time when he is strong enough, prepared enough, and willing to confront this insight. Dissociated handwriting is one such procedure.

Dissociated Handwriting

In Chapter 7, Projective Hypnoanalysis, the technique was widely employed in the treatment of Patient X. It can be initiated as follows: The patient is first hypnotized. An anesthesia is thon suggested in his writing hand. "Your hand is becoming stiff and paralyzed. It is getting completely numb, so that it has no feeling in it. It is no longer a part of you. It is separated from your body at the wrist." If the patient is highly hypnotizable and able to enter a fairly deep hypnotic state he is told, "Open your eyes and look at your hand. You will see that it is just floating in space and that it is no longer connected to your body at the wrist. Notice that because it is no longer a part of you, you have no control over it. You cannot make it move, and you cannot stop it from moving if it wishes to. You are free now to close your eyes or to keep them open and watch the movements of the hand over which you have no control."

By removing feeling from the hand we have changed it from "subject," hence, from part of "the me" into "object", a "not me." "Not me's," being outside our self, are not subject to our control and censorship. They do what they want and say what they want, even if this means revealing secrets we prefer to conceal from ourself or others. If the patient chooses to close the eyes it probably means that he doesn't want to read what might be written. If he keeps his eyes open it may mean that either he is prepared to become informed about the message, or that he is so deeply dissociated that he will not be able to remember what he saw on being alerted from hypnosis.

We next put a pencil in his hand and paper under it and suggest the following: "Your hand is like another little person. It knows many things, perhaps things you do not know about yourself. It will begin to write and say whatever it needs to." Quite often "the Hand" does not move at all now. It holds the pencil and is still. Since we are suggesting that it can "reveal secrets" which the patient does not want to uncover this quiet period is only a symptom of the resistance. The movements of "the Hand" must be removed still further from conscious observation and control. "The Hand" may need to be warmed-up into action on innocuous material. We proceed as follows: "The Hand seems to be moving a little, just a little. Maybe it wants to move up or down. Its movements are slight, but they will become greater in time." One watches carefully and encourages some slight movement, any movement, in "the Hand." Prodding may require some time. This is a period when "the Hand' is becoming increasingly dissociated from controls.

As soon as "the Hand" begins to move we say: "Perhaps 'the Hand' will draw a letter, any letter?" This warming-up period may take some time, but with perseverance by the therapist a letter usually appears. It may be printed or in cursive writing. When it appears we continue: "Good! Now maybe 'the Hand' will write another letter. Fine. Now another. And another."

One usually finds that in a little while the "letters" begin to form words. Communication begins. Sometimes the words are negative, such as "I don't want to write." or "It's none of your business." In one case "the Hand" made scribbling marks and then wrote "Jumble, jumble, jumble" (See Chap. 7, Figure 7:2). All this is to be considered as part of the warming-up period and as resistance. When permitted expression, resistances tend to wear out, and that which is being resisted comes to the fore. This is quite in line with the often-noted psychoanalytic response that when one side of a conflict is expressed, in time the other side will become manifest. If an angry spouse is encouraged to ventilate his/her hostile feelings and disparaging comments about the other, there comes a time when the person says, "Well, he isn't always bad. Sometimes he's sweet." That is why we "wear-out" resistance by encouraging its expression.

Responses from "the Hand" should be treated the same way. When using the dissociated handwriting technique we are concerned with getting communications about inner conflict through the censorship of the ego. Analytic use of dissociated revelation does not eliminate resistances or their appropriate handling, but it often does make easier the securing of pertinent information about a patient's conflict.

One of the drawbacks of dissociated handwriting is that it takes much time, both in the warm-up period and afterwards. Also, if the patient's eyes are closed his pencil will frequently run off the edge of the paper. The therapist will have to adjust the hand on the paper continuously and put new sheets of paper under it. Furthermore, it takes a deeper degree of hypnotic involvement to get such involuntary, dissociated movements. Some patients are quite passive, and the hand does not move no matter how much urging. "Hallucinated" dissociated handwriting may then be a better choice.

Hallucinated Dissociated Handwriting

Since a deeper degree of hypnotic involvement is required to suggest motor movements we may choose to keep the responses entirely in the field of perception. This, however, does require that the patient be able to talk while hypnotized. Such a procedure might be initiated as follows:

"You are walking down a street. Can you see the cars passing by? There is a school up ahead; you are going into it. You proceed to a very special class and sit down. You can learn some very important things here. As you sit at the desk you look around the room. Can you describe how it is furnished."

All this is a kind of warm-up in getting the patient to fantasize images. We are also planting the following suggestions indirectly: "You are going to a school to learn. This is a very special school, hence, you will learn something very important to you. Confirm to me that you are really imaging this situation." The suggestions are both dissociative and projective. We now zero in more closely on what we seek.

"Notice the blackboard up ahead. If you look at it carefully you will see a hand with a piece of chalk on it. The hand is writing something. Tell me what it is writing."

This is like many of the projective techniques described in the last chapter, but it taps in to the same material which we probably would have had revealed if we had actually dissociated his hand physically and then asked "projective" questions. The hallucinated hand may have to be "warmed-up" and urged in the same way that the patient's physical hand required. The two techniques may be combined if the patient can actually write with a dissociated hand. He may be instructed to read what is written on the board and told that his own hand will copy the writing. There are innumerable variations which are possible as we seek to get revelation of unconscious material and wish to place "distance" between what the patient is communicating and what he understands and is aware of concerning those communications.

The finger communication procedure described by Cheek (1962) is also a variation of the dissociated hand technique. (See Chapter 9 in Volume 1.) It has the advantage of asking for only minimal movements, hence, merely lifting a finger. It can also be used frequently without a formal hypnotic induction and thus may involve lesser degrees of dissociation. However, it is limited because questions must require a "yes" or "no" answer with possibly an "I don't know" or an "I don't want to answer."

In good hypnotic subjects, those who have spontaneous dissociative abilities, communication may be established through "automatic writing." which has had considerable study (Messerschmidt, 1927-1928; Mühl, 1968). It is simply script that is spontaneously produced involuntarily and in some instances without conscious awareness. While it is quite similar to "dissociated handwriting" we prefer to reserve that term for writing by a hand which has been specifically dissociated hypnotically by the therapist. "Automatic writing' occurs spontaneously and without a prior hypnotic induction, even though the therapist may have encouraged it. Early examples are the "spirit" writings of various "mediums" (Christopher, 1975; Lambert, 1971). For a survey of experiments in this area see Chap. 7 in Hilgard (1986).

Mühl found that automatic writing helped her patients to unearth hidden conflicts, obtain access to early childhood thought forms, discover latent talents and organize their personalities more effectively. She placed their writing arm in a sling so that it was suspended about 1 inch over the table. She would sit behind them and whisper questions into their ears. Sometimes she had them read so that their conscious mind was districted. She reported that often the first communications were simply wavy lines or single letters. By repeating what they had written she found that letters began to form into words. Sometimes communications were in a code difficult to decipher. Some of the time she also used hypnosis which would then make her procedure more like the "dissociated handwriting" that we have described. She noted that the communications could be divided into two general classes: fantasy and actual recall. While some subjects (especially those who are given to "doodling") may write naturally without using the sling others may require the freedom of movement offered by the hand and arm being lifted off the desk. However, many clinicians may find this arrangement cumbersome and prefer the "dissociated writing" technique using hypnosis.

Although this writer tends to use hypnosis one patient brought in automatic messages which he would write in the school library while sitting in a "kind of fog" state. These said to me, "You good Daddy. You take care of me. I love you" etc. Through them a child ego state was discovered which proved to be a significant element in his problem and which was dealt with by "hypnoanalytic ego-state therapy" techniques. (See Chap. 9). Flexibility, a willingness to experiment with different approaches, and acceptance of whatever covert communications the patient offers will best facilitate therapy. Some patients communicate better through projective techniques, some through dissociative procedures—and others through a combination of both.

The Treatment of Dissociative Reactions

The hypnotic treatment procedures which we have just described rely on controlled dissociation for their efficacy. Certain mental illnesses, primarily amnesia and multiple personality, are the result of spontaneous and uncontrolled dissociation. The hypnotic modality is well suited to treat such disorders.

Amnesia

Although amnesia seems just "to happen," if not organically determined, it is the result of an unconscious conflict which protects the patient from the awareness of unpleasant and derogatory self motivations. We might say that such a person "commits amnesia." Originally classified as a type of "hysteria" dissociative reactions were considered as quite amenable to hypnotherapy. However, like the other main branch of hysteria, "conversion reactions," they are often quite resistant to hypnosis. If they are based on the need to conceal certain conflicts from conscious awareness, and if hypnosis is an approach which threatens to break through that wall, then it would be most logical to expect such resistance. This was the case with Richard Billings (pseudonym), who developed an amnesia for his entire life after suffering a combat breakdown. (For a detailed report on this case see Chapter 11 in Watkins (1949).

In the Army hospital Richard stared blackly at the floor, wandered about in a daze and appeared, not only to forget all of his prior life, his wife, child, parents, but even his own name. Almost no responses could be evoked during psychological testing with the Wechsler Bellevue Mental Ability Test and The Rorschach. One response on the Jung Verbal Association Test (1976/1921), Evil—"Mine, Act." suggested an underlying guilt. Repeated attempts to hypnotize him failed. Even interviews under sodium amytal gave us no information. He moved directly from light relaxation through heavier narcosis into a deep sleep without responding to suggestions.

He was sent home on furlough in the hope that familiar surroundings would return his memory, but he did not recognize the town or any of his family members. This is a rather profound amnesia, since many such patients flee their surroundings in a fugue state, assume other identities, and maintain the changed identity in another location which has no reminders of their earlier life.

We were desperate, and so used a powerful motivation to try and induce hypnosis—fear.

"Richard, you went home on furlough, and you still were not able to regain your memory. Now you've come back to the hospital. You'll have to stay here until you get your memory back. If, after treating you here, we still cannot bring your memory back, it may be necessary to use very drastic methods. You may have heard that people sometimes recover their memories if they are taken back to the place where they lost them. If there is no other way to get this memory back, it may be necessary for us to send you back into Germany, back to the combat zone, into battle, in order that you can get your memory back where you lost it. We hope this won't be necessary, but we have been thinking about it."

Imagine the effect of this on a neurotic patient who has broken down under the stress of combat, and who has escaped from it all by a thorough-going amnesia. Of course, such things are not done with neuropsychiatric patients, nevertheless, the implied threat was there. In the Army men became accustomed to the idea that almost anything might happen, and a tremendous fear was evoked in Richard, a fear which could be strong enough to break through his amnesia. The ethics of such a maneuver are certainly debatable, but at the time we perceived the problem as a need to rescue the patient from himself and send him home. Perhaps reality would reward a more normal adjustment.

The next induction attempt, using a postural-sway technique was successful. Richard went into hypnosis which was progressively deepened. Almost an hour was spent regressing him to various periods in his life, from pre-school up to his marriage and entrance into the Service. He re-lived his trip overseas, then his transportation to the front in France.

He was next brought up to the actual combat scene which proceeded his breakdown, and he abreactively re-lived it. He began to writhe and twitch.

"They're shooting. They're shooting all kinds of shells. It's just hell. I'm scared to death, but I've got to go on—I've got to go on. Hey, they've got our range. Look out! That one was close. They're all too damned close! They hit on both sides of me. Huh—that's funny. I don't know much. Everything's black. All in a daze. Like I'm in a dream. I can see myself going back to hospital—hospital—hospital."

Other than the need to escape from an intolerable combat situation we had no other data to suggest underlying dynamics of such a profound amnesia. We had hoped to do more analytic exploration, but the requirements that men be discharged from the service as soon as possible mandated his release. We had relieved his presenting symptom, amnesia, by a pressure tactic (fear), had worked-through the apparent precipitation trauma, but we knew little about his personality structure.

I wrote follow-up letters to many of my former patients to try to check-up on their post-discharged adjustment. Many months later I received the following note: "Dear Sir: My husband received your letter some time ago, but refused to answer it." (Obviously! Richard had not forgiven us for "dragging" him back to reality.) "So I will. He is just fine, has no trouble at all. Maybe a few headaches when he first returned, but that is all. I think drinking was mostly the cause of them. You see my husband is mean, *very* mean. Those who are good have to suffer. He went to a specialist. The Dr. found nothing wrong with him. His mother tells me that he is just a well as he was before he entered the service." Signed, his wife.

Would the patient, his family and society have been better served if we had let the amnesia be? He could have spent his days in a veteran's facility, and his family would have received a pension.

A much later case afforded the opportunity to relieve a stubborn amnesia, and by uncovering underlying dynamics, work-through to a more permanent and happy resolution. It also taught us better techniques in dealing with amnesias.

Will walked into my office. "You do hypnosis?"

"Well, yes, sometimes," I replied.

"This memory—it's all gone. I was in motorcycle accident, but I don't remember being in it. I've also got a plate in my head," remarked Will, as he rubbed the left side of his skull. "My head got bashed in quite a bit."

With a left parietal injury it was not surprising that he also manifested considerable aphasia. He understood everything said to him, but could not think of or speak many specific words. Will had had much medical treatment plus failed efforts at rehabilitation. No other neurological studies were currently contemplated, and he had been written off as a stabilized, organic "vegetable".

A new graduate class in hypnotherapy was just being started at the University. Will agreed to being treated with a video camera "piping" the therapy to the class in another room. This was the first of 10 sessions, during which his amnesia was resolved and a satisfactory work and life adjustment established. In view of the severe known organic pathology no such outcome was envisioned at that time. But Will was motivated and most cooperative.

"Will, have you been able to work since the accident?"

"I haven't had a job. No."

He then described how he existed on a small pension, didn't go to movies and didn't go out with friends. He just sat at home. As he gloomily said it was, "A real dull life."

Some 35 minutes were spend in hypnotizing Will, and he was regressed to a time prior to his accident, two years earlier when he was in the Navy.

"Will, you're forgetting all about what year it is and how old you are. You're going back to a time when you were in the Navy. You're on ship. What can you see?"

"Water." (His first memory.)

"You're talking to a friend. What is he saying?" (a projective technique).

"Hey Mac, how's the guns holding up?" (Will was a gunner's mate.) Will then described his interaction with this buddy in some detail. There is a "warming up" in the memory recall.

From this point we proceeded to his visit to San Francisco, how a bar wouldn't serve him a drink because of his age, and his "liberty" in Sydney, Australia. He described that "pretty thing" over the harbor but because of his aphasia couldn't use the word "bridge" until it was called to his attention. We tried to stimulate recall first. If not successful, recognition could often be secured.

"Did you go to a night club? Meet any girls?"

"Oh, yes. There were plenty of girls," recalled Will with a grin on his face.

At this time his flat, listless features became more animated. He remembered going to Saigon, then to Hong Kong where he described the floating restaurants and the "Tiger-Balm Gardens." Next, he recalled his travels to Honolulu. He waxed eloquent over the fact that they could "surf and surf and surf."

He was next regressed to the age of 7 where he named the teacher and a number of his classmates in the 2nd grade, and after that to the 5th grade at age 10 where he also named his teacher. This suggested that he was not mentally retarded and had progressed through school normally.

He then re-lived other events in his life, at home, playmates and in high school, where he described his graduation. By now we had "sampled" a wide number of times and events in his life which he had successfully recalled. The amnesia had been breached on a broad front, and he was asked the following:

"Will, when I count up to five would you be willing to become alert and remember everything we have talked about, your service in the Navy, San Diego, San Francisco, Sydney, Australia, Hong Kong, Honolulu, your school days in the 2nd and 5th grades, your friends and playmates, and your graduation. Would you be willing to remember all these things?"

Without hesitation Will said, "Yes."

"O.K. You can remember all these things, and you can remember a lot more."

Will emerged from hypnosis in astonishment and with the utmost excitement.

"Egad. I can remember. I really can remember. Egad."

He then proceeded to recount the many details which had been recovered under hypnosis. He also expanded his memory and described many other events in his life. The amnesia had been broken. However, it had all been through suggestion. Could there be other, psychodynamic reasons which were involved in this symptom—besides the known brain trauma? He left filled with happiness. This was the 2nd session.

At the beginning of the 4th session Will startled the therapist.

"I got my driver's licence."

"You got your driver's licence?" I could hardly believe it. He hadn't driven for over two years, but after only three sessions of suggestive hypnosis he had apparently, not only recovered his memory, but his helpless, dependent behavior had also disappeared. On his own he had gone out, volunteered for the driver's licence test, and passed it— albeit after first failing it twice. Never had I seen such a profound recovery in so short a time. These things rarely happen to a psychotherapist. I could not get over it, but kept returning obsessively asking the same questions about his recovery. The videotape was reviewed again and again. His aphasia remained, but not the amnesia, nor the passive, defeatist attitude.

We continued this 4th session, and he was re-hypnotized. In the 3rd session Will had told me that his accident occurred when returning home from attending the funeral of a buddy, Ivan, who was killed in a motorcycle accident three days before. He was now regressed to the funeral.

"You're at the funeral, Will. What's happening?"

"My buddies are there. It's quiet. There's a body in a funeral case in front. We're all praying for him."

"You're feeling just like you did at the funeral." (An affect bridge). You're thinking out loud. What are you thinking?"

"My God! Why in the hell do I have this motorcycle? Get rid of the damn cycle—or it'll be your death.

The therapist repeated, "Get rid of the damn cycle, or it'll be your death."

More rumination by Will. I then tell him that we're at the end of the funeral and ask what will happen next.

"We're going to bury him."

"He's being buried. There goes Ivan. There goes Ivan. What are you thinking, Will?"

"I wish I could be in his place."

"Why?" No answer. "We're going home now. Where's your cycle?"

"Just off the burying ground."

Will gets on "his cycle, " holds his hands in front of him as if guiding the handle bars. He sadly talks about Ivan. When asked, he indicates what street he is on. Suddenly he comes up behind a truck which has stopped.

"Damned truck."

He "darts out" to pass the truck, faces another truck coming the other way and manifests extreme anxiety.

"What's the matter?"

"I'm having an accident."

"Look out! Look out!"

Will suddenly slumps back into his chair and is silent. I wait awhile, and then say, "Good morning, Will. How are you feeling today?.," talking as if I were visiting him in the hospital.

"I wasn't even paying any mind. That accident shouldn't have happened."

After some reassurance I ask if he would be willing to remember the entire incident clearly when I alert him. He agrees. I count up to 5 and bring him out of trance.

"Egad! I had a dream about the accident. It's so firm."

He proceeds to describe the accident in great detail and ends up noting that the next thing he remembers is waking up in the hospital. We review over many details of his early life. I re-hypnotize him and he tells me, "Who's going to like me now?" I ask "Why," and he says, "Who's going to like a dumb nut."

"So you think you're a dumb nut?"

"No. That's just *the way I act*."

"Do you always have to act that way?"

"NO! NO! I don't have to act that way." Will is almost jubilant at grasping this point. He laughs with animation at his new insight. I bring him out of hypnosis with the reminder, "which will stick in your mind" that, *"you don't have to act that way."*

During the 6th session Will brought out additional information. He was hypnotized and asked to dream about a situation. He then revealed that the motorcycle gang was also a homosexual gang. He had had heterosexual experiences and was deeply disturbed over his membership in this gang. He recalled that he had been arrested just before the accident in a homosexual bar and was to come before a judge the next Monday. He said under hypnosis, "They're going to hang me."

Ivan's funeral was the previous Saturday. He badly needed relief from his punishing guilt. Earl was hypnotized, asked to "go to sleep" and "have a dream" about his problem. In a few minutes he reported he was dreaming about the motorcycle gang and their activities. I asked him how he felt about them, and he replied that at first he thought that what they were doing was "all right." Later, however, he felt differently and said that for 3 months prior to his accident he was "mixed up" and had a "feeling of disgust inside me." Through a "Socratic" method of questioning under hypnosis I pursued the possibility that he was suffering from considerable guilt at the time of his accident.

"When Ivan was killed what were your thoughts?"

"I thought, 'look, if you get killed what the hell would your mother do?"

"Why did you think you might be killed?"

"Well—" Will was evasive.

"Was Ivan killed by chance, bad luck or for some necessary reason?"

"I think there was a reason."

"Because he was bad?"

"Yea. That was probably it."

"Do you think that if people are bad they get punished."

"Yes, I do."

"Was Ivan punished?"

"Yeah."

"And how was he punished?"

"He had an accident."

"Do you think that people who are bad might be punished by accidents?"

"Uh huh."

"Then how about you?"

"I had an accident."

"What does that mean?"

"It means I am bad."

"Do you think that maybe if a person has one accident that pays enough for being bad?"

"Yeah."

"They don't have to pay anymore. They've paid it off."

"Right.—That's right," beamed Will as if suddenly coming to life.

"Then the slate's clean," I suggested. "You're not bad anymore."

Like a sudden burst of sunshine during a gloomy day, sheer joy swept over Will's face. "Yeah. Well that's all right."

"And after a person's paid off his debts he's free to be anything he wants. It's a fresh start."

Will exploded into almost a paroxysm of ecstasy, "Egad. A Brand new start. This dumb nut not to realize that—Egad."

The therapist continued, "And he doesn't have to stay home does he?"

"That's right!"

"And he doesn't have to be, as you say, 'a dumb nut' anymore?"

"Oh, for crying out loud. Oh Jese. I've been such a fool all of this time."

"You have been punishing yourself."

"Yes, and there really isn't any need. Oh for crying out loud."

These expressions of surprise, amazement and insight continued for some time as Will became deeply involved in reorganizing his self-perception.

"Would you like to open your eyes, remember all these things and think them through? If you want to be a free man now you can. Everything's been paid off."

Will emerged from hypnosis in a universe of magnified joy. "Oh God, Doctor."

He described the change in his feelings. "It's as if a great weight was lifted off me."

I mentioned that Vocational Rehabilitation had contacted me renewing its offer to re-train him and help him get a job. On that high note he left.

The feeling of exhilaration when a repression is lifted or a dissociation re-associated has been noted frequently by psychoanalysts. This represents a freeing of repressive energies which then are available for other ego activities—a kind of new-found wealth of energy. Also, previously repressed material seems quite familiar once it has been re-assimilated back into the ego. Stekel (1943c) stated that after having recovered a previously forgotten (repressed) episode in their life patients would remark, "I guess I always knew that. I just didn't pay attention to it." The same thing occurs when a multiple personality alter is reintegrated. It now is no longer an object, but a subject representation. Accordingly it is experienced as self. Rhonda (Watkins and Johnson, 1982) when asked several years later about "Mary," her previously tormenting alter, said simply, "She was me."

In the 8th session under hypnosis Will relived the accident, this time reporting that at the last minute he had specifically turned his wheel into the truck, not away from it. After 10 sessions Will felt he did not need to return, but it was left open if he needed us. He was followed for six years. He reported no more difficulty other than continual residuals of his aphasia. He became self supporting, got a job and held it. At our last contact he was leading a normal life.

We learned much from this case:

1. Just because a patient has severe, known brain damage (even when manifested by aphasia and a plate in his skull) it does not mean that other symptoms, including amnesia, are irreversible, untreatable. We should not give up. Psychotherapy sometimes works surprises.

2. Even though amnesia can sometimes be relieved by hypnotic suggestions, deeper and more analytic probing may be essential if the gains are to stay and be translated into continued better adjustment. Witness the difference between the case of Richard and the case of Will. Contrary to the usual order in Will's case the eliciting and working-through of his repressions followed the suggestive elimination of his main symptom rather than preceding them. Had we been content with the elimination of the amnesia after the second hour we might have missed the opportunity to help him reach a new, significant and permanent life adjustment. "Hypnoanalysis" improved on "hypnotherapy."

Principles in Treating Amnesia (as illustrated in the case of Will.)

1. After hypnotizing go back to non-traumatic events, i.e., before the trauma.

2. Start with tiny experiential details and expand into broader areas later: e.g. "Water." "Guns."

3. Then approach the trauma slowly, in great detail, as at the funeral. Get the person into the scene. e.g. "Watch the funeral; what's happening now?, etc."

4. Suggest affect present at the time of the trauma. "You're getting to feel and think just as you did then." Use an affect bridge.

5. Repeat important sentences: "Get rid of this damn cycle." "I wish I could be in his place."

6. Get patient to express orally what he's thinking: "Think out loud. What are you thinking?"

7. Use repetition and promote build-up of feeling state: "There goes Ivan!"

8. Involve yourself and develop a "we-ness." It allies the therapist's ego with that of the patient and gives support: "OK. Let's go get the cycle." "Where are we now?"

9. Build up tension with your voice (as in abreactions): "What's happening?" "Look out! Look out!"

10. Respond to expected behavior. When Will was silent after the accident the therapist assumed he was in the hospital and said, "Good morning, Will."

11. Review remembered material under hypnosis. Review it out of hypnosis. Repeat at later sessions. Don't let material slip back into amnesia.

12. Talk at the level of the patient in vocabulary and thinking (and at the level of his various child states when using regression).

Multiple Personality

The essence of this complex and baffling disorder has been described in the DMS-III-R (see American Psychiatric Association, 1987) as "the existence within the person of two or more distinct personalities or personality states." The key mechanism is "dissociation," that is, the separation of one personality segment from another by a relatively impermeable barrier. There is often a shifting from one state to another. The primary or "executive" personality is generally unaware of what has happened when one of the secondary or "alter" personalities has emerged and taken over the behavior and thinking. The patient may report no memory of what transpired between certain hours or days. While the primary personality is usually not aware (at least before treatment) of the thoughts and actions of the alters, the alters are often quite aware of everything said and done by the primary state. Sometimes they will communicate with the primary personality through dreams or "internal voices."

Almost invariably patients suffering from this disorder report much abuse during childhood, physical, sexual and/or psychological. The abused child learns that the expression of anger back at the abusers (frequently parents) only results in more abuse. Accordingly, she (more commonly female than male) creates imaginary playmates, who serve as receptacles for dissociated anger. This permits the primary personality to maintain a good girl or good boy role in the hope of receiving better treatment. If early dissociations are effective in adjusting to a punishing home situation still more may occur as new problems are met by the creation of new alters. Most multiples manifest two to fifteen different alters. However, some cases have been reported as exhibiting many more, perhaps even 100. Intensive case studies of multiple personality which have been published include the well-known ones by Prince (1906), Thigpen and Cleckley (1957) and Schreiber (1974).

Cases of multiple personality have been reported as far back as medieval times, but then it was usually considered "demon posses-sion." For reports on historical cases see Ellenberger (1970) and E.R. Hilgard (1986). Recent theoretical conceptions, diagnostic criteria and treatment procedures are surveyed in Beahrs (1982), Bliss (1986), Braun (1984,1986), Hilgard (1986), Putnam (1989), Ross (1989), and Watkins and Johnson (1982).

In the past, multiple personality was considered to be a "rare" disorder. With better understanding, newer diagnostic tools and recent research we now know otherwise. These cases have suffered greatly from mis-diagnosis and mis-handling, and the average spe-cialist in this area usually gets contacted by patients only after a long record of their having been diagnosed as schizophrenics, manic-depressives, sociopaths, and having been in and out of many clinics and hospitals. Many recent clinical reports and research studies are now available. Boor and Coons (1983) have published a comprehen-sive bibliography of literature in the field which lists over 250 items. Since our concern here is with hypnoanalytic techniques in treating such conditions we will not attempt to replicate these extensive reviews of the literature.

A brief case will be described to illustrate some of the hypnoanalytic treatment procedures which may be used.

Jamie, age 38, clutched a pillow and a small doll when I first saw her in the hospital. She looked like a frightened 3-year old—which in fact she was at that time, "Little Jimmy". As I gained her confidence a mature personality emerged and described many instances of being abused as a child. There were also numerous blanking-out periods throughout her life. Gradually I became acquainted with other per-sonalities: Jill who was forthright, strong and friendly, Megan an idealized mother state, who pontificated as mothers often do, Betty, who had good, common sense, was jolly and knew what was going on inside of Jamie, and a hint of a more malevolent personality, Jeri, who would cut Jamie with knives or broken glass.

One often tries to find an ally inside the patient who can furnish reports of what is happening, the relationship of the various alters to the primary state, to each other, and to the world, and who can make therapeutic suggestions,as well as describe the effect of therapeutic maneuvers—which sometimes backfire.

Most important of all is to make friends with each of the alters, especially the more destructive ones. An alter which has been angered by a therapist, who perhaps has inadvertently or innocently trans-mitted a message that he/she might like to eliminate him, can easily sabotage the entire treatment. This therapist has made that mistake as is well described in Watkins and Johnson, (1982). Many errors occurred before I learned to correct my ways and turn the malevolent alter into a friendly, cooperating "co-therapist."

Accordingly, after each of the alters had been interviewed in detail Betty became my internal intelligence agent.

"I think Jimmy is very angry at Jamie's mother but is afraid to say so," remarked Betty.

Jimmy was activated under hypnosis by simply asking for her. Her doll and pillow were placed conveniently near, and while she clutched them I tried to talk to a frightened, angry, little 3-year old.

"Jimmy, You're scared aren't you?"

Jimmy eyed me suspiciously and then nodded a cautious "Yes."

One must be close enough to give support but not so close as to frighten.

"You're been hurt, haven't you?"

Again a nod, this time more definitely.

Slowly and hesitantly Jimmy began to talk to me. Gradually we steered the conversation into the times where she had "been hurt." First, incidents of humiliation at home, then more severe ones of slappings, then beatings, and even molestations where her attempts to inform her mother were met by accusations of lying. In time, a full fledged abreaction emoted as Jimmy strode about beating the walls. I did not interfere hoping to exhaust this childish rage. I left the hospital feeling we had made progress.

But as so often happens in the treatment of multiples one makes two steps forward only to find a step or more backwards the next day.

"Last night Jamie broke a light bulb and cut herself," reported the nurse the following morning.

Sure enough here was Jamie, her arm bound up, but it was really Jimmy clutching the doll and the pillow. We had released much anger, but not all of it. This, plus the guilt for attacking "Mommy," had provoked the suicidal gesture of an attack on her own self. Here we see the dangers to a therapist (Watkins and Watkins, 1984, 1988). Abreactions are needed to relieve the anger, but once the anger is dislodged it can turn back on the patient or others. Such patients can become both suicidal and homicidal, and the protective environment of a supervised hospital setting may be required. Out-patient treatment can often be hazardous. If the release of dissociated rage becomes too threatening, a procedure proposed by Kluft (1988) which is a slow release or "slow burn" approach is recommended. It permits the escape of the anger more gradually and spreads it over a longer period of time (See Chapter 4. Abreactive Techniques).

Since Jamie was in the hospital, and since her eligibility for paid hospitalization was limited, we decided to continue the more violent abreactions but keep her under close observation to protect her from self-mutilation.

Numerous abreactions were initiated about different frightening and abusing episodes in the life of "little Jimmy." However, when possible we would induce "Jimmy" to "share" or "give-back" her memories and feelings of these early experiences to Jamie. We have found that when working with multiples this is the most effective approach. It was the destructive environment (people, events) which beat upon the child Jamie in the first place. This caused her to "create" a dissociated "Jimmy" who could serve as a kind "garbage can" for anger that could not be expressed without inviting more abuse. That is why it was stored up in "Jimmy." Accordingly, it should be released in the reversed order. Jimmy should release it back into the primary personality, Jamie, through their internal boundary. Jamie should then be the one to abreact it out into the external world, hence, "telling-off" the mother of her childhood. This procedure requires a close, supportive relationship with her therapist who will "protect" her from retaliation by the angry mother—that is, the mother-introject inside which she must confront, not the outside mother.

We do not encourage the grown patient to confront or attack the parent in reality. The problem is internal now, no longer external. It must be solved in therapy.

So it was with Jimmy-Jamie. Jimmy existed to absorb the mistreatment, dissociate Jamie's anger, and protect her from further abuse. As the rage was released and dissipated the need for a separate "Jimmy" no longer exists. She can be "integrated."

But as also happens in these cases their were many traumas and abusing incidents, and more than one "alter" split off. Soon another state, called "Becky," appeared. She, too, was loaded with anger but apparently split off at an older age, when Jamie was about 9.

Again, Betty became our source of information as to how well the abreactions had relieved Jimmy's rage, what were the "back-fire" behaviors, the possible dangers, like who was planing suicidal or homicidal actions, and what should be our next therapeutic step. The cooperation of such an internal entity (termed "internal self-helper" or ISH by Allison, 1974) is a valuable resource to the therapist and should be located if possible.

Becky reported the existence of another "malevolent" personality, called Sue. We use the word "malevolent" to indicate that its present behavior was destructive, but therapists should remember that every alter or dissociated state was created to *protect* the patient. It emerged to improve survival—a better option than childhood suicide or psychosis, as could have occurred. Viewed this way destructive alters can be treated as potential allies. (Watkins and Watkins, 1988) They came to protect, only their "protection" is now both ineffective and maladaptive. We must get Becky's cooperation.

"Becky, would you please come out and talk to me."

"What do you want?"

"I want to understand you and help you if I can."

"Jamie is no good. She's bad, and I'm going to kill her."

Becky looked most unfriendly, "And besides you don't want to help me. You just want to get rid of me like all of the others did."

One assumes that when Becky was "out" the patient was viewed with great rejection by her family since rebellious Becky was not the smiling, acquiescing Jamie. We repeated the same therapeutic strategy: Making friends, then inducing release of anger through abreactions, strong-immediate or controlled-flow, just as we had done with Jimmy. It is not at all uncommon that as one begins to release rage and "integrate" one personality the battle-ground will shift to another, all of which makes the treatment of dissociative disorders a most demanding and thankless task.

In addition, one does not always have the cooperation of other medical personnel. Many physicians (and even many psychiatrists and psychologists) refuse to accept the reality of a multiple personality diagnosis. They haven't seen one perhaps, because MP patients do not reveal their multiplicity to clinicians whom they perceive as unbelieving and lacking in understanding. The American Psychiatric Assoc. recently held a debate on this matter (See Kluft, Frankel, Speigel & Orne, 1988).

The same is true with nurses. In the case of Jamie one psychiatrist, with whom I had worked earlier, was most understanding and took the necessary medical responsibilities. A few of the nurses were also supportive. However, I often had to hear from the patient that Nurse "X" told her, "You're just putting on an act, being exhibitionistic, and if you'd only straighten up and behave yourself all would be well."

"Contracts" not to engage in suicidal or self-destructive behavior are often used in mental hospitals. Unfortunately, the staff seldom realized that such a "contract" signed by Jamie did not commit "Jimmy," "Becky," or any of the other personalities to such control. When subsequent suicidal attempts were made Jamie was then accused of "lying," not keeping her word, etc.—just as her parents had done many years before.

Because a primary personality, like Jamie, may be sweet, compliant, friendly and look so normal, not hallucinating nor manifesting deep depression, mental health personnel who have little or no experience with multiples are easily convinced that it is all an act. One often spends as much time educating the hospital staff as treating the patient. Resistance to the therapy may be as great in the staff as in the patient. ("You're just pampering her.")

In the case of Jamie after 40 hours of hospitalization with frequent abreactions, self-cuttings, new insights and "integrations" she was discharged. Her alters emerged rarely and generally only under hypnosis. They appeared like normal "ego states." These personality segments will be discussed in greater detail in our next chapter. Jamie's adjustment was now such that she could return home, hold a job, and take care of her children as a single-parent.

A wide variety of abreactive, projective and dissociative procedures were employed. Transference reactions were noted and often interpreted. Resonant-support by the therapist was constantly required. We cannot speak of a multiple personality as being "cured," at least not until good adjustment has been confirmed over several years. There is always the possibility of a relapse or a new dissociation occurring in response to a new environmental stress. However, such patients are not untreatable, as previously believed.

Before leaving the hospital Jamie made a plaque in occupational therapy. It read:

"To Dr. Watkins. How do I thank you for bringing me through a time of fear, confusion and pain? Your kindness, consideration and help will long be remembered with fondness.

Thank you,

Jamie."

On the back side it was signed by: Jamie, Jimmy, Betty, Megan, Jill, and Becky, plus "Sue" and "Brenda", two alters whose roles we have not described here.

Only Jamie continued to emerge spontaneously. Some alters remained as covert "ego-states," and a few disappeared entirely. Time alone can test how stable her future will be.

"Integration" vs. "Fusion"

We do not believe that "integration" is the same as "fusion." Integration means making the boundaries between the various alters permeable, increasing communication and cooperation, then returning the various sub-personalities to the status of "covert" ego states—which cannot be contacted except under hypnosis. We feel it is unnecessary to attempt to "fuse" them into a unity, since this is not the structure of "normal" personality. Normal personality has its "hidden observers" (Hilgard, 1986) and is divided into covert segments for the purposes of adaptive differentiation similar to mood states. Alters in multiple personalities are much more resistant to treatment if they are threatened with "fusion." In our therapy with multiples they can (if they wish) continue to exist as normal, adaptive ego states with loss of independence but still retain their identity. In the patient's internal "Civil War" the "states" (like Alabama and Mississippi) have returned to the "Union" as normal personality segments, but have not lost their identity within a "Federal jurisdiction" of self.

Strengthening an Alter

In unity there is strength; in division, weakness. When a personality has been Balkanized into numerous weak fragments separated by relatively impermeable boundaries each state, when it becomes executive, has very limited energy resources to confront the problems and stress of living. It needs help. Helen Watkins has developed a technique which can often significantly change an alter or ego-state's outlook, especially when it is lonely, depressed and perhaps suicidal. It might proceed as follows:

Erika, a previously alcoholic alter in a 30 year old woman who had been "rehabilitated," emerged during a depressed spell in the patient. She was discouraged, lonely, felt isolated from other people on the outside and had virtually no contact or communication with other alters. She had suffered beatings by her husband plus a steady stream of criticisms from him. Erika worked hard cleaning the house and cooking meals for her family. In fact, she was an excellent cook who had once prided herself on her meals. It was the beatings which had driven her several years earlier to alcoholism and for which she had been hospitalized. However, she had not emerged overtly now for many months. She stated that life was not worth living, and she was ready to "give up," meaning suicide.

She was my patient. However, Helen Watkins, my wife and colleague, was sitting in during this session to act as co-therapist. Without an hypnotic induction Helen asked Erika to imagine "being in a peaceful, quiet room, just the three of us." Through half-closed lids Erika nodded she could see this. Helen then continued as follows:

"Erika is very lonely, and she needs help. She works hard taking care of the children, cleaning and cooking. She is very tired. Is there anybody there who will help out. Will somebody who is willing to help Erika please come into the room."

Some time was spent in urging before Erika reported that somebody was entering.

"It's Alexandra, and she is holding out her hand."

Alexandra was also an alter who hadn't been heard from for many months. She was the artistic one and delighted in decorating the home pleasingly.

"Alexander wants to be your friend, Erika. Do you know her."

"Yes I know of her. We have often worked together about the house side by side. But we never spoke to each other.:

"Ask her if she will be your friend."

"She doesn't say anything, but she's still holding her hand out."

"Why do you think she wants to help and be your friend?"

"Alexandra is humiliated the same as I am. Her husband makes fun of her art just like he's always finding fault with my cleaning and cooking." He tracks the house up with mud just after I've cleaned it and then makes fun of me. Alexandra is so talented and artistic. I'm no good and don't have anything to contribute."

"But Erika," Helen objected, "You are an artist too. You cook fine meals, and that's being artistic in your own way. The two of you would make a fine team. Why not reach out and take her hand?"

"I'm afraid," said Erika timidly.

"What are you afraid of? She won't hurt you. Besides, Alexandra may be afraid too. Let her know you want to be friends. Reach out to her."

Erika "reached out" to Alexandra, and the two of them came much closer together. Now they could be allies in coping with an abusing husband. They could share support and energies. Erika was not so lonely and isolated now, and they had moved toward "integration."

This technique of asking for someone to come in and help can be used in normal ego-state therapy (See Chapter 9) as well as in the treatment of true multiples. I asked Helen what she would do if nobody came. Her reply, "It's never happened."

Strategy in Treating Multiple Personalities

1. Interview each of the major alters to determine its purpose and function in the whole psychic economy. Determine how it regards itself and how it views the main personality and the other alters. Find out its assets and liabilities for building a more integrated person.

2. Formulate some general plan of treatment. What are the support and stress factors in the patient's environment? Which alters will you work with first? Which ones are probably the most integratable? What dangers to the patient, to the therapist and to others are possible—suicide, homicide, etc.? Can the individual be treated as an out-patient, or will hospitalization be required? What cooperation will be needed from allied professions: medical, psychological, social, etc.? Do you have other therapists available if needed?

3. Erode the rigidity and increase the permeability of the boundaries separating alters from each other and from the main personality.

4. Increase awareness and communication between the alters.

5. Encourage alters to "cooperate" with each other in meeting their needs.

6. Suggest that alters "share" their symptoms, strengths, memories and feelings with each other and with the main personality.

7. Make friends with all alters, especially the more malevolent and destructive ones.

8. Release dissociated fear and rage by abreactions.
   a. Insights must be experiential, hence, affective, perceptual and motor, not merely cognitive.
   b. Wear-out dissociated affect by repeated abreactions, hence, re-experience, re-experience, re-experience.

9. Strengthen the main personality.

10. Seek integration of alters with each other and with the main personality.

Specific Tactics for Implementing the Above Strategies

1. To erode boundary rigidities name and talk about other alters when communicating with any alter and with the main personality. Educate each about the nature and purpose of others. Try to get alters (and the main personality) to resonate

with the feelings and needs of the others. I often speak of them as "my friends," perhaps telling "Jamie" just how "my friend, Jimmy," feels about a recent event. ("You'd feel burned up, too, if you had to take everybody else's anger shoved off on you, because they didn't want to handle it.")

2. Increase awareness and communication by suggesting that alters talk to one another or communicate their thoughts and feelings to the main personality through internal voices, dreams, written notes, etc. Suggest to the main personality that he/she call upon various alters and put questions to them? ("Jeri, how do you think we should handle this situation?")

3. Encourage cooperation by suggesting that one personality help another. ("Diana, Alex is getting very bored. He thinks nobody pays any attention to him any more. Why don't you take the children on a picnic to the park and let Alex teach Billy, (the patient's son), how to play baseball?) Such activities may meet the needs of both "Alex" and Billy. Or suggest to an alter, "Georgia," (the main personality) "has to go to court tomorrow because of that speeding ticket. You know, she's scared to death. How about you and Henrietta (another alter) giving her some backing at that time?"

4. Sharing strength, symptoms, memories and feelings. "You and Mary have some of the same ideas. Why not share your ideas as to how you can best deal with Father?" Or, "Make her" (the main personality) "take back and share some of the pain she's been giving you over the years. Why should you have to be the one that gets all that anger-garbage? Open up the door (inside) between your room and hers. She really needs to be aware of how tough it's been on you."

   And to the main personality, "Jimmy has been a real heroine. She's taken all the pain from Father's beatings for years. Don't you think it would be fair if you took some of it back and shared a few good feelings with her?" The patient emerges from hypnosis, reports some depression and "bad feelings." She is not happy about getting them back but can often understand the necessity. Little Jimmy reports feeling better and is less suicidal.

5. Multiples are often aware of a precursor to switching states. It may take the form of a sudden headache, feeling dizzy, having a hard time "keeping it," etc. These will frequently occur during therapy when one personality is being pressed too hard by the

therapist to understand or accept some unpleasant interpretation. Shortly after the warning sign the alter abdicates, and there is a shift to another state.

When patients come to recognize this warning they can protect themselves from a possible switch to a destructive alter. E.g. the patient is under some stress, perhaps during an argument with a spouse. A warning sign appears. She feels dizzy, indicating that the current executive state can no long accept this stress and is about to abdicate, perhaps to be replaced with a suicidal or homicidal one. Recognizing this danger the current executive personality breaks off the argument and goes for a walk, so that she can "calm down." The patient has learned a defensive behavior designed to protect her and others for the time being. Therapists should point out this precursor to the patient—and if the stress is being caused by an offending interpretation, layoff, unless a forced change of state is desired.

6. Establish your fairness and benevolence toward each of the alters but concentrate especially in winning over the "bad" ones. A destructive alter is usually a very frustrated and hurt child state. How does one win over an angry child? At heart, it wants acceptance, understanding, and affection. Keep building up your relationship with this "friend." A 3-year old, furious little girl was partly won over to the therapist when she brought the little alter a small teddy bear. After that she was never angry at the therapist again. The prerequisites for a constructive abreaction and a building of new, less angry attitudes were laid. Never indicate that you are out to "eliminate" a malevolent alter. As your enemy he can completely sabotage your treatment. (Watkins, J.G. and Watkins, H.H., 1984,1988).

7. Release bound-up fear and anger through abreactions (See Chapter 4). This is, perhaps, the most potent technique of all, especially if it is followed by true experiential, affective insight. These may range from a few tears, through angry exclamations,up to beating on walls and smashing furniture. Once started the patient must not be released until the rage has exhausted itself. If you or the patient cannot stand the violence release it over a period of time with the "slow-burn" approach. Try "poison-pen" therapy, pounding or sobbing into pillows at home when alone, etc.

The best procedure is to ask the alter containing the rage to release it into the main personality through their internal boundary. Get the main personality to take it back, and then do the abreacting. This releases it in the reverse order from which it came in the first place. The child was abused. It dissociated into an alter, withdrew itself from perception of the abuse, thus "anesthetizing" the pain, and shoved the pain down into the dissociated alter. The alter must now give it to the main personality who then releases it back into the outer world through crying, shouting, cursing, pounding, etc.

We have found this format for the abreaction more effective than simply activating the alter and letting it abreact. However, it is possible to initiate the abreaction in the alter and then ask it to give "that anger and pain" back to the main personality including the memories of the original events (beatings, molesting, etc.). The main personality may emerge angry at you for having to experience the dissociated feelings, but unless you have confronted it with more than it could handle it will forgive you in time. In one case (See Watkins and Johnson, 1982) the patient regressed into a temporary psychotic-like 3-year old state. But when she returned to "normal" in a few days demonstrated a profound, constructive change, almost a recovery.

8. Find an internal "volunteer," some one to come and help a distressed alter or the primary personality.

9. Seek integration, not "fusion." Integration means returning the various alters to "ego states," (see Chapter 9). They become a part of normal differentiation and adaptation. They exist in the sense that they can be re-activated hypnotically, but they no longer emerge overtly, spontaneously. They report, We aren't separate persons any longer. We are just parts of 'her.'" Nobody wants to be eliminated, whole people or alters. When they are threatened with "fusion" their resistance to the therapy is greatly increased. We promise them they will not be eliminated; they can stay and retain their uniqueness if they want to—but as "states" within a "Federal" self-jurisdiction.

When one has worked for a long time with a multiple it is usually quite easy to activate an alter merely by asking for it. Accordingly, one tends not to "bother" doing a hypnotic induction first. However, the activation of an alter non-hypnotically may not be quite the same as making it overt under hypnosis. Whenever I did an induction first it seemed as if there was more progress. Perhaps hypnosis renders the boundaries of the alters more permeable, the communication between them facilitated, and the moving of their contents from one to another easier. Cornelia Wilbur, in her account of the treatment of Sybil (Schreiber, 1974), reported that while much of the therapy was conducted with traditional psychoanalysis, when she shifted at various times to hypnoanalysis the work progressed more rapidly.

Comstock (1986) sees spontaneous abreactions occurring following "signals" of their approach, such as visual, auditory and kinesthetic hallucinations, and self mutilating behavioral patterns. She believes they have three major purposes: 1. To inform (concerning past abuse), 2. To educate (such as the victim's recognizing she was not at fault during a molestation, and 3. To release the repressed effect.

In a more recent paper Wilbur (1988) has called attention to the fact that "each alter within the MPD complex develops its own transferential relationship with the therapist." This means that one alter may be manifesting positive feelings at the same time that another is hostile. Or, hostile behavior may stem from different alters for entirely different reasons, greatly complicating the treatment. The therapist needs to be familiar with the process of transference and sensitive to the many changes in it which characterize the therapy of a multiple. The analysis and interpretation of transference reactions is of equal if not greater significance in the therapy of dissociative disorders as in any of the neuroses. However, we will defer discussing this aspect until Chapter 10 on Transference.

Integration

Although every case is different there are certain general stages which the treatment of multiple personalties seem to go through. First, the therapist and the various alters get acquainted with each other. The alters may reveal themselves spontaneously, or the therapist may activate them. ("Is there somebody there whom I have not talked to?" or "Is there somebody who can give me information about why Jan feels so depressed?") These queries can be made either to the conscious, executive personality or made under hypnosis. During this initial period (which may take many months—or even years) the therapist discovers who are the major players in this internal drama, the patient's age and the event at which they first appeared. It may be somewhat like taking a social case history, but with different "people." An assay of the attitudes of the respective alters is done, which ones can be counted on for constructive help and which may be destructive. Other data desired includes: The likes and dislike of each, how each regards itself, the main personality and the other alters—and who is aware of whom. Patterns of likes and hostilities are determined. Gradually the social structure of the condition is determined.

Simultaneously the alters are each "sizing-up" the therapist and building attitudes of like, dislike, trust, suspicion, hostility, willingness to cooperate—and even affection. All of this is not really treatment but a pre-requisite to serious therapeutic work. It is in this stage where the therapist may establish the relationships which will move toward success—or ruin his chances of helping the patient, perhaps permanently.

"Iatrogenic" Alters

The phenomenon of multiplicity is always fascinating, but new therapists sometimes become so involved in "discovering" another alter and exploring it that this initial stage goes on interminably with the patient producing more and more minor personality segments as the therapist reinforces these productions with tremendous enthusiasms. ("Oh, so you're not Geraldine. You say you are Marcia. How great to meet you, Marcia. Tell me all about yourself.") One wonders if many of the cases which some therapists gleefully report are not partially iatrogenically created ("I had a patient with over 65 different personalities.") One should afford every opportunity for important ego states to emerge, but one does not reward simply for the production of every new one. It is our experience that a limited number of alters (or closely-bound clusters), perhaps 7 to 15, will account for most of the variance in the patient's behaviors. The resolution of the conflicts between them and an "integration" which results either in their independent dissolving, or their close communication and cooperation through highly permeable boundaries as they become normal, covert ego states, should be sufficient. It is not necessary to resolve every minor dissociation to achieve a functioning individual. All of us have repressions and dissociations—even the most "well-analyzed."

During the second stage "diagnostic evaluation" has, for the moment, become sufficient. The real therapy begins. The therapist will have a fairly-good map of the condition's structure and have formulated a general therapeutic strategy. He will have established the best communication and relationship possible with each of the alters (including the most hostile and destructive ones).

Every alter was established as a protective and survival measure. At heart, each wants to survive—even the most suicidal. One can appeal to the angry suicidal one as follows: "Marianne, you came to protect her back there when father was beating her. That was a fine thing to do, and you deserve a lot of credit for your courage. You also took all her hurt and anger then, and you shouldn't have to do this alone. I understand your hurt. Will you let me be your friend?"

In this second stage of the treatment the defensive structure is threatened by the therapist (in the eyes of the affected alters). Like a rickety old house which needs to be demolished and then rebuilt the multiplicity has served a purpose. However, its inhabitants will strongly resist change. The patient knows no other way of coping, and fears that giving up these dissociations will re-activate the brutality, pain and anger originally suffered. One can let "Mary" and "Meg" out of the basement hypnotically, but they may come charging upstairs wreaking their newly-released violence suicidally or homicidally. This is the most hazardous period of the treatment (Watkins and Watkins (1987). The therapist should be prepared for dangerous acting-out. Close relationships, constant communication and supportive gestures toward aggressive alters, sometimes periods of hospitalization as the patient releases the fear and bitterness. Alliances with constructive alters and encouraging their (sometimes life-saving) interventions may become the order of the day. The therapist may find himself in continuous crisis therapy, perhaps for several months.

In time, the dissociated affects are released. Bit by bit memories re-appear, and little new insights manifest themselves. The patient less frequently threatens suicide, violence toward others, or less often abuses her own children. The time for integrations approaches. We use the plural, "integrations," because it rarely happens that all the alters suddenly disappear into one great "ah-hah" experience. Rather, alters who have much in common begin sharing their thoughts, feelings and act in concert with one another. The therapist can encourage this under hypnosis ("Why don't you open the door to your room, Jean, so that you and your friend Dorothy are free to go back and forth to each other's room." Don't try suggestively to force them into a union for which they are not ready, e.g. "When I count up to five you will wake up. Jean and Dorothy will not be separate any more but will have fused into a single person." If they are too far apart a new split may take their place—or the patient will "split" from the therapist.

If personalities A and B are very much alike they should be integrated first. A patient of mine had two attorney alters. One did the research on legal cases; the other presented in court. After a while the need for such a separation no longer existed. They could be easily integrated.

With A and B integrated one might turn attention to C and F who have suffered from the same abuser or have much else in common— but not entirely different agendas for meeting that problem. If C and F don't spontaneously integrate the therapist can give a "gentle nudge" under hypnosis. Now we have an AB alter, a D alter and a CF alter. The patient is reducing the number of conflicting states, strengthening those which remain, building internal communication, cooperation, and developing whole-person responsibility for memories, affects and behaviors that emerge in the "body."

For the therapist the key therapeutic motivation should be "commitment," for the patient it is the increased willingness to take "responsibility for self." As each learns and practices these the patient slowly moves toward integration, mastery of his/her internal world, adaptation to the outer world and new-found mental health.

The stress on the therapist has been great, but it is rewarding to re-affirm one's therapeutic self and see the fragmented pieces of a dissociated human being come together to form an integrated, adapting person—who is usually very intelligent, talented, and a contributor to society.

Summary

Amnesias and multiple personalities represent pathological forms of dissociation. Hypnosis is a controlled dissociation which can be employed in both diagnosis and in therapy.

"Dissociated handwriting" is a procedure whereby the hand is removed from conscious control and by writing can reveal unconscious or pre-conscious material. A variation is "hallucinated dissociated handwriting." Instead of hand movements the subject sees a "dissociated hand" writing on a blackboard and reports what it says. "Automatic writing" is similar but is done without prior induction of hypnotic state.

Amnesias are susceptible to treatment by hypnosis, but when the symptom is removed simply by suggestion it may not remain eliminated permanently. When symptom removal of amnesia is accompanied or followed by hypnoanalytic resolution of underlying unconscious conflicts recovery without substitution of other undesirable sequelae is more likely.

Multiple personalities are difficult and time-consuming to treat, and are often accompanied by risks of suicide, homicide or other violent behavior toward the patient, the therapist and others. They require much clinical sensitivity and skill in working with them.

Alters are resistant at attempts to eliminate or "fuse" them. Accordingly, the integration can be more expeditiously done if the boundaries between them are made more permeable, and there is an exchange of communication and mutual awareness without their complete elimination. In this case the alters may continue to exist as covert entities within a normal personality structure, such as is found in the "hidden observer" or ego-state phenomena.

By reinforcing the appearance of each new alter the therapist may "iatrogenically" stimulate the patient to keep creating more minor dissociations.

Recovery depends greatly on the "commitment" of the therapist and the willingness of the patient to "take responsibility" for his own feelings and behaviors. Abreactions of dissociated rage are almost an essential in the treatment strategy.

Chapter 8. Dissociation

Outline

1. Dissociated handwriting.
    a. Hallucinated dissociated handwriting.
2. Amnesia and multiple personality as pathological dissociation.

3. Hypnosis as controlled dissociation.

4. Amnesia treated by hypnosis.
    a. Through suggestion.
    b. Hypnoanalytically.

5. Multiple personalities.
    a. Origins and pathology.
        (1) Etiology in child abuse.
        (2) The protection of dissociation.

b. Hazards in treatment.
c. Use of abreactions.
d. "Integration" vs."fusing."

Chapter 9

Hypnoanalytic Ego-state Therapy

Ego-state therapy is a sophisticated form of hypnoanalysis whose practice requires a new theoretical rationale in order to comprehend its operation. Originally stemming from psychoanalytic concepts proposed by Paul Federn (1952) and elaborated by Edoardo Weiss (1960) the theory has been modified and further developed by me and my wife, Helen, who has contributed many of the specialized treatment techniques. (Watkins, J.G., 1978; Watkins, J.G. & Watkins, H.H., 1979, 1981, 1982, 1986). In this endeavor we have drawn both from our experience with multiple personalities (1984, 1988, see also Watkins & Johnson, 1982) and our experiments with normal, hypnotized volunteers (Watkins and Watkins, 1979-80, 1980).

Subject-Object

My arms is me. My leg is me. My thought is me—or is it if I am hallucinating? Subject-object, what is within my "self", and what is not, is a most significant area of human experience. It has been largely neglected in behavioral and experimental psychology, but is often addressed by psychoanalytic theorists (Greenberg & Mitchell, 1983).

Perceptions refer to mental images and sensations which are normally elicited by objects outside the body. However, a stone in the stomach, and an infection in the blood stream are also "objects." An arm is normally considered as "subject." But if it is paralyzed and devoid of feeling and movement then it, too, is an object. An idea is normally subject, ("my" thought). But an hallucination is an idea which is perceived as coming from the outside, hence, not part of "the me." It is therefore an "object."

Accordingly, the body cannot be the criterion for distinguishing between object and subject. The entity which does so discriminate is "the self." That which is *perceived* as outside "my self," whether it is within the body or not, is "object." That which is *experienced* as within "my self," hence, part of "the me" is subject. The "self" and not the body is the distinguishing agent, and the difference is judged by our *feeling of selfness* when becoming aware of it.

The Self

Just what constitutes "self" has been the subject of many theories and scientific controversies. Freud (1933) postulated a state of "primary narcissism," an inherent condition in the original child. Later, he viewed the ego as a structure within the mind which was equated with the self. Hartmann (1958) regarded the ego, hence the self, as not only an inherent structure, but partly determined by the impact of the real world on the developing infant. Other object-relation analysts, such as Winnicott (1965) held that the self and its feeling of self-existence came about as the mother, who acts like a mirror, reflects back to the child his own experience and gestures. The child then believes that, "When I look, I am seen, so I exist." When the mother resonates to the child's needs the latter becomes aware of them. This awareness then slowly evolves into a sense of self. The concept of "resonance" is discussed in considerable detail elsewhere (Watkins, 1978, Chap. 15). Mahler (1972) emphasized the maternal role in developing the child's self through a "separation-individuation" process by which he comes to know himself. As he interacts with the mother he separates himself to develop a unique identity and sense of selfness.

Jacobson (1954) wrestled with the conflict as to whether the self is to be equated with the ego or whether it is an image or mental content within the ego. She apparently did not arrive at a conclusion. Hartmann considered the "self" as a "representation," an experiential construct similar to an "object representation." Another theorist (Kernberg, 1976), building on Hartmann's formulations, reserved the term self to "the sum-total of self-representations." By this he apparently meant that certain experiences, feelings and images which were endowed with self feeling interacted with other images and sensations that were felt as "not-me, but were also "represented" within the mind. This interaction was clearly embedded within the ego and constituted the self.

I proposed a similar view (Watkins, 1978, Chap. 6) that "existence," occurred only when an object, "a not-me," impacted a subject, "a me." This was in line with Fairbairn's formulation (See Guntrip, 1961) that ego and object are inseparable. An object is not significant (e.g. does not exist to its perceiver) unless it has a bit of the ego in contact with it.

The original, classical theory developed by Freud posited that the individual was born with innate "drives," sexual and aggressive, and that it was in the satisfaction or frustration of these that personality structure and neurotic conflicts developed. Drive model analysts operate from this basic assumption. The theorists just quoted: Hartman, Mahler, Kernberg, Jacobson, Winnicott and Fairbairn are considered members of the "relational" model school, who have increasingly emphasized the role of inter-personal relationships in shaping human development.

Kohut (1971, 1977) is one of this group who has departed most from "drive theory." In his *Psychology of the Self* (1977) Kohut assigned the classical functions of ego, super-ego and id to the self. He held that this entity was developed by the infant's internalization of "selfobjects," meaning the significant people in his world, usually his parents. Though their empathic responses to his needs they provided the experiences necessary for the development of his "self". This is an extension of Mahler's concepts, but unlike her Kohut broke more definitely with the drive theory, since he perceived the self as almost entirely a product of interpersonal relations. The self expresses a need for contact with others, not sexual or aggressive drives, as its basic motivation.

The object-relation theorists, because of loyalty to Freud, the founder of psychoanalysis, and because of their wish to be identified within the body of classical psychoanalysis, kept trying to reconcile their new concepts (derived from clinical experience) with classical drive theory (Greenberg and Mitchell, 1983). They all were inhibited to some degree in proposing concepts of personality development which departed too widely from accepted theory. Innovative psychological theories which deviated too radically from Freud's, such as

Adler's (1948), Jung's (1916) and Rank's (1952) had resulted in the past with their author's being "drummed out of the corps." Kohut's views, the most progressive of these object relation theorists has moved closer than any of the others to the earlier views of Paul Federn, a close associate of Freud and one of his most loyal friends.

The Ego Psychology of Paul Federn

Federn was one of the first to join Freud's group and developed innovative techniques for treating psychoses. As early as 1927 he proposed many concepts advocated later by object relation theorists. However, his work was relatively unknown and almost completely ignored in the current controversies between drive model and relational model theorists. One gains the impression that they have never read Federn, and it remained to Edoardo Weiss (who was analyzed by Federn and trained by Freud) to publish an English compilation of his papers.

This relative ignorance of Federn's contributions probably stem from two problems. Federn wrote primarily in difficult and long-winded German sentences. Weiss (who was this writer's analyst) once said to me, "Federn is very difficult to understand. That is why I had to write an introduction to his book to explain him." (See Federn, 1952.) At that time in my analysis with Weiss I had not yet acquired the courage to say, "But Dr. Weiss, your writings are also hard to understand."

The second reason for the apparent ignorance of Federn's views in psychoanalytic circles is probably because he proposed concepts which 20 years later object relation theorists were mentioning with the greatest of caution so as not to attack the drive model theory of Freud and become alienated from acceptance within the psychoanalytic movement.

A third reason may have been that Federn used a somewhat different terminology to refer to psychoanalytic structures and processes than were currently in vogue. In fact, Federn himself was not fully aware of the extent to which his view departed from Freud's. At any rate his theories have not been widely read and understood. They do provide a foundation for "Ego-State Therapy," a form of hypnoanalysis which I and my wife, Helen H. Watkins, have been developing (Watkins, J.G., 1978; Watkins, J.G. & Watkins, H.H, 1979, 1981, 1982, 1986).

Ego-state Theory

Freud, it will be recalled, based much of his theory on the displacements of a single energy, libido, which originated in the id. Fairbairn (see Guntrip 1961) suggested "the attribution to the ego of its own energy rather than energy siphoned off from the id." Hartmann (1955) alluded to a "primary ego energy," not derived from instinctual (libidinal) energy, but he did not pursue this idea further. Freud, himself, (1953c) felt the need to hypothesize two variants of libido: "narcissistic libido," and "object libido." Yet this still represents primarily two different allocations of the same basic energy, not two different "kinds" of energy. Jacobsen (1964) suggested an initial state of undifferentiated energy, which acquires libidinal or aggressive qualities. Kohut (1971), while attempting to remain loyal to Freud's drive theory, proposed that libidinal energy could be divided into two separate and independent "realms,"narcissistic libido and object libido.

All of these psychoanalytic object-relations theorists apparently felt that Freud's single energy theory (libido) was not adequate to account for the phenomena which they observed in their patients. Their tortured writings show many efforts to force these phenomena into a single energy (libido) mold. Yet Federn much earlier, 1927, had broken with that position and clearly formulated a two-energy theory which resolves many of the conflicts in understanding psychodynamic processes and provides a rationale for therapeutic interventions (See Federn 1952a). It also provides a rationale for hypnotherapy and hypnoanalysis, a consequence not envisioned by either Federn or Weiss.

Ego and Object Cathexis

Federn hypothesized two different energies, one which he initially called "narcissistic or ego libido," the other, "object libido". Later, he more frequently called them "ego cathexis" and "object cathexis". He apparently used the term "libido" out of loyalty to Freud and to gain more acceptance from libido theory advocates. However, the term "libido" as formulated by Freud meant an instinctual "sexual" energy emanating from the Id. It was also an "object" energy, since it could be displaced to various objects (such as a patient's mother) who then became an object of erotic interest. The term "libido" was further extended by Jung (1966) who regarded it as a life energy. To avoid confusion let us follow Federn's (and Weiss's) later terminology and speak only of "ego and object cathexes."

"Cathexis" can be defined as the investment of a quantum of energy to activate a process. A motor is "cathected" with electricity and then runs. Ego cathexis is the energy which "cathects" or activates the ego. It is the energy of the self. In fact, it *is* the self. Self is an energy, an organic, life energy, not a compilation of feelings, thoughts, behaviors, etc. Ego cathexis has one basic quality, the *feeling of selfness*. If an arm is invested or cathected with this ego energy, then I experience it as "my" arm. If a thought is invested or activated with ego cathexis then I experience it as "my" thought. It has become part of "the me," and I regard it as within "my self." By calling it "ego cathexis" and not "ego libido" we no longer confuse it with an instinctual, sexual and object energy.

Federn's second energy was "object cathexis." It is qualitatively very different, being a non-organic energy, much like electricity, radiation, etc. It also has one basic quality. Being an energy it, like ego cathexis, can activate or make a process go, but any process (or body part) so cathected is not experienced as "me." It is sensed or perceived as an object, hence, outside "my" self.

In his earlier formulations Kohut (1971), apparently unfamiliar with Federn's contributions, "introduced his theoretical and technical innovations within the framework of classical drive theory by positing a division of libidinal energy into two separate and independent *realms: narcissistic libido and object libido." (See Greenberg and Mitchell,* 1983, pp. 357-358.)

However, Kohut and other object relations theorists did not seem prepared then to challenge Freud's drive theory to the point of eliminating the concept of a single "kind" of cathexis, called "libido." Instead, he modified this concept of the *manner* of cathecting by a single energy which determined whether a representation became a "true object" or a "self object."

Federn's concept of two different *kinds* of energy directly challenges Freud's basic views regarding a single, unitary "libido." As such, it has been ignored by current-day psychoanalysts and was dismissed by Kohut (1978) in a single footnote (Vol.1, p.429) as "hard to integrate with the established body of psychoanalytic theory."

Neither ego cathexis nor object cathexis are to be equated with consciousness. If my arm has been hypnotically anesthetized, paralyzed, and removed from my self control its ego cathexis has been removed. The arm is now experienced by me as "an it," an external object and outside of "my" self. If the paralysis is hypnotically removed, and the "feeling of selfness" restored, that is because we have invested it again with ego cathexis. From this perspective *hypnosis is a modality for directing the various displacements of ego and object cathexes.*

Existence is impact between object and subject, so consciousness in ego-state theory is an economic matter. When the impact of an object-cathected element on an ego-cathected boundary exceeds a certain magnitude we become aware, hence, conscious of it. This depends both on how highly cathected the object is and how highly cathected the ego boundary is. We can become aware of strongly cathected (energized) objects even if the ego boundary is lightly cathected. And the impact of a low-energized object may become conscious if the receiving ego boundary is highly cathected. If you stroke my hand lightly I may not feel anything. If you slap it strongly I become quite aware of the touch. And the analyst with a highly tuned listening, ego boundary, hence, a sensitive third ear (Reik, 1948), may become quite aware of an unconscious and symbolic communication from his patient which the more obtuse practitioner will completely miss.

Introjection and identification depend on the allocation of object or ego cathexes. When I introject an outside person, perhaps my father, I have erected a mental image, a replica or representation of my father based on my perceptions of him. This "introject" is an object because at this time it is invested with object cathexis. If my father was a critical person at the time that I introjected him I will feel (perhaps unconsciously) the lash of his criticism within, which I may simply experience as depression. It, a "not-me," is critically and harmfully impacting "the me."

An old American political slogan is that "if you can't lick 'em, join 'em." Psychodynamically we call it "identification with the aggressor." Accordingly, to escape from the internal criticism which I am experiencing as depression, I may "identify" with my father. That means I remove the object energy from this representation and invest it instead with ego cathexis. I infuse the representation with the feeling of selfness. The introject is no longer a "not-me" object but instead has become a part of "the me." I experience it as being within my self. I am no longer depressed by my father's introjected criticism; but I am now critical of my own children. The content of the "introject" has not been changed. It has now become an "indentofact," a part of "my" self. I have become like my father, and the neighbors say, "He's a chip off the old block." According to object relations terminology we might note that what had been an "object representation" has now become a "self representation." Yet this same maneuver is possible with hypnotic intervention since through hypnotic suggestion ego and object energies can be manipulated (See the subject-object techniques described in Vol. 1, pp. 156-159).

Federn did not theorize as much on the development of the self as on its composition and structure. For example, some object-relation theorists use the term "self-object" to mean an undifferentiated representation in the psychotic or in the infant who has not learned to distinguish between self and object (Blanck and Blanck, 1974: Kernberg, 19872).

Kohut (1971,1977) appears to define the term like what earlier psychoanalysts called "introjects" of significant others which at first are objects but later may be changed into identifications. He held that such entities are necessary even in adults.

According to Federn's Ego Psychology the term "self-object" is contradictory. A representation of a significant other constructed within the individiual will either be activated by object cathexis (like an introject) or energized by ego cathexis (like an identification). Granted that the child's "merger" with such "self-objects" may be gradual, a "representation" cannot be both "self" and "object" at the same time since this is determined by the quality (the nature) of the activating energy. It cannot be experienced as "me" and as "not me" simultaneously.

The Development of Personality

Personality develops through two basic processes: Differentiation and integration. Put more simply we grow by separating psychological items and by putting them together. The child learns that cats are different from rabbits, hence, he "differentiates" them from each other. He also learns that they are both called animals, hence he "integrates" them. Through integration and differentiation he develops an increasingly complex personality structure. When the separating (differentiation) becomes excessive and maladaptive we call it "dissociation" as exemplified in multiple personalities.

Complex configurations of psychological elements may be integrated into a single pattern which is then differentiated from other such configurations within the individual. We call these patterns "ego states" (Watkins, 1978).

Ego States

The second major contribution of Federn was his conception of "ego states." He held that perceptions and images which are ego-cathected are organized into internal patterns of self behavior and experience. Ego cathexis is the unifying energy which binds these items together. These configurations are enclosed within ego boundaries. When one of them is activated, the individual then behaves and experiences according to the contents of that "ego state." Ego states can be created through identification with significant figures in one's life. For example, if I introject my mother an object representation of her will be formed around my perceptions of her. That object representation may be changed into an identification through its investment with ego cathexis, then a mother ego-state will have been created within me. When that ego state is activated I will experience and behave toward the world like my mother—or at least as I had perceived she would. The mother ego state then becomes "executive", hence, "the self in the now".

Federn considered only elements that were ego-cathected as belonging in an ego state. However, since experience consist of both ego representations and object representations interacting within a cohering pattern we have defined ego states more broadly. *An ego state is an organized system of behaviors and experiences whose elements are bound together by some common principle and separated from other such entities by a boundary which is more or less permeable.* One ego state might be organized around being six years old. When hypnotically activated and regressed to six the subject behaves like a six year old. Another ego state might be organized around the concept of reaction to authority figures. It becomes executive when dealing with teachers, bosses, etc. It contains within it those ego and object cathected elements which are relevant to dealing with authority figures.

Ego states may be large, encompassing broad areas of behavior and experience. Or they may be small including very specific and limited reactions. They may overlap. For example, a six-year old child ego state and a "reaction to father" ego state both speak the English language. They can range from minor moods to true overt multiple personalities, the difference being the permeability of their separating boundaries.

Ego-State Boundaries

Most psychological processes exist on a continuum. We do not experience either anxiety or no-anxiety, depression or no-depression. There are many degrees of each. So it is with the separating process which divides ego states from one another. Near one end of the continuum the boundaries are so permeable that they are almost non-existent. The individual's behavior is very much the same from time to time. The difference that does occur is generally adaptive, and we call it normal differentiation. As the ego state boundaries become increasingly rigid and permeable. intra-personal communication is impeded so that behavior becomes less adaptive. When we approach the end of the continuum the boundaries are very rigid and impermeable, the behavior is maladaptive, and we call it "dissociation". At this extreme end of the continuum the various ego states no longer interact with one another or communicate with one another, and the individual suffers from a true multiple personality if more than one becomes energized enough to temporarily assume the executive position..

In between these extremes lies a body of ego states which may act like "covert" multiple personalities, but which do not spontaneously become overt. However, they can be activated hypnotically. (See Figure 9:1.) Hilgard (1986) tapped this area of personality organization when he discovered the "hidden observer" phenomena.

The Hidden Observer Phenomena

While demonstrating hypnotic deafness before a class of students Hilgard was asked by a student as to whether some part of the apparently deaf subject might be aware of what was going on. Hilgard then said to the subject, "Although you are hypnotically deaf, perhaps there is some part of you that is hearing my voice and processing the information. If there is I should like the index finger to rise as a sign that this is the case." To his surprise the finger lifted. Later, he discovered that individuals similarly reported being aware of pain in a hypnotically anesthetized hand. Hilgard ascribed this phenomenon to a cognitive structural system which he called "the hidden observer."

We (Watkins and Watkins, 1979-80, 1980) have replicated Hilgard's techniques using volunteer subjects from introductory psychology classes and former ego-state therapy patients. We found that when "hidden observers" were activated (both with auditory deafness

Ego States

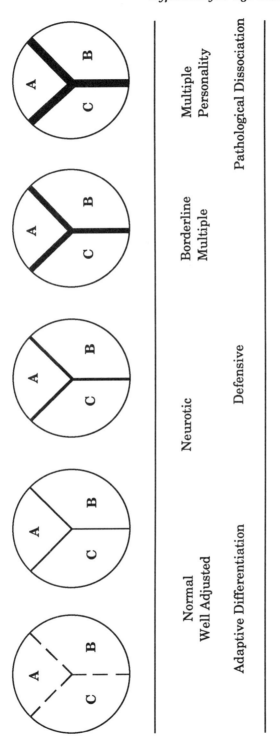

Normal Well Adjusted		Neurotic		Borderline Multiple		Multiple Personality
Adaptive Differentiation		Defensive				Pathological Dissociation

Differentiation-Dissociation Continuum

Figure 9:1

and with pain analgesia), and then interviewed, they proved to be the same covert ego states with which we had been working therapeutically. Apparently hidden observers and other partially-separated personality segments exist as ego states within the middle of the range on the differentiation-dissociation continuum.

The Characteristics of Ego states

Ego states should be regarded as part-persons. Except in the case of a true multiple personality they do not normally appear overtly unless hypnotically activated. There is too much evidence to the contrary to impute them simply to therapist-created artifacts since they often differ widely from therapist expectations. Some act like rather complete "persons." Others appear to be very limited personality fragments, perhaps created for a specific purpose. They may have quite differing interests, purposes and values, even as do the various alters in a true multiple personality. Accordingly, it is not surprising to find them often in intra-personal conflict with one another, creating tension, anxiety, psychosomatic symptoms and maladaptive behaviors. As one ego state put it, "I make her eat because if she is overweight men (who are dangerous) will not be attracted to her." Covert ego-state conflicts may create headaches, just like the quarreling of multiple personality alters who struggle to emerge and take over executive control of the body.

The Origin of Ego States

We hypothesize three most likely origins of these "part-persons."

1. Normal adaptive differentiation. Even as a society divides into individuals who farm, teach, market, etc., so also may an individual separate and assign to various personality segments different responsibilities in adapting to the world. If external pressures require more drastic defensive operations the "normal " ego state (such as a temporary imaginary playmate in a lonely child) may develop more rigid boundaries. Under the impact of severe traumas it may become an alter in a true multiple personality—a situation which occurs infrequently. It has then moved along the differentiation-dissociation continuum from adaptation through maladaptation to pathology.

2. Splits may be caused by traumas, which result in ego states that can play a good boy or good girl role toward punitive parents in order to placate them and avoid further punishment. They may be created from a need to dissociate the body when being molested, perhaps to avoid pain or to disavow guilt.

3. The introjection of significant individuals (and experiences). Ego states can be built around an introjected parent, thus creating an internal "mother" or "father" representation—or both. The *drama* regarding them can also be introjected. If they were perceived by the child as in conflict with one another the two introjects may continue the battle intra-psychically. The individual (perhaps now an adult) may report headaches concerning whose origin he is ignorant. Parent ego states are basically child ones since they represent the child's *perception* of his parents when they were first introjected.

Federn considered an ego state as only a self representation, hence ego-cathected. However, we prefer to use the term to represent the body and content of the entity. When the state is invested with ego-cathexis then it is "me" to the individual who behaves and experiences according to its content as part of his own self. When it is object-cathected then the individual experiences it as an "it," outside the "me" and interacts with it in pleasant or painful ways. The sensory, experiential and behavioral contents of the entity remain the same, only its experience of selfness has been altered.

This changing of a state from an ego representation to an object representation and vice versa by the infusion of the other form of energy (ego or object cathexis) happens all the time during the operation of normal introjecting and identifying processes. It occurs spontaneously in multiple personalities as the various alters take turns being executive. And these alterations can often be therapist directed through relationship, especially with hypnosis.

Ego-State Therapy

Ego-state therapy is the use of group and family therapy techniques to resolve conflicts between the various ego states which constitute a "family of self" within a single individual. It may employ any of the directive, behavioral, cognitive, psychoanalytic or humanistic procedures, but these are directed toward the "part-persons" represented by "ego states" and not toward the whole individual. While it is possible to practice ego-state therapy in the conscious condition, dealing with them under hypnosis is generally preferable. This is because ego states, unlike true, multiple personality alters, do not usually become overt spontaneously. They require hypnotic activation most of the time. Since this text is about hypnotic therapy we will not describe non-hypnotic techniques for activating ego states. Helen Watkins, however, has developed a "chair technique" for activating ego states in subjects who may not be very hypnotizable, (see Watkins, J.G. and Watkins, H.H., 1981, pp. 257-260; 1982, pp. 144).

Ego-state therapy is a form of internal diplomacy. It has been found useful in treating a wide variety of behavioral and psychosomatic disorders, ranging from study habits, stop smoking, anxieties, phobias, conversion reactions, and multiple personalities. The important element is that the problem involves conflicts between ego states, often at the covert, and hence at the unconscious level.

Transactional Analysis

Transactional Analysis is a variant of ego-state therapy proposed by Berne (1961). However, the "Ego-State Therapy" which we are describing here differs significantly from it, although both stemmed from the contributions of Federn. In T.A. three basic ego states are hypothesized: Adult, Parent and Child. Conflicts are presumed as resulting from dissonance between these three. In our ego-state therapy we do not suggest any specific number of states but rely on the patient to inform us what states he has. Ego-state therapy has no preconceived number or content. They may be 3, 4, 5 or any number, and they may not be conveniently identified as simply "adult," "parent" and "child." Ego-state therapy differs from transactional analysis also in that the treatment is primarily done under hypnosis, which apparently is not used in T.A.

Ego-state therapy as a treatment modality may be compared to multivariant analysis in the field of research. In research we isolate a number of independent variables and ascertain the effect each has on the dependent variable—and their interaction with one another. In ego-state therapy we isolate various personality segments to determine what effect each has on the total behavior and personality of the patient—and how these various ego states interact with one another.

Therapists usually proceed on the assumption that "the patient" they interview at one session is the same one who appears at a later one, or that the same patient is present throughout the entire therapeutic hour. Experimentalists make a similar assumption in their testing of "subjects."

I once suggested to an experimental colleague that many if not most "research subjects" could have different "ego states" within them, which are factors that are never controlled. And I asked, "What would be the research situation if ego-state A of a subject took the base measurement. Ego-state B showed up for the application of the experimental procedure, and the terminal evaluation was adminis- tered to ego-state C." In shock he replied, "My God! You have just invalidated 90% of all psychological research." If the subjects were recognized as true multiple personalities this error would not be permitted. Yet in the case of "covert" ego states, which often exist within subjects, this factor is never considered or evaluated.

The activation of ego states during treatment is usually accom- plished by inquiring of the hypnotized patient whether, "There is a part of John who knows about the cause of his headaches." etc. The inquiry may be combined with Cheek's finger signal technique (see Vol. 1, p. 216). For example, the previous question might be followed with, "If so, lift the index finger of the right hand." Or, "if there is such a part please come out and say 'I'm here'."

We never suggest a name, nor do we press for "a part." While we may ask if any "part" knows something different about the patient, or is responsible for some symptom or behavior, we always say that, "If there is no such part, that is O.K., too." It is wise to be very non- directive to avoid suggesting artifacts. One wants to activate what is there, not create something which was not there.

Hypnosis in Ego-State Therapy

Hypnosis is of value because the hypnotic modality is a focusing procedure. It enables us to ablate temporarily other segments of the personality and concentrate on one ego state. However, it should not be used suggestively to create entities with specific boundaries and contents. The therapist, while establishing conditions which permit or encourage states already present to become manifest, should be very careful that these are not formed at the time by the patient merely to please the therapist.

As in the treatment of multiple personalities each ego state is interviewed (and perhaps psychologically tested) to determine where and when was its origin, what is its role, and what are its goals. A strategy of constructive suggestions, exchange of communications and reconciliation between the various ego states is then formulated.

Sometimes an ego state may be exerting an influence as "object" on the primary individual. In which case we might say, "I would like to talk to that part (we don't use the term 'ego state' with patients) of Mary Anne who has been compelling her to over-eat," (or who knows about her over-eating.) A communication back from such a "part" commonly results. The content of this "part" is often at considerable variance with the therapist's expectations, contra-indicating the notion that these ego states are only artifacts created to please the therapist.

Ego states, being only "part-persons" often think concretely like a child and must be communicated with accordingly. Sometimes ego states appear during sleep or under hypnosis like dream figures. The same general strategies and tactics used in treating multiples (see Chapter 8) apply when working with the more covert ego states, except that they must usually be preceded by a hypnotic induction.

Ego-State Therapy as an Internal Family or Group Therapy

Ego state therapy sessions typically resemble family therapy in that one member speaks, another is asked to respond, and an exchange of communications begins. Sometimes it is necessary to call on specific states to come out and speak. At other times they will emerge spontaneously. Or one will abdicate if pressed too hard, and another will appear. The important point is that the therapist think of talking to a multiplicity and not a unity, even though a single body is in view. What one says to one ego state may well be heard by others who can take offense and oppose one's treatment efforts.

The clinician operates like a group therapist. Any therapeutic maneuver, such as suggestion, ventilation, desensitization, abreaction, free association, interpretation, reinforcement, clarification, etc., which is a part of one's therapeutic armamentarium, may be employed. And these can be utilized within the basic theoretical orientation of the clinician. However, they are applied under hypnosis and to the various personality segments rather than to the entire patient.

Sometimes the awareness of what has been has done with an ego state may be brought to the attention of the conscious person. At other times efforts will be made to strengthen some of the more constructive ego states. Occasionally an ego state can be found which may serve as an auxiliary therapist, consulting with the clinician about strategy, advising of the effects of earlier maneuvers and helping in planning future steps. We have taught ego states, who at first were destructive, to become behavior modifiers after constructive relationships had been established with them. (See Watkins, H.H. in Watkins, J.G. 1978, Chap. 22). In one case Dark One, previously "the Evil One," provided systematic desensitization to a child state in helping to eliminate its phobia of being in an oxygen tent.

We try at all times to discover and meet the needs of each ego state. Where they are conflicting, modification, negotiation and compromise are indicated. The therapist's role is frequently that of communicator and mediator between clashing states. For example, "George," (a teenager ego state) was asked, "would you be willing to do your home work during the week if "Father" (a parental ego state) doesn't bug you about playing on week ends?"

It should be remembered that ego states, like multiple personality alters, originated for defensive or adaptive purposes. It is therefore unwise to eliminate "bad" ones. Rather, one can avoid much resistance if he treats all ego states with the utmost courtesy and respect, secures their cooperation, tries to meet their needs, and plays the role of a good friend to each. Attempts to eliminate a state mobilize much resistance which can sabotage the treatment.

Perhaps the role of the therapist in reconciling ego-state conflicts can be described by presenting segments from a significant treatment session.

The Case Of Mikale[1]
Therapist: Helen H. Watkins

This individual, who had suffered for 1 1/2 years with depression and insomnia, was referred to me (HHW) after she reported hearing "voices in her head." She also suffered from allergies and specifically a recurring rash on her thighs and buttocks. Her mother apparently was a very strict and controlling individual. Mikale reported being molested by a man in the basement, but when she told her mother, she was not believed. During the first session three ego states were located: a mother figure, a hurt child, and a "Silent Center" who listens as the above two argue.

In Session II she described her rash, and on being hypnotically regressed to the basement scene she cried, "He is touching me there, and it hurts," referring to her buttocks.

By Session III the rash was gone; however, she now discussed her fear of the wind. At the age of 3 her mother during a storm had locked her out of the house for misbehavior. She was rescued by the return of her father. Following the re-living and abreaction of this incident she was given suggestions that she would never be afraid of the wind again—and also that she was not bad.

In Session IV the "Mother " ego state emerged and revealed that she had started the allergies as a punishment for Mikale. "Mother" agreed to work on getting rid of the allergies. The next week a most important session resulted in a compromise between the three major ego states, and subsequently a considerable improvement in the symptoms. The following recorded excerpt from that session illustrates interactions typical of ego-state therapy.

"Compromise With Mother, Mike and Misha"

Session V
(Hypnotic induction ends.)

Therapist-Patient Interaction	Therapist Reactions and Theoretical Notes
T. And now I would like to talk to just part of you, and the part that I'd like to talk to again is the part that I talked to the last time. I'd like to talk to Mother, and when Mother is there just say, "I'm here."—You don't want to talk to me?	*Shakes head.*
Pt. I'm here. No, that was Mike or Misha or whoever she is. She wanted to talk but...	*Mother ego state has the voice of a child pretending to be her mother.*
T. Oh, She wanted to talk, the Little One?	
Pt. Yes.	
T. Ok. Maybe I'll talk to her later. I'm glad you told me. Tell me what happened. You told me you were going to work on her allergies, and apparently for several days it was much better, and then she spent some time with her mother and then all of a sudden the	*Need internal information.*

allergies became worse. Tell me, how you perceive this.

Pt.   Well, I did go home, and I did the thinking like I told you I would.

T.   Umhum.

Pt.   And I decided maybe you were right. I was being a little overly harsh in my punishment. Umm...and so I started, and it seemed to work. She was feeling better, and she was sleeping better, but when we got there it was like I just lost control, kind of. Strange...

Softening of mother ego state.

T.   It isn't like you to lose control, is it?

Pt.   No. It was like the real mother had more control over what was going on than I did, and she just kind of took over, and I tried to stop it, and I managed to keep it at a semi-flat level until Saturday, but I couldn't fight anymore.

T.   And you don't know why, is that it?

Pt.   I don't understand why. I don't understand how she on the outside could have more effect than I do on the inside. It just don't make any sense, but it wasn't me doing it. I was trying not to do it.

I don't understand that either, so let's find out.

T.   Umhum. Well, maybe we could find out from other parts in there what's going on, and maybe they had something to do with it. I don't know. Do you think that'd be alright if I try to find out for you?

Getting Mother's permission is an expression of respect. Important therapist attitude.

Pt.   Yes. I don't understand this, and I'd like to know.

T. Well, why don't you stay where you are. You can stay in the room, and I'm just going to call on someone else, but you can listen in. OK?

Want open communication

Pt. OK.

T. Alright. The part that I'd like to talk to is Little Misha, and when she's there just say, I'm here.

Since Misha is anxious to speak, I call on her first.

Pt. I'm here. I'm here.

T. Oh, you're happy to be here.

Pt. You should go faster down those stairs though, because I wanted to run down the last part...it's like (pants)

The concrete thinking of an energetic child.

T. I didn't realize you were there.

Pt. Well, I was.

T. OK.

Pt. I took 'em slow but I didn't want to.

Descending stairs: Hypnotic deepening technique used.

T. OK. Well, next time I'll pay attention to you. OK?

Pt. OK.

T. Alright. Do you know anything about these allergies, Misha?

Pt. Well, you said something that was really interesting earlier. You said guilt and that fits.

Misha not only plays; she thinks and ponders.

T. Oh, it does?

Pt.   Yeah, because Mommy always told me I was a bad girl and I should feel guilty and I would, but I didn't like it.

T.   I see. That doesn't feel good, does it?

Pt.   No. It made my tummy hurt.

At age 7 recalls taking ulcer medication.

T.   Oh, sure.

Pt.   They also fit last night. We also had this naughty dream last night. Well, it wasn't real naughty because nothing happened, but, it fit. It's really strange.

T.   Tell be about it.

Pt.   The dream?

T.   Yes. Whatever you want to tell me about it.

Pt.   Well, it's real strange because, because the big person, the one on the outside, well, she's been having problems with her sex life because something's been holding her back, and she had this dream last night, and she kept kissing her fiance, and it felt so good, but they kept stopping because she was like afraid to push too far and that's why because she feels so guilty. She's not supposed to feel like that because Mom doesn't like her to feel like that.

Child state regards main personality as "the big person."

T.   Oh.

Pt.   It's not right to have those type of feelings.

T.   Oh, she shouldn't feel sexual. Is that the idea?

Pt.   Yeah. Because they're naughty feel-
       ings.

T.   Oh, I see.

Pt.   And she even calls them naughty feel-
       ings, kind of, but I think it's because
       she feels guilty.

T.   That's very good thought on your part.   *Sincere compliment to*
                                                 child state helps her
Pt.   I don't know where it came from, but it   *self-esteem.*
       fits; but don't tell Hardnose over there.

T.   Who, Mother?

Pt.   Yeah. She's grumpy. She'll tell me I'm
       wrong. She always does.

T.   Well, I think that sounds like a very...

Pt.   I like the feeling like that.

T.   Well, sure that's normal and natural.

Pt.   But I'm not supposed to...but I think
       that's how come, we can't, because we
       feel guilty.

T.   You know what, maybe it's ok now.   *Purpose: to alleviate*
       Maybe it's ok now to feel that way. You   *guilt in child state.*
       know you're kind of growing up your-
       self. You're having some fine ideas.
       And maybe your ideas are better than
       what Mother on the outside used to
       say. Because you're just acting nor-
       mally and naturally and healthy like.
       Maybe it's ok to feel those feelings and
       to let the grown up part feel those
       feelings. After all, those are just nor-
       mal feelings, and she's going to be

married pretty soon, and it's no good to have all those guilt feelings about sex when you're married. You're not free to be happy with your sexuality.

Pt.   Well, I try, but Hardnose always goes (yuck).

T.   Ohhh.

Pt.   That's Hardnose. I always wonder who did it. But it's Hardnose always.

T.   Oh, you're talking about Mother.

Pt.   Yeah. Whatever her name is. She doesn't have a name, she doesn't like names. She's above names. So I call her Hardnose.

T.   I see. You have a good time, don't you? Well, tell me what do you know about the allergies?

Pt.   Well, I don't know much about them. They itch.

T.   Well, you don't have anything to do with it, huh?

Pt.   Nope. I don't like them.

Misha is not the culprit.

T.   Mother inside would...

Pt.   They're kind of disgusting (interrupted)

T.   Yeah. She was trying to stop, and then all of a sudden she found out that the Mother on the outside had more influence than she did, and she was very surprised, and I thought, well, I'd talk to you and see if you know anything about it.

Pt.   It probably has to do with guilt, but I don't know I would tend to think it would have to go through Hardnose...I don't like guilt. I'm the one that makes us do things we end up feeling guilty for.

Child state blames Mother introject for guilt but accepts responsibility for the cause.

T.   You're the one that's fun, huh?

Pt.   Yeah.

T.   You like that.

Pt.   I feel pretty good too.

T.   That's nice.

Pt.   After you rescued me, I feel much better, or after Mike rescued me, I feel much better.

T.   Good. Now you're out of that basement. You don't have that rash anymore either, do you?

Pt.   We itch, but that's because we got sunburned.

T.   Oh, sunburned. That's a good reason to itch.

In hypnotic regression to age 4, I 'rescued' her from molesting stranger in basement. Then Mike volunteered to take her to a safe place. Present symptom: rash on buttocks and thighs where he grabbed her. Rash disappeared after abreaction.

Pt.   We're going over that too.

T.   Well, I'll let you go play and do whatever you want to do, have fun and...

Pt.   Those stairs.

T.   Oh, those stairs.

Pt.   I want to run down 'em.

T. Yes. I'll have to remember, but not everybody can run as fast as you can. That's
the only problem.

Pt. Ok. Ok.

T. Ok. Alright. Now you go where you need   *Dismissing an ego*
to go or want to go, and I'd like to talk to   *state.*
any part of the personality that knows
about the allergies and what happened
this weekend.

Pt. I think I did it.   *Another spontane-*
                                                    ously appears

T. Who are you?

Pt. I'm Mike.

T. Oh, you're Mike. Why did you do it?

Pt. Well, I don't know for sure. Misha was
having a good time, and she was trying to
avoid unpleasantness which is Misha's
purpose, I guess.

T. She's a child, and she wants to have fun.

Pt. Yeah. And Mother was doing things that
were, you know, this Mother.

T. The inside Mother or outside?   *Clarification*

Pt. Yeah, the inside Mother.   *The introjected*
                                                    Mother.
T. OK.

Pt. Was doing things that were contradictory to what normally happens. Like, you
know...She was fighting the outside
Mother, and I guess I got to feeling bad,
and I let them come back.

T.   The allergies? Oh, for what purpose? I'm kind of confused. (pause)

Pt.   It was so different, and I was afraid that if things changed they're gonna get worse. At least with them being the same, I know how to deal with that.   *Change is unpredictable and therefore scary.*

T.   I see. In other words, you could predict. You knew what to do.

Pt.   Yeah.

T.   I see. Sometimes you got to take a little risk. There is risk in change, isn't there? You don't know what's going to happen; you got a little scared, huh? Do I have it right, you're 19? Do I have that right? (Nods assent) Well, Mike, you did a nice job with the Little One, and I really appreciate that, but you notice how that change that you promoted and that you helped me with, that change was for the good, and Misha is much more predictable now, much more fun, much more willing to play but no more rash anymore. But that was a change, and you were part of that change.

Pt.   I'm afraid she's going to do something. Even now I'm afraid. I don't want her to do something that's going to hurt us.

T.   How can you get hurt?

Pt.   She may do something that somebody on the outside doesn't approve of.

T. So? Neither you nor her nor Mother inside need to be so concerned about what
other people think. What other people
approve of or what they don't approve of.
You realize that the main personality is
an adult. She's, I guess, what, 22 years
old? The main personality. Ok. Well, she's
going to get married. She can make decisions for herself. She doesn't have to do
what the outside Mother says anymore.

Pt. But Misha is so unpredictable and so
carefree now, and the other Mother is
acting really strange. Normally she's the
one who keeps Misha in line, but she's
not keeping Misha in line anymore.

*Result of last
session's softening
of introjected
mother.*

T. Wonderful.

Pt. But, but somebody's got to, don't they?

T. Do they? You know you have to have a
little trust in the main personality who's
now an adult. She can make judgments
for herself or what behavior is appropriate or not appropriate. I haven't seen
Misha do anything crazy, inappropriate,
wild, dangerous. She's just a delightful
kid. I think you need a little more faith.

Pt. Could be.

T. And she really doesn't need the allergy.
That main personality doesn't need that
allergy. I'll tell you that, and besides it
doesn't stop Misha anyway.

Pt. That's true.

T. I think you can let go and just trust the
process a little more. And, of course,

*Therapy can
change introjected*

Mother has been changing. She was a little confused. She tried so hard to get rid of those allergies, and all of a sudden she didn't know what happened. It got worse and she thought it was because of the outside Mother. She didn't understand why but now I think...I asked her to listen in so she could hear what was going on, so she could find out what was going on. And I appreciate your listening, and do you think maybe you could let go a little. Do you think you could let the process just happen and not worry so much? Just trust the main personality. Really.

Mother if not original, real Mother.

Pt.   I'll try.

T.   Ok. I would appreciate that. Now you go where you need to go, and you can certainly listen in. You don't have to go away. You can listen in, and I would like to talk to Mother again.

Continued open communication between Mike and Mother.

Pt.   Yes.

In a "motherly" voice.

T.   Did you hear what Mike had to say?

Pt.   It's interesting, very interesting.

T.   Umhumm.

Pt.   But why would she try to take over my position?

T.   Very interesting, isn't it?

Pt.   I don't understand it. Usually she's so noncommittal to anything. You know, she's like Silent Center. It's really strange. I kind of understand why she did it. I understand how she did it, but I don't understand the motivation, I guess.

T.   I think the motivation is, if I understand it correctly, that you have been kind of, as Misha calls it, hardnosed.

Pt.   She can be a little insightful, but she's probably closest to correct.

T.   And you have been controlling, you see, the little one, so then Mike has not been doing much as you call the silent cent - noncommittal. So, all of a sudden you changed, and the little one changed, and she got all confused as to what the rules were and what she was supposed to do, and then all of a sudden the allergy went away, and she didn't know what to do. And of course the allergies were based on guilt from starting at age 16 as you told me the last time. And so with the guilt there, in a sense, but not there, not a physical manifestation of that guilt, she just didn't know what to do.

Explain to Mother, to reinforce our colleague-type alliance.

Pt.   Yeah. I can kind of see that.

T.   She got kind of confused as to what the rules were. In other words, when you feel guilty you're supposed to have an allergy.

Pt.   And I wasn't creating the allergies.

T.   That's right.

Pt.   But the guilt was still there, so the allergies had to be there. So she let them in. That makes some sense.

T.   Ok. But now that she understands this, and I ask her (I'm sure you heard) to have a little bit more faith in you and the main personality, there's no reason for the allergy. In fact, there's no reason for the guilt. I mean, after all, the main personality is a grown woman, and she can do what she wants in term of decisions in her life and her wedding, and she doesn't have to feel guilt about what Mother says. That's from the times past when she was young, and she needs to get away from that. And as I told the main personality...I don't know if you heard me or not...did you hear me say she needs to accept the idea that the real Mother will not change?

Pt.   Yeah, I heard that.

T.   Alright. Now acceptance doesn't mean she has to like it, but she needs to face that, that she can't change the world or change Mother, and that's just the way it is. And I thought the behavior of the main personality in terms of dealing with Mother is really quite adult. What do you think?

Pt.   Yeah. I think...Yeah, she's starting to catch on.

T.   Yeah. She didn't have a tantrum or acting like a little kid, and I was wondering if you had anything to do with that?

Pt.   Well, it's really strange. It's like Misha and I both kinda met in the middle instead of arguing.   *Cooperation!*

T.   Oh, I see.

Pt.   And so we kind of decided on a line of   *Less separation of*
      action that was neither of us but a com-   *boundaries.*
      bination of the two.

T.   That sounds great. I see, and that's why
      the Silent Center, as you called it before,
      and she calls herself Mike, didn't have a
      function, didn't know what to do.

Pt.   Well, Misha, I guess, Misha and I aren't
      used to dealing with her because she's
      like you said, the Silent Center and so
      we're used to fighting, and now we're
      cooperating. You're right. She doesn't
      have much of a function.

T.   But maybe she needs a function.   *"She" = Mike*
                                                  All ego states want
Pt.   That's what I was thinking, but I don't   *a purpose.*
      know what kind of a function, you know.

T.   Well, what kind of a function do you
      think she had before?

Pt.   Well, she would take...well when Misha
      and I fighting all the time, we would fight
      and whoever was the strongest, that was
      the decision made, and she would kind of
      implement it.

T.   Oh, I see. She would just do it for you.

Pt.   Yes.

T.   Seems to me she had to do a lot of hard   *Confrontation.*
      work, and you two didn't take much re-
      sponsibility for the behavior.

Pt.   Ohhh, probably true.

T. Doesn't feel good, does it?

Pt. No.

T. ...to admit it. Maybe we ought to ask...why don't you ask Mike to come in where we are, and maybe we could ask her what she'd like to do in the future, what kind of function she would like to have. Why don't you bring her into our room. Are you there, Mike?

Respecting the opinion of Mike so that co-operation is feasible.

Pt. Umhum.

Mike activated.

T. Have you heard what we were saying what Mother and I were talking about...we'd like to hear from you, what kind of a function would you like to have. I'm sure you heard that Mother and Misha got together in the last few days, since the last time I saw them, and instead of being separate and arguing they kind of got together, and so I guess you weren't needed at that point.

Pt. I guess I've really never been needed and I don't know why I'm here.

T. Umm. Well, you were the arbitrator I guess in a sense or you had to listen to both sides and then, I guess, whoever was the strongest, said mother, you did that particular behavior. I wonder the function you would like to have now that maybe that's not necessary.

Better to find a new function for an ego state than threaten its existence when the previous function no longer needed.

Pt. I felt bad when they went around me.

T. Ohh.

Pt.   I guess I feel that should still be my job now, but now in a positive sense. I wish, you know, instead of them meeting and going out if they would of come to me.

Feeling left out with no purpose.

T.   You'd like to be a partnership, a part of the group.

Pt.   Yeah. Yeah.

T.   Ok. Mother why don't you talk to her and say whatever you want to say about the idea of being part of the three of you.

Dialogue between two ego states.

Pt.   Well, it's going to take some work...Umm, especially with cooperation. But I think we can try. Well, we can try. I don't think, I know we can try. Maybe a little rough on all of us for awhile, and maybe some unpleasantness as we're working all of this out, but I'd be willing to try.

T.   Mike, what do you think?

Pt.   I think it'd be fine.

T.   And let's bring Misha in here too. Misha, I'd like you to come back. I'm not sure if you heard what the other two were saying, but I'd like to hear from you.

Misha must also be consulted to effect a compromise.

Pt.   I was listening. I think it'd be great 'cause then I wouldn't have to think anymore.

T.   Well, good.

Pt.   Then I can play, and she can think.

T.   Who's she?

Pt. Mike. Then she could do the thinking.

T. Oh, she can do the thinking.

Pt. 'Cause right now I have to think, be-   *Interesting perspec-*
cause I have to take what I'm doing   *tive.*
and feeling and kind of convert it into
words, so that what's-her-name up   *Points to left posterior*
there...   *area of brain. (Misha*
    on right side; Mike,
T. Mike?   *the Silent Center, in*
    the middle—from
Pt. Mother.   *another session.)*

T. Oh, Mother.

Pt. Mother can understand me.

T. Oh, I see.

Pt. But if I funnel it all into Mike, then
Mike can do the thinking, and I can do
the fun.

T. How about that! Whee!

Pt. I better put the brakes on. I better be
careful (tips chair back).

T. (laugh) I wouldn't worry about that.
OK. Well, now that sounds like a good
idea. Mike, did you hear what Misha
had to say? She'd like you to have an
important function. She'd like to funnel all the thinking into you. Mike,
how would you like that?

Pt. I would like that a lot.   *Now Mike has purose.*

T. Great, then you'd have an important
function.

Pt.   Yeah.

T.   Ok. Now, Mother, what about you...What
      do you think about that idea that you just
      heard?

Pt.   Well, yeah, Misha's thinking isn't always   *Mother hates to*
      real logical. She's a little young, but I   *give the child*
      think it will work. Yeah.   *credit for logic.*

T.   Well, Mike is older anyway.

Pt.   Yeah. Quite a bit older. Misha's not real
      old sometimes.

T.   She's around 4 or 5. What is she?

Pt.   She doesn't stay the same age.

T.   Uhhuh.

Pt.   From 3 to 6

T.   Oh, I see.

Pt.   She's....

T.   She's up and down. Anyway, she's young,

Pt.   Yeah.

T.   Well, that sounds like a pretty good com-
      promise. And now maybe with the two of
      you working on the allergies, I have a
      feeling you can get rid of them.

Pt.   I do, so do I. I'll stop letting them in.

T.   Mike's talking huh? You say you're going
      to stop letting them...who's talking just
      now?

Pt.   That's me. I'm Mike.

T.   Alright, I know Mother agrees, you agree, so that ought to work out very well and I appreciate the cooperation. Ok. Now I want to talk to the total personality. In a moment I'm going to count up to 5, and when I count up to 5 you will be wide awake, fresh and alert. Coming up now at the count of 5...1,2,3,4,5.

T.   Now, what do you remember?

Pt.   That's weird, they're both talking...all three of them...Sometimes I wish I could just turn my eyes around and see what's going on.   *Concrete thinking of the adult state.*

T.   Strange, huh. Well it sounds like a compromise. That should give you a little peace and get rid those allergies.

T.   Yeah.

T.   OK.

After 12 sessions the depression and insomnia ceased, and the treatment was terminated. There was no return of the allergies, and she no longer heard "voices" in her head. The boundaries between the ego states became more permeable, and they were more "integrated" with one another. However, when she was serious she spoke in a "Mike-type" voice. A nurturing "Mother" voice appeared when she was taking care of a neighbor child, and a "Misha" voice when engaged in playful activities.

Summary

Hypnoanalytic ego-state therapy was derived from the study of multiple personalities and experiments with normal, hypnotic subjects. These include the work of the Hilgards with "hidden observers."

The theories of Paul Federn served as an origin for its conceptual structure. However, we have elaborated on his original formulations and altered them in certain significant areas based on our experimental studies and clinical experience.

Its essential element is the recognition that the "separating function" in the formation of personality structure (like almost all psychological processes) exists on a continuum, ranging from normal, adaptive differentiations, through defensive operations, to maladaptive dissociation as exemplified in true multiple personalities.

Ego-state therapy may use any of the directive, behavioral, cognitive, analytic or humanistic approaches to treatment. But it applies these to personality segments (part-persons) and not to the entire individual, and generally does so under hypnosis, since covert ego states do not ordinarily appear spontaneously without having been hypnotically activated.

Our orientation here is eclectic-psychoanalytic, hence, we have termed it "hypnoanalytic ego-state" therapy. However, a therapist with a different theoretical orientation might prefer to practice a "hypno-behavioral ego-state therapy," applying his interventions to part-persons, e.g. "ego-states," rather than to the entire individual.

It appears to be a very potent treatment procedure because it zeros-in on the specific areas of the personality which are most relevant to the presenting problem. This tactical advantage is valuable, not only in dealing with true multiple personalities, but extends to a vast array of neurotic, psychosomatic and behavioral disorders, ranging from simple stop-smoking and weight reduction problems, to severe phobic and anxiety cases. When utilized skillfully it can suggest approaches for handling borderline conditions, or in fact in any case where some measure of dissociation, mild or severe, is found.

Chapter 9. Hypnoanalytic Ego-State Therapy

Outline

1. Ego-state therapy developed from the theories of Paul Federn.

2. Subject-object.

3. The self.
   a. Object relation theories.

4. Ego and object cathexis.
   a. Existence as the impact between an ego state and an object-cathected item.

5. Introjects as object-cathected.

6. Self representations as ego-cathected.

7. The interchange of ego and object energies.
   a. The creating of "identofacts" (identification).

8. Ego states.

9. Ego-state boundaries.
   a. The continuum of ego-state boundary permeability.
   b. Adaptive differentiation vs. pathological dissociation.
   c. Multiple personalities as the extremes of rigid boundaries.

10. Hidden observers.

11. The characteristics of ego states.

12. The origin of ego states.
    a. Normal differentiation.
    b. Traumas.
    c. The introjection of significant others.

13. Ego-state therapy
    a. Internal diplomacy.
    b. Hypnosis in ego-state therapy.

Footnote
1. Scripts and/or recordings of other ego-state therapy cases can be found in Watkins, J.G., (1978), (1978a): Watkins and Watkins (1980), (1981), (1982), (1986).

Chapter 10

Hypnotic Transference and Counter-Transference

The Nature of Transference

Transference is a phenomenon which occurs with all people. In the analytic situation its understanding and interpretation provides a powerful therapeutic leverage. It refers to the process by which an individual experiences feelings and attitudes in relation to a present-day person or situation that were originally acquired much earlier toward another.

Commonly, a patient will "see" in his therapist traits which he originally perceived in a parent when he was a child. Thus, if a daughter had been rejected by her father she may have the feeling that her therapist is rejecting her, when in reality he has done nothing of the kind. She "transfers" onto him the image of her father and attributes to him her father's characteristics. She feels the kind of emotions toward him which she once felt toward her father, and which she now retains unconsciously. In fact she may accuse him of precisely that. "You don't really care anything about me. You would like me to go away and not bother you."

In the psychoanalytic situation, where the analyst has been sitting quietly and patiently behind a couch on which the patient reclines, he is in a position to point out to the patient that her view of him is in contradiction with his true behavior. He "interprets" her transference reaction. This forces her to confront the discrepancy between her perceptions of him (which have been contaminated by her early perceptions of her father) and the analyst's reality behavior. Since he had not behaved in ways to justify her feelings they must be re-examined and their true source determine. In this way she acquires "insight" and come to realize that perhaps her feelings that he (and all men) reject her are not justified. She takes a step forward toward maturity, e.g. perceiving, feeling and behaving realistically toward the real world.

The term transference has often been used erroneously to mean all feelings which a patient has toward the therapist. The clinician may say, "She has a positive transference toward me," when the feeling does not stem from some early childhood learning experience but from good impressions which are realistic and result from their normal interaction with each other. The term transference should be reserved for those feelings and attitudes which (positive or negative) come from experiential patterns learned toward earlier significant figures in the patient's life.

Before investigating transference in hypnoanalysis let us consider how it was originally acquired. As a child develops, it experiences different feelings in reaction to its perception of the world and the important people in it. If mother is rejecting, given to much scolding and "discipline," then the child may develop a constant fear toward her. This fear may be re-initiated when he contacts a person in later life who reminds him of his mother. Perhaps he was ambivalent toward his mother. On the one hand he loved her and needed her. On the other, he was afraid of her criticisms and punishments. Because of his need for her he may marry a woman who somehow reminds him of her. (As an old song said, "I want a girl just like the girl who married dear old Dad."). The cue which brings back this reminder may be a personality trait which both the mother and the wife possess. Or it could simply be that one or more physical features of the wife (hair color, size, posture, face, etc.) are similar to his mother's. This constitutes the source of the attraction which draws him to her.

We must remember that the image of the mother that is preserved in the unconscious of the individual is not that of the old lady of the present but that of the young woman who gave birth to him and governed his early years. This may well have been a woman whose age would not be greatly at variance to that of his betrothed. However, after the marriage, now that he has an opportunity to live with her and interact with her more closely, he begins to feel, rightly or wrongly, that she also has the critical traits which characterized his mother and which he did not want to recognize. He develops fear toward her and anxiety in the relationship. This may result in many different symptoms, such as sexual impotence, anger flare-ups, psychosomatic reactions, etc. Because she reminds him of his mother on the one hand he chooses her and needs her. On the other hand, (also because she reminds him of his mother) he gets the feeling that she is critical, rejects him and punishes him, whether or not she actually does so in reality. It is in such transference situations that Freud's classical "Oedipus Complex" may be revealed. The foregoing is a very elemental explanation of transference, which is well known to analytically-oriented practitioners, but is presented here so that we can agree on the basic phenomenon before extending it and showing its uses in hypnoanalytic treatment.

There is another way by which we can explain transference. Our perceptions of the real world and our understanding of it stem from two sources: the stimuli coming from that world, and the distortions and interpretations which we place on those stimuli that arise from our own memories, feelings and attitudes, hence from an amalgamation of outer and inner stimuli.. The resulting "experience" is like a photograph of the outer world but colored and changed by our own earlier encounters, wishes, hopes, fears and motivations. Furthermore, from all such experiences we form inner replications (images and memories). As discussed in Chapter 9, when these inner memory images are replications of significant people they are called "introjects" or "object representation." We "introject" a parent and form an internal replica, a "object representation" of that parent, which acquires a kind of life of its own. If the parent has been a nagging, criticizing parent we may go through life feeling constantly depressed because this inner "introject" (self-object, ego state) continues a barrage of unconscious criticism which is consciously experienced as lowered self esteem.

We not only introject a significant person, we also introject "the drama" around such a person. This drama may continue to be enacted in later life. Thus, if one introject or "object representations " stems from our original perceptions of mother, and if another was developed from our early perceptions of father, and if mother and father were constantly arguing, we may repeat this confrontation unconsciously in our own head—and wonder why we suffer from frequent headaches. Then, if a new person in our life reminds us of mother or father the conflict between these two object representations may be reactivated, and we begin to suffer from "transference headaches" whenever we are around that person.

Transference, therefore , may occur whenever perception of something or some person in the real world is "contaminated" with a "memory something" or person from the past. Perception and reaction to the real world is probably "contaminated" with inner "memory-perceptions" for all people, even the most "completely analyzed" individuals. However, the aim of psychoanalytic therapy is to reduce the influence on a patient's behavior and experience from contaminating unconscious memories or inner feelings stemming from the past, and to increase the correctness of perception of the "real" (external) world.

While the goal of analysis is to increase realistic perception and behavior, the goal of all therapy is to improve the adjustment and happiness of the patient. There is an implicit assumption among psychoanalysts that these goals are the same, hence, that a well-analyzed person will be more happy, successful and symptom-free because he/she now experiences and behaves more appropriately toward the real world. This assumption may not always be true. In fact, there is no reason that a happy, optimistic, giving person, who radiates good will to others, and continuously enjoys life, should undertake analysis and submit to change simply because psychoanalytic theory says that he is living in "a fool's paradise." based on repression.

Consider also the case of people in love (perhaps a transference love). Because of their affection they may overlook flaws in each other and enjoy a very happy life together. The problem arises, not from an adjustment based on repression or other defenses, but it only becomes overt when that adjustment breaks down because of great disparity with reality.

In our previous discussion on Hypnosis in Dentistry (Vol. I. pp. 333-334) a technique was suggested for helping a patient to relieve the strangeness in the feel of new dentures. The "memory" of how the original teeth felt is hypnotically reactivated and tied to the stimuli received from running the tongue over the new denture. In other words, the reality perception of the new teeth is "contaminated" with a past memory of what one's original teeth felt like. This is transference hypnotically activated and manipulated to alter an unpleasant sensation in present reality. If successful, the patient becomes adjusted to the newly-acquired prosthetic device and is the happier thereby.

While the foregoing examples are presented to point out that human happiness and reality orientation are not necessarily identical, still we must assume that in most cases the long-term well-being of an individual is generally enhanced if transferences are analyzed and resolved than if they are reinforced and maintained. Accordingly, hypnoanalytic therapy primarily will be devoted to the same goals as psychoanalytic treatment: the uncovering of unconscious processes, the resolution of unrealistic transferences, and the promoting of maturity and reality behavior.

The human personality is a dynamic system of equilibrium with both input and output. We have mentioned "input" in terms of the internalization or "introjection" of outside people and situations, and the building of replicas of these within the self which then acquire object (not me) characteristics and thus can become almost autonomous.

The other side of this equilibrium is the "output." The personality externalizes or "spits-out" from itself these same replications through a process termed "projection"—a form of transference. In its extreme form projection is at the basis of paranoid reactions. The individual, unable to face his own hatred, "projects" this out onto another and accuses the other of hating him. Freud (1953c) explained this mechanism in a paranoid individual as transforming latent homosexual feelings toward another male ("I love you.") first into its opposite through reaction formation. This feeling then becomes an "I hate you," which itself not being acceptable is reversed and project onto the other as "You hate me" before it can come to consciousness. Freud felt this accounted for the patient's delusions of persecution.

Transference may be considered as a special form of this projection. The internalized replica, perhaps of the patient's mother, is projected out onto the person of his wife. He figuratively has garbed the perception of his wife with his mother's attributes. He looks at his wife, but unconsciously he sees his mother and reacts toward her as he once did towards his mother—be it with affection, fear or hatred. This mechanism may also be recognized and interpreted in dreams. Hypnosis gives us much flexibility, not only in deciphering images but in altering them, manipulating them, and intervening in their internalization or externalization.

Transference and Hypnosis

The relation between transference and the hypnotic modality has been the subject of conjecture and study for a long time. The major theories of hypnosis emphasize inter-personal suggestion, regression and dissociation (See Vol. 1. Chap. 2.). Yet each of these are essential components of transference. Suggestions given by one individual (a hypnotist) to another (a subject) are generally rooted in the established patterns of feeling and behavior acquired in their respective childhoods toward others. Regression means a return to earlier patterns of feeling, thinking and reacting—which is precisely what is involved in transference. And dissociation is invariably a part of transference since to manifest it an individual must dissociate to some degree his perception of the present in order to accept one acquired in the past.

Schilder & Kauders (1926) spoke of hypnosis as an "adaptive regression," hence, one controlled by the subject and consciously reversible. Brenman and Gill (1947) emphasized the relationship aspect of hypnosis. Watkins (1954, 1963) first considered hypnosis, itself, as a special form of transference behavior, and then later held that its induction, deepening and termination reflected transference and counter-transference needs within the two participants, hypnotist and subject. Shor (1978) proposed that hypnosis consisted of three essential factors: role-playing, trance and "archaic involvement", by which he meant transference. Smith (1984) examined the hypnotic relationship from an object relations theory viewpoint. Murray-Jobsis (1988) has proposed an integration of adaptive regression, dissociation and transference to form a more comprehensive theory of hypnosis. While most contributors emphasize that hypnosis is founded on parent/child transference Meares (1976) disagrees. He based his theory of hypnosis on "atavistic regression" (See Vol. 1, Chap.2), and affirmed that this regression is to a primitive (prehistoric) mode of behavior, not to the parent-child relationship. Parent-child transferences can arise during hypnosis but they are not basic to the hypnotic modality itself.

Brenman and Gill (1947) made a clear distinction between "the changing transference manifestations which take place during the course of the therapy and the relatively constant transference relationship which we assume to underlie the hypnotic state." In fact, they held that the "hypnotic state" should be termed a "hypnotic relationship", a view with which many hypnotic experimentalists would not agree, since research studies require an effort to minimize or control the relationship factor. In this respect Brenman and Gill believed that hypnosis takes place because it is the gratification of unconscious fantasies or wishes in the subject. Later, they (Gill and Brenman, 1959) extended this position to maintain that hypnosis must be viewed as a two-way (transference-countertransference) relationship in which the overt behavior of the one is the covert fantasy of the other. E.g. if the subject overtly is passive and acquiescent the therapist then behaves in a dominant manner. Simultaneously, the dominant behavior of the therapist may be a reaction formation against his own passive-dependent needs—which he gratifies by resonance with the patient. The patient likewise is resonating with the aggressive, dominating therapist and satisfying his covert desires for omnipotence.

Even more significant are the data these two analysts (Gill and Brenman, 1959) present concerning the interactions between transference and the depth of the hypnotic state/relationship. The ability of the patient to enter hypnosis, and how deeply, varies with changes in the transference-countertransference situation. When resistance to hypnosis changes, interpretations of the negative transference are often followed by more rapid inductions and regressions into deeper hypnotic states. Gill and Brenman said they did not normally interpret the basic transference which underlies the hypnotic contract between a given therapist-patient unit, but did so for changes of transference manifestations which arise as they normally do in traditional psychoanalysis. They preferred to leave the underlying constant transference situation alone. One might suggest that if this is based on "fear," or if it is interfering with the hypnotic induction or the therapy, then it warrants interpretation.

They reported that brief hypnotic states often appear during traditional analysis when transference changes occur. The patient is momentarily glassy-eyed and manifests other trance behaviors. They held that this happens when there is a change in the impulse/defense balance. Transference then becomes an equal precursor for induction with "attacks on the sensori-motor level" (such as eye-fixation, postural-sway, hand-levitation, etc.).

Hypnotherapists who have worked for some time with a patient may find that lengthy, formal inductions are no longer necessary. Just a simple request, "Please go into hypnosis," is sufficient. The underlying transference-countertransference relationship is so developed that sensori-motor level changes are automatically triggered by it.

During the early stages in treating a young woman with multiple personality, if I wanted a particular personality, I would hypnotize her and ask for it. Later, I would simply say, "It's been a long time since I conversed with Meg. Would you please come out, Meg, and talk to me." The patient would respond with the requested dissociation, although some coaxing might be required if "Meg" was angry with me at the time. The close transference relationship made unnecessary formal induction procedures. Here the equivalence of "dissociation" with "hypnosis" becomes quite clear (Hilgard, 1986).

Fromm (1968) in a very readable paper describes a number of transference manifestations which occur in hypnosis, such as Oedipal and sibling. She recommends that in hypnotherapy the transference be "utilized" and not necessarily "analyzed," and she gives the example of a patient who competed with her by reporting that self-hypnosis was deeper than that induced by the therapist. Instead of analyzing this transference reaction Fromm suggested that the patient use her self-hypnosis to unearth more material for hypnoanalysis.

Gill and Brenman conclude that hypnosis is a modality by which the therapist (and patient) can regulate the amount of closeness or distance between them. They noted the resistance encountered when an attempt is made to analyze and interpret the "meaning" of hypnosis to the patient. Both consciously and unconsciously patients generally show that they want this area left alone, and therefore it is probably best to accept and work with its transference meaning than to remove it by interpretation—which might then render the patient unhypnotizable.

Another example of utilizing or manipulating the transference is as follows. A 28-year old patient reported to me that he was very much afraid of his father, but that when accused of being like his father he would feel "strong" and not block. Under hypnosis he was asked to image a stage with a man and a boy on it. He was told to "fuse" with the boy and identify with him. He then manifested much fear. When asked to describe the theater he blocked and was unable to talk well. It was then suggested that he remove himself from the boy and approach the man, "fusing" with him. His blocking ceased, and his speech cleared. Here we have changed an object representation hypnotically (the boy) to a self representation (me) and then reversed them again by making "the boy" object and "the man" self.

After some exploration to determine what negative traits might be acquired by identifying with his father, the "fusing' was fixated post-hypnotically by suggestion. He emerged from trance with no speech blocking. The clearing of the speech was not permanent following this first session. However, after a number of repeats the blocking apparently disappeared and did not return. Here the transference was not interpreted but utilized in a subject-object suggestive approach to treatment. In object relations theory terminology his father object representation had been turned into a self representation—an introject into an "identofact."

As in psychoanalysis the successful resolution of a transference reaction can be the significant turning point in hypnotherapy. This will often concern a block in the treatment related to the specific emotions (fear or love) which are evoked in the patient by the hypnotic relationship. Lazar and Dempster (1984) described a case in which a woman who had been sexually abused by her father reported an "overwhelming sexual desire" toward her male therapist. He correctly recognized this as a transference related to her father and informed her that "she was entitled to help and no further payment was needed." Her first reaction was indignation, and she regarded it as a rejection. However, she soon came to see that the sexuality was a way of continuing contact with her "therapeutic father," since she had "given" sex to her original father to reduce his abuse. Following this she began to feel that the therapist truly "loved" her in a way she had not previously experience, and the treatment progressed to an effective conclusion.

When blocks to progress do occur the therapist will be wise to consider carefully the transference (and counter-transference) situation, and to resolve them through proper interpretation. This is especially true when a previously hypnotizable patient suddenly becomes resistant to hypnosis. Not only does the patient manifest transference reactions, but the therapist also is subject to distortions of perception and behavior which stem from his or her own childhood experiences with others. This is called counter-transference.

Counter-Transference

Analysts are human too. Feelings and attitudes can be stimulated in them also by interactions in the therapeutic relationship. Many of these are quite normal. When challenged we may become competitive. When approached seductively we may develop erotic feelings. These are often termed "counter-transference" since they are developed as "counter" to those initiated by the patient—the reactions of an object to the patient's subject. Even though therapists commonly refer to counter-transferences as any feeling state initiated in them by the patient, strictly speaking this term should be reserved for only those therapist feelings and behaviors in which the patient's actions have served as stimulus to activate a re-experiencing in the therapist of patterns he learned toward early significant others.

Stein (1970) suggests items by which a therapist might recognize his own counter-transference. These include alterations in usual fees,

signs of familiarity, overlooking failures to take prescribed medica-
tions, allowing telephone abuses, neglect of history taking, and
repeated discussions regarding the patient with colleagues.

Gruenwald (1971) noted that the manner of a hypnotist, aggressive, seductive, etc., may often represent counter-transference. Fromm
(1968) held that such reactions are all counter-productive therapeutically, and that unless they are understood and resolved the therapist
will be unable to help the patient. This view seems a bit extreme since
all people are subject to counter-transferences, most of which are not
analyzed and resolved. By such a yardstick most therapists could not
help people. In some cases the natural counter-transferences of the
therapist may actually be helpful to the patient by fitting in with the
patient's needs even though based on distortions of perception. Perhaps we should take the position that counter-transferences *may*
interfere with therapy and should optimally be understood, analyzed
and resolved. However, "helping-humans" do not have to be perfect.

Counter-transference can, not only impair therapists' reactions to
their patients, but, also may be an equally distorting factor in the
interactions of experimentalists with their research subjects. This
possibility is never controlled for in the design of studies in hypnosis,
or other experiments (Watkins, J., 1989).

In Chapter 2. the Psychodynamics of Hypnotic Induction, we have
already given considerable attention to the effect of transference in
initiating an hypnotic state. Our emphasis here will be the consideration and use of that process in dealing therapeutically with patients
who are working within a hypnoanalytic relationship. In psychoanalysis the purpose of having the patient recline in a passive
condition and concentrate on his internal processes is to encourage a
regression in which transferences may become manifest (Menninger
and Holzman, 1973.) In hypnoanalysis we establish the regression
more directly by the induction of a hypnotic state. This brings the
patient more rapidly into contact with childhood behaviors and
experiences.

As the patient sinks into a deeper and deeper trance reality
perception fades and regressive material becomes more evident.
However, this does not give us permission immediately to interpret
the transference. Conducting analysis in the hypnotic state does not
mean that resistances are removed, that the hypnoanalyst needs less
skill and sensitivity than the psychoanalyst. Quite the contrary. Even
though the hypnotic modality has given him access to regressive
processes more rapidly, and offers more leverage in managing them,

it does not indicate that resistance disappears, and that we can immediately interpret the transference and achieve genuine insight. If we now interpret directly while the patient is in the hypnotic state we may find that upon emerging from hypnosis he has "forgotten" what we said, re-repressed it, or merely recalls an "intellectual" interpretation. He does not at that time fully recall "the experience." It is like confronting an alcoholic with his intoxicated behavior later when he is sober. He will either not remember it, remember it vaguely, or perhaps simply deny it. ("That wasn't me. I was drunk and not responsible for my behavior then.") We say that the experience has not been "egotized."

We can give the transference interpretation ("You are reacting as if I was your father") under hypnosis and find that it is not well remembered subsequently, or not re-experienced and integrated. Or we can interpret it after he has emerged from hypnosis. Then, the transference interpretation cannot be compared with the conscious reality perception, because the interpretation is no longer tied to the "experience" which he had under hypnosis. The "experience' of the transference, the reality perception, and the interpretation should be tied together—hence, experienced simultaneously.

This is the objection classical analysts have to hypnosis, and it is not without merit. However, all is not lost. The experiencing of the transference under hypnosis may be considered as a fore-runner or precursor of its full experience in the conscious state later. Even as the experiencing of the transference in psychoanalysis may come first of all in dreams and only later in the relaxed (semi-hypnotic) state which is normal on the psychoanalytic couch. The next time the experience is re-activated hypnotically it will be closer to "the surface." Like a dress rehearsal in a play the elements are approaching "the real thing." This is the leverage which the flexibility of the hypnotic modality offers to the analyst. He can not only elicit repressed and dissociated material, not only vivify this into affective experiencing, but he can also to some extent control the state of the patient's ego for its reception, acceptance, and integration. He can have the remembering and experience occur in deeper to lighter stages of hypnosis and thus approach the fully conscious, egotized state. "Working-through" may still be required, but it can be done in less time when using hypnotic interventions.

In psychoanalysis the tendency is to try to get the patient to focus transference on the analyst. This has considerable advantage since the crucial experiences which compare a fantasy from the past with the reality behavior of the present are immediately available and being experienced within the analytic hour. Since the analyst has always acted in an objective and neutral way the behaviors and attitudes imputed to him transferentially by the patient are more easily demonstrated as false.

However, there is also a restricting effect by this great concentration of inducing the transferences to manifest themselves on the person of the analyst. Transference is operative in almost all life relationships, and it often takes a long time before these are projected onto the analyst. That is one of the reasons why psychoanalysis is so time-consuming and expensive—thus limiting its availability.

The hypnotic modality, in addition to stimulating such reactions earlier, makes possible greater attention to the analysis of transferences which occur *outside* the analytic hour because of its ability to alter both object and self representations. The great impact of transference interpretations occurs because of the disparity between an externally perceived reality and an inner experienced fantasy-reality. There is no reason why the individual (analyst) who makes the interpretation must also be the same one on whom the transferences are targeted. Freud discovered transference when as an outsider he observed its projection onto Breuer by an hysterical patient.

The important point is that to be believed an interpretation must be given by one whom the patient trusts. While the analyst's objectivity helps build that trust, a person who is actively our friend and supporter may be able to make suggestions and interpretations to us with enhanced credibility. Interpretations concerning transferences which are being manifested toward other relationships *outside* the analysis that are made by analysts who have real, positive rapport with their patients may be more effective than those voiced by a completely "neutral" analyst. The clinician, not being a party to the *outside* transferences, can utilize the continuous, underlying positive rapport that is indigenous to his credibility regarding these outside transferential manifestations.

Today, the positive relationship aspects of good therapists are being increasingly emphasized by object-relation theorists and others over the "objective" manner—which sometimes is perceived by the patient as cold and rejecting. This is especially true in the treatment of psychotics and borderlines. The comparative values of an "objective," neutral analytic attitude with a more warm and supportive approach needs further research in our efforts to reduce the time of analytic treatment.

The first impressions that a patient gets of his analyst are both real and "transferred." This is because the analyst is relatively unknown to the patient then. As the two work together, more material emerges, and the patient "works-through" transference manifestations. However, he is also gathering more real perceptions, and his analyst or therapist is becoming better known to him. Simultaneously, as time passes there is less and less new material left to be transferred. Even though he is behaving non-directively and minimizing his "real" presence, as advised in classical psychoanalysis, the analyst cannot escape becoming more and more a real object to the patient.

As the psychoanalysis (or hypnoanalysis) progresses this is not necessarily bad. Personal comments about himself by the therapist will not have the distracting effect they would have had earlier. They now permit the patient to make him gradually into a "real" person. When the termination of a successful treatment arrives there is no further need of the patient to use him as a transference target, and he *should* become a real object.

In the earlier days of psychoanalysis this change from analyst to friend was celebrated by a "rite" of great significance to both parties. The analyst invited the analyand to dinner. This signified the transition in their relationship from analyst/patient to friend/friend in which both became reality objects for the other. Since this usually occurred with analysands who were undertaking a "training analysis" it meant that the two were now colleagues. This delightful and meaningful event is rarely practiced today, partly because now we view the treatment as "taking analysis," not as completing *an analysis*. It is never finished, since analysis is not a discrete undertaking but a continuing growth process carried on in self-analysis by the "patient" who is no longer in face-to-face contact with his analyst.

Transference in Hypnoanalysis

Transference can be worked with, managed, or interpreted. In working with a transference, usually a positive one, we may recognize its transferential nature but choose to keep it and utilize its motivation to achieve symptomatic and behavioral changes. As long as the transference remains positive the patient (for love of the therapist) tries to please and works hard at the treatment. As pointed out earlier (Vol. 1, Chapter 8) there is nothing wrong with symptomatic change if the patient is improved thereby, and if the underlying conflict needs are not so strong as to render the improvement only temporary.

Sometimes for good psychodynamic reasons constructive symptomatic improvement becomes permanent. Analysis is unnecessary and economically contra-indicated.

If the positive transference becomes highly sexualized, a situation which can threaten both the therapist and the treatment, then it requires special attention. Soskis (1986) lists a number of warning signs to the clinician which should alert him to this problem. They include finding the patient unusually attractive or appearing in the therapist's sexual fantasies or dreams. Other alerting signs are a patient with a past history of sexual relationships with clinicians or teachers, one who emphasizes the erotic aspects of the hypnotic relationship in discussions or who acts in sexually provocative ways. Freud (1924) discussed this problem at considerable length in his "Observations on Transference Love," and warned the young analyst against being entangled in it.

The analyst risks being caught up in a dilemma. If he rejects the patient's overtures she/he may turn against him and discontinue therapy—or even sue and make allegations that he did seduce her. On the other hand if he/she succumbs to the temptation and "acts out" the situation then the possibility of ever interpreting this transference to disentangle the patient from an early erotic transference on a parent is forever lost. When resistance arises in the therapy the patient will seek a repeat of the sexual affair, the treatment will fail, and the lives of both therapist and patient eventually become miserable.

If it is essential to keep the transference positive and not to analyze its source then its sexual aspects can be minimized by interpretations like this: "You are indeed a very attractive person. But you have come to me to help you with your problem (illness). An affair might be very pleasant temporarily, but it would complete spoil our efforts to help you in therapy. Lovers are easier to come by than good therapists. I respect you and care too much about your welfare to ruin it in this way. Let us keep our relationship on this level of high regard for one another." Interpretations in such a vein are usually sufficient to retain the positive transference and not let it degenerate into a treatment-destroying sexual affair. If the therapist's erotic counter-transference toward the patient is too strong for him to accept a stabilization of the relationship at a "respect and caring" level then the patient should be referred to another clinician.

Wilbur (1988) warns especially of this hazard when treating a multiple personality. One alter may be very seductive toward the therapist. Another also has an erotic transference toward the therapist.

Another also has an erotic transference toward the doctor but manifests it by a denial and hostile defense. Interpretations which resolve the transference when dealing with one alter may still leave a sexual transference masquerading in another. The transference situation becomes extremely complex when treating a multiple with many alters (Watkins, J. & Watkins, H., 1990).

When simply managing the transference the therapist is aware of the changes in its manifestations and adjusts the therapeutic interventions for maximum impact. No attempt is made to resolve them by interpreting their origins. Alexander and French (1946) have described many cases of psychoanalytic therapy where the transference was simply "managed" or at least given minimal interpretation. They did not use hypnosis, but did achieve significant symptomatic improvements with few sessions.

It is when transference interpretations are employed to counter resistance and reveal underlying conflicts that we can truly speak of the therapy as being "analytic." Let us consider techniques for implementing this within the hypnotic modality.

The Interpretation of Transference in Hypnoanalysis

A dissociated patient, having experienced both the pain and subsequent relief in previous abreactions, reacted to a new induction with considerable resistance ("I don't think I can be hypnotized today."). I replied, "You act as if you are afraid of me." To which she responded, "Yes, I seem to be very afraid of you right now." She was permitted to enter hypnosis in her own way (non-directively), and soon she was re-living scenes where her father molested her. (Like him, I had given her pain.) Transference interpretations (both under hypnosis and afterward) brought relief from "the fear," and a renewal of the positive transference.

That dreams often reflect the current state of the transference between doctor and patient has been well documented by psychoanalysts. Often, the analysis of a dream through hypnosis will permit a transference interpretation that removes a block and significantly moves the treatment forward (Kline, 1967). In hypnoanalysis the patient who reports a dream that probably stems from transference can be hypnotized and its meaning more easily divined than in the conscious state. However, the hypnoanalyst often discovers that the resistance in a negative transference dream may be manifested by greater difficulty in hypnotizing the patient at that time. The resistance to induction is, itself, evidence that the dream represents a negative transference manifestation. The resistance will require interpretive removal before the content of the dream can be activated and analyzed.

Psychoanalytically-trained practitioners will find that the principles they learned for interpreting transference manifestations apply equally well in hypnoanalytic therapy. The hypnotic state does not basically change them but does add more options and flexibility. E.g., interpretation of negative transference is commonly followed by a change to the positive and vice versa. Interpretations generally require a subsequent "working-through," hence, repetition and elaboration. Interpretations are most effective when given at the time that the transferred affect is strong. However, the ability of hypnosis to manipulate the amount or degree of ego participation adds a new dimension for control.

In the traditional psychoanalytic situation hypnosis is involved but usually unrecognized. The patient reclining on the couch is instructed to concentrate on his inner productions and to report them without alteration or censorship. Both relaxation and attention to inner processes, especially fantasies, are in themselves induction techniques. So it is not surprising that many psychoanalytic patients do their "couch work" in a light hypnotic state controlled only by their own internal and transference processes.

The hypnoanalyst recognizes the presence and potentialities of transference. He interacts in ways to control this factor so as to optimize the balance between the uncovering of repressions and the ego integration of material so elicited. It is customary during psychoanalysis to wait until the transference feelings are quite strong and the ego is conscious and highly alert. Thus, Fenichel (1945) states, "The fact that the pathogenic conflicts, revived in the transference, are now expressed in their full emotional context makes the transference interpretation so much more effective—."

For best ego-integration this is true. However, the hypnoanalyst accepts this fact that the relaxed patient on the analytic couch is probably lightly, and sometimes more deeply, hypnotized (through self induction). Accordingly, what appears overtly to be a genuine re-experiencing of conflicts "in their full emotional context" may be less than psychoanalytic theory holds. The "ego" is not fully conscious and alert, but partially so. This may be one of the reasons why the psychoanalyst frequently has to make his transference interpretation more than once, and why it often requires more substantial, subsequent working-through.

The hypnoanalyst, therefore, by controlling the depth of hypnosis, from hypnoidal, to light, to medium, to deep, to profound, is simply optimizing a level of ego participation which in the traditional psychoanalytic treatment is left uncontrolled. One might argue that the patient is best left to setting his own hypnotic (ego-participating) level for uncovering and integration. However, patients, left entirely to themselves, seldom analyze, work-through and become free of their conflicts without professional assistance. The question is not whether to intervene or never intervene, but rather how much and when therapist intervention is required.

If interpretations are given when the patient is deeply hypnotized they will probably require much repetition and working-through in subsequent, lighter states. If the interpretation is made when the transference manifestations are "almost conscious," hence, in a light hypnosis, less repetition will be required to meet the analytic criteria of "genuine insight." In general, the hypnotic interpretation will have some effect in moving the patient forward. However, occasionally the premature hypnotic interpretation may alert defensive processes. The patient then resists hypnosis, and interpretations must be directed against these blocks (the defense transference) before a return to activating and interpreting the original conflict transference. Handling this transference resistance is quite important and in fact has been termed by Fenichel as "the core of analysis."

Hypnoanalysis with Psychotics and Borderlines

Classical psychoanalytic theory held that psychotics could not be analyzed because of their inability to establish a stable transference onto the analyst. Other writers (Kroger and Fezler, 1976) have stated that, "presence of a severe psychosis is a prime contraindication to hypnoanalysis." However, much recent thinking (Baker, 1981, 1983; Copeland, 1986) holds that psychotics and also borderlines do establish transferences, even though unstable and vacillating between externalizing and internalizing their representations.

The literature in this area has been reviewed by Baker (1983), Scagnelli-Jobsis (1982), Pettinati (1982) and Lavoie and Sabourin (1980). Baker notes that psychotics have now been found to be as hypnotizable as any other patient population, and that apparently the same techniques that are employed with other conditions can be applied to them. There is still continuing research and controversy about the hypnotizability of psychotics (D. Spiegel, 1983; Scagnelli-Jobsis, 1983). However, many workers are now reporting success using hypnosis with psychotics and borderlines personalities.

Baker asserts that hypnosis could be a modality for stabilizing this transference onto the analyst. Biddle (1967) found the hand levitation induction effective with psychotics. Beahrs (1986) describes the dramatic disappearance of psychotic symptoms in a severe schizophrenic after a single brief treatment by hypnosis. These reports suggest that we need to take a good second look at treating psychosis hypnotically.

This chapter has been essentially about transference and its manifestations in hypnoanalytic therapy. However, since the problems of treating psychoses and borderlines depend so much on the ability to establish, elicit and work with transferences this seemed an appropriate point to consider these conditions.

A great difficulty in psychoanalytically treating psychotics and borderlines is that they have generally not established stable object relationships early in life. Accordingly, they cannot usually start treatment by introjecting the analyst and thus form an object representation of him/her. Baker (1981) utilizes hypnosis in the early stages of therapy to help the patient establish such an object, a therapeutic object with which he can interact. This may be considered as a "transitional object" (Winnicott, 1965). Since the psychotic did not establish object representations because the objects (parents) in his early environment were not accepting and nurturing he cannot distinguish an object from subject, external reality from self.

If we have been through an experience ourselves it is easier to resonate and understand another in a similar situation. A very excellent therapist with psychotics, whom I know, has herself been through a psychotic episode. This enables her to understand deeply many communications of her patients which most clinicians would miss. However, therapists generally have not had this experience personally. But when sleeping and dreaming we do exist in a temporarily "psychotic," internal world. The boundaries between "the me" and external reality are at that time laid aside, and we cannot differentiate between self and object representations. Like the psychotic or borderline who has not established ego boundaries we, too, may have difficulty in the middle of a dream pulling ourselves out unless there is some "transitional object" embedded in reality to provide the needed stimulus for re-cathecting our ego boundaries—like an alarm clock or the voice of another person.

If you are accustomed to sleeping soundly throughout the night (though perhaps with dreams) try an experiment. Determine that you will awaken at 3:00 A.M. without an alarm clock. Often you will fail and continue to sleep until your accustomed time for arising. Even if you are successful you may find yourself in a great struggle desperately trying to pull yourself out of a dream and re-establish contact with an external world in which the touch of bed sheets provides only a very weak "transitional object." Perhaps in such an experience you can appreciate the difficulty facing the psychotic or borderline patient who is trying to regain contact with external reality.

Psychotic and borderline patients are often in a conflict between wishing to merge with a loved object (therapist) and fear of being engulfed and destroyed by one. Copeland (1986) used hypnosis to regulate the amount of "distance" between therapist and patient so as to optimize motivations for the patient to establish an object relationship with her. This takes advantage of the focusing ability of hypnosis.

It has been said that psychosis is like an individual turned inside out. In neurosis the "Id" is repressed, and the ego contacts the outside world. In psychosis it is the reverse. The "Id" is released to interact with the outside world, hence, the hallucinations and primitive behavior. On the other hand it is the ego which is repressed and which needs to be contacted.

Margaretta K. Bowers, one of the early workers in using hypnosis to treat schizophrenics (1961), held that schizophrenia is actually a defense. She used hypnosis to contact the "little me," or "inner self" of the patient. Bowers believed that the schizophrenic uses auto-hypnosis to ward off an outer reality and to maintain an inner reality, which was less threatening. Object relation theorists (Winnicott, 1965) point out that the patient needs a "transitional object" to make contact with the outer world again.

The therapist can help this type of patient by becoming for him a transitional object which gives a sense of some external, anchoring reality that can later be extended to significant others in his world. In this respect Bowers used herself as such an anchoring object, reaching out to contact "the little me" of the patient. However, she warned that sometimes the schizophrenic would "merge" with the therapist in a symbiotic relationship, which, if reinforced, might continue indefinitely. In this case the patient fails to establish a self/non-self boundary that is achieved by most children in relation to their mothers during the "separation-individuation" development stage, and which is normally completed by the age of 24 months (Mahler, 1972). Bowers believed that this was one of the greatest hazards in treating schizophrenics.

But sometimes a real relationship with a live person, like a therapist, may seem too threatening to such a patient. Then, even a teddy bear or inanimate object may be less fearsome, enabling him to establish some contact with external reality and start the process of differentiating self from non-self. Teddy bears (or even ragged fragments from a security blanket) should not be taken from young children until their "objectivity" has been extended to include other people and things.

A middle-aged, professional woman was so detached from her world that she existed only in a schizoid fog. Though successful in her occupation she never had a sense of reality. She lived in a kind of dream world. Hypnosis is a focusing process. Accordingly, I (See Watkins, 1978, Chap. 4) used this characteristic to mobilize her self energies (ego cathexes) and focus them all on her fingertips, a small area of her physical ego boundary. She was then given a pencil. In a flood of tears she exclaimed, "For the first time in 30 years I'm feeling something real." For her, the differentiation between "the me" and "the not-me" was started. She had experienced an external object, if only a pencil.

This was the beginning of an extended treatment which I called at the time "existential hypnoanalysis," (Watkins, 1967). It aimed to establish "meaning" to self and to external reality as they impacted one another. First, she impacted a pencil, next the therapist, then other people in her world. Finally, a normal (neurotic) transference could be established permitting therapy to continue along more traditional analytic lines. Existential hypnoanalysis will be discussed more in Chapter 11.

Federn (1952) distinguished between "estrangement" and "depersonalization." Estrangement means the inability to sense the external as real. Today, we would call it a deficiency in forming "object representations." By "depersonalization" Federn referred to the inability to experience one's own self—the inadequate energizing of self representations. In his theoretical conceptions estrangement meant the lack of the object cathexis vested into the perceptions. Individuals feel "depersonalized" when they cannot cathect self representation with "ego cathexis" because of weakness or lack of self energies. However, the two are interactively related. For us to have the impact of reality an object representation must be innervated by a certain quantity of object cathexis in contact with a minimally energized ego representation (Watkins, 1978, Chap. 6). Unless object plus ego cathexis add up to a certain quantum the"experience" does not take place—or does so only at an unconscious level. As an analogy unless the magnitude of light from an object plus the degree of sensitivity of the retina exceed a certain threshold, vision does not take place. Hypnotic suggestion can be used to focus object and ego energies on different physical or mental points of contact.

Baker proposed several hypnotic techniques for building self and object representations. First, the patient was asked to visualize an image of self accompanied by a pleasant feeling. Second, the patient was instructed to open his eyes and see the therapist, then close them again and return to the image of self. Next, the patient was helped to visualize an image of the therapist, a step that borderline patients often found difficult. The hypnotized patient was then asked to alternate between the images of self and those of the therapist. Next, the two would be pictured together letting the patient set the distance between them. And finally, fantasies would be developed involving the patient and therapist in parallel activity and in interaction. As ego functioning stabilized, the process was extended to include other significant objects and to integrating positive and negative images. In this way the therapist was first established as a transitional object followed by a strengthening of the patient's ability to form other object relations.

Federn (1952) did not use hypnosis. However, he had an ingenuous way of teaching his patients to establish boundaries between the self and outside reality. When psychotic patients would report that their hallucinations were "real" he would not contradict them—as so often is done. He would say, "Yes, I agree, but there are two kinds of reality. You can see me sitting here in front of you. Let us call that reality A. You can share Reality A with others. But when you see those people who are persecuting you that is Reality B. Reality B is a kind of private reality for you. If you try to share Reality B with others they will not be able to perceive it, and they will say you are crazy. Now, whenever you experience anything I want you to tell me whether it is Reality A or Reality B."

Federn claimed that the patient could always tell the difference between Reality A and Reality B. In other words, the psychotic is aware of the difference between object representations which are initiated by stimuli coming through the senses from the outside world and those which emanate from unconscious processes (the id) and create an internal "object," even though both are experienced as objects. In fact, Federn might even tell the patient that if he would always keep Reality B to himself, and never mention it to anyone, he could leave the hospital.

At first glance, this seems like showing the patient how to conceal his psychosis. However, Federn was teaching him to distinguish between hallucinations and reality. As the patient practiced this discrimination he was strengthening the ego boundary. Federn claimed that in the course of time Reality B receded and was no longer experienced consciously. This meant that because of the focusing of attention (and hence energy) toward Reality A, Reality B was being de-cathected. In working hypnotically with patients we use its focusing ability to direct energies toward Reality A and away from Reality B.

Much of Federn's treatment of psychotics was in collaboration with Gertrude Schwing (1954), a motherly nurse, who provide the "holding environment" which Winnicott (1965) described as being an essential feature in helping psychotics to establish a stable object representation. Federn also believed that the analyst-patient transference should be kept positive and be interpreted only when it becomes negative. There seems to be no reason why Federn's techniques could not be applied more effectively using hypnosis.

In using hypnosis with psychotics it should be noted that the activation (or only the memory enhancement) of psychotic dreams or other regressions will likely re-precipitate the psychotic episode associated with them. Accordingly, the "analytic" methods of free association and dream interpretation are contra-indicated. Interpretations should center on blocks to ego control and the development of defenses, not on remembering and releasing primitive (id-related) drives. The psychotic patient's ego has already been overwhelmed by such. It needs integration and building-up, not tearing down. In fact, since psychotic and borderline conditions represent developmental failures Brown and Fromm (1987) have suggested that the therapy should be "hypno-integrative" rather than "hypnoanalytic." Fromm reported a patient who, using hypnotic visualization, conceptualized himself floating inside a protective bubble which protected him from merging with the therapist and which could establish the safest and most acceptable distance from outside people. In the early stages of treatment the bubble would break-up easily, but as the patient's boundaries became more stabilized it would burst only under intense emotional interactions (a precaution to note if treatment becomes too abreactive).

Scagnelli (1974, 1976, 1977, 1980) has developed effective procedures for using hypnosis in treating psychotics and borderlines. She recommends auto-hypnosis since patients are less fearful when they are not forced into a one-to-one close relationship with the therapist, and because they are more in control of their own therapy. Apparently, most of her patients used hypnosis for ego strengthening and the formation of self or object representations and not for uncovering, although a few borderlines did do uncovering. She also recommended autohypnosis for the therapist, a state in which she reported being better able to concentrate and be more sensitive to her patient's needs. Scagnelli was most empathic in co-experiencing with her patients. This is similar to "resonance," a term which will be discussed more in Chapter 11.

Biddle (1967) in a early treatise on the hypnotic treatment of psychoses reports the case of a young woman who developed a sexual ("hebephrenic") fixation on him. When he refused to gratify her erotic overtures she became paranoidal and would have nothing more to do with him—truly a case of "—no greater wrath than that of woman scorned". He did not interpret her changes of transference, but he refused to accept the rejection, and for "several weeks" continued to see her on the hospital ward. Eventually, a more realistic relationship was achieved, and the treatment progressed favorably.

I, too, had a dissociated patient (Watkins and Johnson, 1982) enter a psychotic state following several days of severe abreactions. She regressed to the age of 3, carrying her teddy bear around the ward. However, after contacts with her mother, and continued perseverance by the therapist, she returned to normalcy—and with a great improvement in her dissociations. Moral: don't give up. The regression into a suicidal, psychotic or child state may be the most potent, possible request for help and "love" that a patient can make. The therapist who doesn't run, and who meets the challenge, will often be rewarded by the patient's taking a big step forward.

Helen Watkins uses a "safe-room technique" to help the patient restore boundaries and save energy when stress (external or internal) becomes too severe. The patient is taken hypnotically down stairs accompanied by the therapist. At the bottom he is asked to walk along a hallway and visualize a door on one side, "a door to a room of your own choosing in which you will feel safe and comfortable. Look at the door and tell me what it looks like. Have you ever seen this door before:?" (This question is designed to elicit possible past associations.) She then continues, "Would you like to enter this door alone, or would you like me to come with you? Either way is fine." (The answer reveals the patient's dependency needs.) He can close the door in this place and be "safe" while he rests and restores his self-integrity and his energy.

One patient (H. Watkins, 1978) was pursued by a malevolent ego state, called "the Evil One." At times he would emerge as a full-fledged auditory hallucination. He kept trying to follow the patient into the safe room, shouting and yelling. Helen said she would hold onto the Evil One while the patient went into the Safe Room and closed the door. The patient did so. The hallucination of the Evil One temporarily ceased, and the therapist's role as the patient's protector was strengthened.

Hypnosis and transference are both regressive processes. Normally we think of regression as taking one back to more primitive and child-like behaviors. It is a bit strange, accordingly, to report the reverse. The hypnotic regression took one patient back to an earlier and much better adjusted existence.

Clarence was a paranoid schizophrenic in his mid-thirties. He had been hospitalized for 8 years as a chronic psychotic, plagued by hallucinations of "the It's," a malevolent gang who constantly perse-cuted him—and about whose machinations he continually talked. After working with him hypnotically for some six months, and after having established a good therapeutic relationship, I decided to try to regress him back to a time before he had become psychotic and hospitalized. With some difficulty he was hypnotized, regressed back 9 years, and told that when he emerged from hypnosis it would be 1942 instead of 1951.

To my astonishment he came out of hypnosis and showed not the slightest sign of psychosis. Gone were all his delusions, his halluci-nations and his concrete verbalizations. Instead, I was confronted with a perfectly normal-appearing individual. Hardly believing it, I invited Clarence to join me and a colleague for lunch. My friend knew nothing about Clarence. During lunch he, a very experienced psy-chologist, and Clarence conversed normally, exchanging childhood reminiscences and their impressions of certain communities. At no time did my colleague suspect he was talking to a chronic, paranoid schizophrenic. In fact, Clarence's manner was so completely normal that the only time a puzzled expression appeared on my friend's face was when Clarence mentioned that he was expecting to receive his draft notice soon (World War II having been over for six years then).

Later that day I re-hypnotized Clarence and removed the post-hypnotic suggestion. He immediately reverted to his usual psychotic ideation. My colleague, when asked about the lunch, assured me he had no idea he was talking to a chronic paranoid and hospitalized schizophrenic. A few days later I tried to re-hypnotize Clarence. He was resistant, and after that I was unable to hypnotize him again. Apparently, the paranoid structure had a life of its own and would not accept permanent elimination. Bowers (1961) has observed that, "the schizophrenic who is hypnotized successfully by a therapist whom he is not ready to trust completely" may be "consequently most difficult to hypnotize the second time." Perhaps living in his earlier life of reality was too frightening unconsciously to Clarence, and in suggesting to do so, (even though only for an hour or two) I had stretched the credibility of my relationship with him too far.

A few weeks afterward I was transferred to another Veterans Administration facility and never saw Clarence again, However, three years later on re-visiting the hospital I was observing a group of patients some distance away being taken to the exercise gymnasium. From the middle of the group a hand waived in my direction, and I heard Clarence's voice shouting, "Hey Doc, we got the Its on the run."

I have often wondered what would have happened to Clarence if I had not removed his post-hypnotic suggestion. How long could the regression to "normalcy" have been maintained in the face of the world of reality, and the absence of a continuous hypnotic relationship with his therapist. Apparently he could act the role of a normal individual, but I am certain that the world would not have allowed him to live in "1942." As soon as that point came up, and he had been informed that "now" it was really 1951, his regression would probably have been broken; his paranoid condition would have returned. Nevertheless the possibilities here for treating a psychosis seem intriguing.

Summary

Transference, a common phenomena, occurs when an individual reacts to a present day person (frequently his/her therapist) as if they were a significant person in the individual's past. The interpretation of this transference is a powerful technique in analytic therapies. When the therapist is perceiving the patient similarly, hence, experiencing feelings which stem from early relationships in his own past it is called "counter-transference." The elimination of transferences and the developing of reality perceptions is a basic goal in both psychoanalysis and hypnoanalysis.

Transference reactions tend to be activated sooner in hypnosis.

They can be utilized, manipulated or interpreted. Hypnotizability and resistance may be changes in transferences. The timing and skill with which transferences are interpreted are highly significant in both psychoanalytic and hypnoanalytic therapies.

It had been held in the past that psychotics could not be analyzed because they were unable to establish stable object relationships, and hence, transferences, on the analyst. Newer thinking uses hypnosis to build the therapist into a "transitional object" for the patient. In this way he learns to establish stable object and self representations. These approaches have brought schizophrenia within the possibilities of treatment through hypnosis.

Chapter 10. Transference and Counter-Transference

Outline

1. Transference, the unrealistic projection onto present day figures of feelings derived from experiences with significant people from earlier life.

2. Counter-transference, the same when experienced by the therapist or analyst.

3. Interpretation of the transference as a powerful therapeutic technique in both psychoanalysis and hypnoanalysis.

4. Transference manifestation more easily activated in hypnosis.

5. Similarities and differences in transference analysis between psychoanalysis and hypnoanalysis.

6. Difficulties in treating psychoses because patients unable to establish stable object representations (hence, transferences) onto the therapist.

Chapter 11

Forensic Hypnosis

Forensic hypnosis, or the application of hypnosis to legal problems, both civil and criminal, is a new and controversial area of specialization for clinical practitioners. The law is concerned with many questions regarding sanity, competence, credibility of witnesses, motivation, memory, perception, extent of knowledge, culpability, mitigating circumstances, etc., all of which involve psychological appraisal of defendants, litigants and witnesses. Judges and juries make decisions everyday on any or all of the above, and they must frequently rely on "expert witnesses," professionals who can bring specialized skill and knowledge to assist them.

Mental health practitioners, such as psychologists and psychiatrists, are increasingly being called upon by the prosecution, the defense or the court to make evaluations, prepare reports and testify. Since hypnosis may permit access to personality areas not always overt, such as motivation, unconscious process, memories, etc. it is not surprising that the services of clinicians and researchers in hypnosis have been sought.

However, the credibility of evaluations made with the use of hypnosis has had a spotted history, ranging from complete rejection to limited and restricted acceptance, and the entire domain of "forensic hypnosis" has been wracked by controversy. What can "hypnotic" interviews add to police investigations that will provide more clues for solving a crime or apprehending guilty parties? Are "memories" elicited under hypnosis better, equal to, or worse than those secured from unhypnotized individuals? What are its values, its limitations, and what safeguards must be practiced if it is employed?

Finally, why should a chapter on "Forensic Hypnosis" be included in a book on "Hypnoanalytic Techniques?" While the forensic examiner is not usually concerned with "treating" his subjects, he must often utilize "hypnoanalytic" procedures. Regression, hypermnesia, even abreactions, and dealing with amnesias or dissociations in defendants and witnesses are quite common in this area. Sometimes, under hypnotic examinations, witnesses will "break down" manifesting neurotic (or even psychotic) behavior. The practitioner must be prepared to handle such situations. That is why he/she should first of all be a well-trained and experienced scientist or clinician in the field of psychology and mental health, besides being knowledgeable in the requirements of the law.

Court Recognition of "Forensic" Hypnosis

The history of the field of "Forensic Hypnosis" might be divided into three general stages (with possibly the beginnings of a fourth one currently).

Up until about the 1960's courts simply refused to take hypnosis seriously. In two California cases (*People v. Worthington,* 1894, and *People v. Eubanks, 1897*) they refused to recognize hypnotism as a defense when the defendants claimed they committed the crimes under hypnotic compulsion.

The question as to just how much the hypnotist can influence responses of the subject is highly controversial (See Vol. 1, Chap. 15). Earlier hypnotists claimed to have strong and dominating influence over their subjects. These were exemplified by the dramatic direct-suggestive therapy of Liebeault (1866), Bernheim (1964/1886), and Janet (1907), and by dramatic demonstrations of personal "power" by stage hypnotists. Others, (Erickson, 1939; Conn, 1972; Orne, 1972) have argued that individuals cannot be suggested to do that which violated their own moral principles—such as told to engage in anti-social acts. From that viewpoint, the effects of hypnotic suggestion would seem to be considerably limited. However, in another context Orne (1979) argues that the most inadvertent word dropped before a hypnotic session or the slightest suggestive nuance of emphasis by the hypnotist can influence or modify the testimony of a witness. He believes that the memories and testimony of a hypnotized witness can be very easily contaminated by even the most indirect suggestion. Perhaps a more conservative position lies between these extremes regarding the potency of hypnotic suggestion.

Antisocial Behavior under Hypnosis

This writer had occasion to testify on several occasions in which women were apparently seduced against their will by hypnosis. In one case a police hypnotist induced some 5 different women to permit sexual liberties including intercourse under the guise of treating them for weight reduction. Not only did all five testify publicly against him, but he recorded a seductive hypnotic session with one of them on a audio tape which I heard. His induction technique and his programming of the suggestions were accomplished with extraordinary skill. He was found guilty by an investigating panel and discharged from the police force.

In a second case two different women, unknown to one another, sued the same physician for sexual seduction (and cruelty). I had the opportunity to hypnotically interview each of them some time apart. Their reports on his techniques were similar, as were their memories of the inside of his home to which he took them, hypnotized them and raped them. Both of them sued for malpractice—and each won their suit, the video-recorded hypnotic interviews being presented in evidence. Each woman required many sessions of subsequent therapy (from different therapists) to unto the damage they suffered. Rulings of confidentiality prevent a more detailed report on these two cases.

Several trials occurred during the first half of the 20th Century in which defendants claimed that they carried out their crimes under compulsions induced by hypnosis. Each time the court ruled that there was no evidence that this was possible and dismissed this defense. In a New York case (People v. Leyra, 1951) a defendant after being interviewed by a psychiatrist, confessed to murdering his parents. He claimed that his confession had been secured under hypnosis, although the physician denied using hypnosis. Other psychiatrists testified that the physician used gestures which were hypnotic, and the U.S. Supreme Court finally ruled that the confession was secured under duress.

By the mid-1960's courts were permitting examining doctors to report what they were told by defendants under hypnosis, but direct statements made by hypnotized defendants were still excluded (*State v. Harris*, 1965). A young woman was killed in an automobile accident (Kline v. Ford Motor Co., 1975). Her passenger's memory was refreshed under hypnosis, and she was permitted to testify as to these memories during a suit for damages against the Ford Motor company initiated by the deceased's estate. In California in 1979 (*People v. Colligan*) the victim of a robbery was able under hypnosis to describe her robber and to recall the license number on his car. The defense objected to her testimony on the grounds that hypnosis was used in securing it. These objections were overruled by the court, which held that the use of hypnosis to refresh memory did not invalidate such testimony.

These cases are representative of the attitudes of courts concerning the use of hypnosis during this second period following its complete earlier rejection. Interest in hypnotically-enhanced memories increased, and police examiners were trained in its use (Hibbard & Worring, 1981; Reiser, 1980).

The distortions that can occur in all eye-witness testimony became a matter of experimental research. For example, studies reported by Hilgard and Loftus (1979) demonstrated that the form of a question can make a significant effect on the kinds of responses elicited. Thus, when a hypnotized witness was asked, "Did you see *the* gun?" the individual was much more likely to say "yes" than if the question was worded as follows: "Did you see *a* gun?" These, however, are directive, specific and intended wordings, not inadvertent or "unconscious" cues. Nevertheless, most workers in this field would agree that the hypnotist is in a position to exert influence on a subject's responses and that the greatest care possible must be taken to reduce this influence to a minimum.

This second period of moderate acceptance was soon followed by a third period in which there was a drastic change in attitudes toward the use of hypnosis to enhance eye-witness testimony. In 1979 major hypnosis societies voted strong resolutions deploring the use of hypnosis by police investigators*.

Police investigators, although experienced in interrogation, are not trained in psychiatry or psychology, and might not be prepared to handle emotional disturbances in their witnesses. Moreover, the police are rewarded for apprehending criminals, not necessarily for exonerating innocent parties. Accordingly, there could be much suggestive bias in their questioning under hypnosis where suggestibility is such a potent factor. The weight of professional hypnosis opinion was such that the training of police in hypnotic interrogation has drastically declined. In an attempt to reduce the possibilities of suggestive bias when interrogating witnesses under hypnosis Orne

* (See *Int. J. Clin & Exp. Hypnosis,* Oct. 1979, pp. 452-453).

(1978) proposed minimal safeguards which were filed with the U.S. Supreme Court.

The New Jersey Supreme court (*State v. Hurd*, 1981), held that such memories are admissible providing they meet certain rigorous controls (such as those originally proposed by Orne, 1979). They have been re-stated and expanded in a Wisconsin Circuit Court opinion (*State v. White*, 1979) as follows:

1. The person administering the hypnotic session ought to be a mentally healthy person with special training in the use of hypnosis, preferably a psychiatrist or psychologist.

2. This special trained person should not be informed about the case verbally. Rather such person should receive a written memorandum outlining whatever facts are necessary to know. Care should be exercised to avoid any communication that might influence the person's opinion.

3. Said specially trained person should be an independent professional not responsible to the prosecution, investigators or the defense.

4. All contact between the specially trained person and the subject should be videotaped from beginning to end.

5. Nobody representing the police or the prosecutor or the defendant should be in the same room with the specially trained person while he is working with the subject.

6. Prior to induction a mental health professional should examine the subject to exclude the possibility that the subject is physically or mentally ill and to confirm that the subject possesses sufficient judgment, intelligence, and reason to comprehend what is happening.

7. The specially trained person should elicit a detailed description of the facts as the subject believes them to be prior to the use of hypnosis.

8. The specially trained person should strive to avoid adding any new elements to the subject's description of her/his experience, including any implicit or explicit cues during the pre-session contact, the actual hypnosis and the post-session contact.

9. Consideration should be given to any other evidence tending to corroborate or challenge the information garnered during the trance or as a result of post-hypnotic suggestion. (For a more detailed and up-to-date revision of these guidelines see Laurence and Perry [1988], pp.379-385.)

These safeguards can be highly recommended to the forensic practitioner. They should minimize the suggestive biases which can influence memories during the period of retrieval. However, they cannot always be carried out in practice. It should also be noted that such stringent safeguards are not commonly applied when a hypnotic induction is not used prior to witness interrogation. Hypnotizable and other highly suggestible witnesses can likewise be subject to suggestive bias (Loftus, 1979)—nor can we assure that a presumably "unhypnotized" subject is not in a self-hypnotized state.

However, experimental studies on eye-witness memory and on hypermnesia itself have suggested that even these safeguards may not be sufficient. Memory is "reconstructive," that is, it is not like a tape recording wherein everything that happens is recorded and reproduced when later activated (Bowers & Hilgard, 1988). A "memory" may be part veridical and part fantasy, or it may be contaminated from other memories.

When an event occurs, presumably in the presence of a witness, we can never be sure just how much of it was perceived in the first place. Second, only a part of that which was perceived may be recorded or "encoded" in the nervous system. Finally, not all that was encoded may be retrieved, either by recall or by recognition. Furthermore, at any stage of the process interference from external biasing circumstances, internal fantasies or other memories may result in the emergence of a "reconstructed" memory. This has caused some workers in the field to suggest that hypnosis should *never* be used as the basis for enhancing eye-witness testimony (Orne et al., 1988). This view is supported by a substantial number of experimental studies (See Orne, 1979; Pettinati, 1988; Relinger, 1984). It is this complete rejection of the modality for memory enhancement on the part of many researchers which constitutes the third stage in the history of "forensic hypnosis."

In line with these findings the California Supreme Court (*People v. Shirley,* 1982) reversed a rape conviction based on hypnotically refreshed testimony. It ruled further that *all* hypnotically influenced memory enhancement was lacking credibility and could not be used in testimony. Several other State Supreme Courts followed the lead of the California Court.

Hypnosis has historically vacillated between periods of boom and bust. Forensic hypnosis seems also to be undergoing extreme swings from early complete rejection, to partial acceptance, to new rejection based on recent experimental findings.

There appears to be some evidence of a very recent swing back toward reconsideration of the experimental findings (Watkins, 1989) and a partial acceptance of hypnotic memory enhancement. The U.S. Supreme Court (*Rock v. Arkansas,* 1987) ruled that hypnosis may be used to refresh testimony of witnesses when they testify in their own defense. Other courts have also been taking second looks at this matter. The Idaho Supreme Court (*State v. Iwakiri*) decided that cases must be examined individually to determine whether hypnotically refreshed testimony should be admissible in courts. The Colorado Supreme Court (*Romero v. Colorado v.*, 1987) agreed with the reasoning of the Idaho Court.

Hypnosis in the laboratory is not the same as hypnosis in clinical practice. It may be the "hypnotic relationship" plus the nature of its quality and control that will ultimately determine whether an interrogation under hypnosis is or is not credible.

Since this book is primarily about "techniques" we will not try to review the voluminous literature on this controversy. Readers are referred to the excellent reviews in Pettinati (1988) and in Laurence and Perry (1988) covering the studies on memory and hypnosis. A comprehensive coverage of court decisions related to hypnosis can be found in Udolf (1983), Orne, M.T., Dinges, D.F. and Orne, E.C. (1984), and in Scheflin and Shapiro (1989). See Watkins (1989) for a critique of flaws and biases in many of the experimental studies.

Problems in Forensic Hypnosis

Psychiatrists and psychologists are often called upon to examine and "diagnose" a defendant. The court wishes to know if he/she is "insane" or mentally competent. Also important are the motivations and perceptions which the defendant held at the time of the crime.

Hypnosis may be employed by prison psychologists to evaluate mental status of convicted criminals for the purpose of providing additional information to parole boards. Obviously the same precautions and considerations of the possibilities of securing self-serving "memories" must guide the hypno-investigator as when evaluating defendants and witnesses. This writer, in the role of a consulting prison psychologist found a wealth of data among prison inmates as to the extent to which some form of dissociation is involved in the commission of many crimes.

A black man who had never been in trouble with the law was arrested after he shot and killed a white man under a bridge. He had apparently bought a new pistol and was doing "target practice" at rocks in the river when he was accosted by the victim, who demanded that Joe (the black man) go under the bridge with him. Joe, who was normally a very meek person, acquiesced. The victim then threatened Joe and tried to take his gun away from him. Either on purpose or accidentally the gun discharged killing the white man.

Joe was examined hypnotically in the jail. Under hypnosis a very aggressive ego-state, "Bill," emerged who was entirely different from the Joe personality. Bill said that since Joe was too meek and could never defend himself, especially from white boys, he, Bill, would come out and protect Joe by administering a beating to white assailants. Bill had been "created" when Joe was a small boy.

Joe was found guilty and given a long sentence. I was called in by the prison authorities to assess the possible danger to other inmates, (white "yard bosses") who were fond of picking on Joe because of his mild "Uncle Tom" manner. The hypnotic evaluation suggested that indeed there was danger of further violence if Joe was pushed too far and Bill emerged prepared to violently kill those who teased him. This information brought a reconsideration of ward assignments.

Sometimes the hypnotic evaluation of a subject comes out much differently than anticipated by the subject, the examiner or the referring attorney. I interviewed under hypnosis a defendant who had previously served time for burglary. While in prison he became acquainted with Satanic cults, and was in conflict between this "religion" and his previous Christianity.

The defendant, "Wilson," had entered a woman's apartment, threatened her with a knife, and repeatedly "stabbed" her with small pinpoint (not deep) strokes. When hypnotized and induced to re-live the evening of the crime he reported entering a kind of trance state while sitting in a car and fixating on a flashing beer sign. At this moment a "demon," by the name of "Asmodeus" had come out and urged him to enter the woman's apartment. The small pin-point stabs represent a conflict between Asmodeus, who wanted to kill the woman, and Wilson's Christian upbringing, which was trying to stop the action.

During the hypnotic interview "Asmodeus" emerged and discussed his role in the Satanic hierarchy, naming several other "Demons" that were in Wilson. A library check of Satanic mythology disclosed that "Asmodeus" and the other "demons" mentioned were entities described in medieval lore (Baskin, 1972).

The entire 2-hour session was recorded on video tape. This tape was played to the jury at the request of the defense attorney, who hoped that it would portray his client as a victim of "demon-possession" and increase the chances for court leniency or a psychiatric acquittal. It had quite the opposite effect. Both the judge and jury were scared and horrified at the murderous statements by "Asmodeus." Although he had not actually killed anybody Wilson was convicted of deadly assault, labeled "dangerous," and sentenced to 99 years in prison without possibility of parole.

I was called in March, 1979, to hypnotically interview Kenneth Bianchi, a mild appearing young man accused of murdering two coeds in Bellingham, Washington. He claimed amnesia for the event. With great difficulty he was hypnotized whereupon a dissociated alter, "Steve," emerged. "Steve" not only claimed "credit" for the murders, but also revealed himself as the Los Angeles Hillside Strangler by bragging and pointing out all the girls which he had killed and those which his cousin, Angelo Buono had killed. During a later session in which "Steve" was activated indirectly without a formal hypnotic induction Steve and Ken were given Rorschachs separately, which were totally different from one another, as were their handwritings, their manners, their use of the language, etc.

The prosecution's position was that Bianchi had simulated both hypnosis and multiple personality, and had confessed to ten additional murders in order to establish an insanity defense. In view of the fact that Ken had repeatedly maintained he wasn't "crazy" and had finally agreed to plead insanity only at the insistence of his attorney this position is not very compelling. The controversy about this case has been debated in print (See Orne, et. al., 1984a and Watkins, 1984).

I mention cases like these because in the criticisms of hypnotic hypermnesia and regression the fact that people can lie under hypnosis is emphasized, and it is assumed that they will always try to use hypnosis to "prove" that they weren't really guilty. My experience has been quite the contrary. Hypnotized individuals often reveal their guilt, while consciously maintaining otherwise. Like a naive child they blurt-out a self-incriminating truth. Hypnosis is a regression, and regressed subjects think more concretely—like a child. Hypnosis is also a focused concentration and a restriction of the experiential field. Accordingly, the pre-censoring cautions that might warn the defendant being interviewed not to say something which could later be incriminating may not be operating very well.

Hypnosis is also dissociation, and the recollection regarding one's culpable actions may be dissociated from the defensive controls which would inhibit its expression or produce outright lying. Yes, hypnotized subjects can lie. It is no "truth serum." But hypnotized subjects are probably less likely to lie than unhypnotized ones. Even in the treatment situation hypnosis is used to penetrate defenses and activate repressed material that creates cognitive dissonance and anxiety. It can do no less in the forensic situation where the defenses are conscious.

For example, a defendant, "Henry," while driving on a country road struck another car head on. The wife of the other car's driver was killed. The driver of that car claimed that the defendant was driving on the wrong side of the road. Henry claimed otherwise. I was asked to "regress" Henry to the accident and get him to relive it. Under hypnosis he described in great detail driving down the road, the approaching car, and his reactions. It was clear to me and to Henry's attorney that he was indeed driving on the wrong side of the road. The attorney induced Henry to plead "guilty" and throw himself on the mercy of the court.

In another case a young man, "Ned," had been convicted of murdering a service station operator and had been sentenced to prison. Several years later he applied for parole, and his attorney presented the defense that he had not intended to pull the trigger of the gun, but that it had fired accidentally during the hold-up. Under hypnosis Ned relived the crime with great detail. But just before the shot, as Ned turned toward the victim, he could be heard on the tape to whisper softly to himself, "Kill the son of a bitch." We amplified the sound and played the tape many times over. The whisper was quite clear. The attorney's reaction? "Thank you, Dr. Watkins, we won't be needing you to testify at the hearing."

Sometimes, even in civil actions, the mental status of one of the parties becomes an issue on which hypnosis can throw some light. In one such case evaluated by the writer, a man who had previously been known as an alcoholic ran into another car which was pulling a trailer up onto the highway. He sustained severe injuries, and the woman who was riding with him, as well as an elderly man who was driving the other car and his son, were killed. He was the only survivor of the accident. He claimed amnesia for the entire episode from the day before until several days later in the hospital. Two actions were simultaneously pending in court: 1) a suit by him for damages against the estate of the elderly man and 2) a criminal charge against him for drunken driving. A blood alcohol test made on him in the hospital was inconclusive because the competence of the technician who ran the test was in question.

The defendant was hypnotized and, after being regressed to a number of earlier periods in his life, was brought up to the day of the accident. He recalled drinking a half can of beer and then setting out for a trip to a destination 100 miles away accompanied by the woman. During this hypnotic re-living, he apparently recalled many details of their conversation, the exact turns and buildings that were passed, in a way which evidenced no disturbances of perception, speech or cognition such as might be expected from a drunken driver. The regression was so vivid that he shouted a warning to his companion on seeing the other car drive up onto the road, and at the "moment of impact" he shot out of his seat onto the floor. Many of the details recalled were corroborated by police reports and other observations on his actions prior to the beginning of the trip.

Next week, a group of six lawyers, his own and five representing the estate of the elderly man, together heard the tape recording of the session, at the end of which the estate's attorneys agreed there was no evidence of drunkenness and settled for $10,000 damages. The following Wednesday the criminal trial started. Evidence that the elderly man's estate had already settled for damages was not permitted. I was asked to describe what had been reported and "re-lived" under hypnosis, but a playing of the tape was not allowed. The jury chose to believe the controversial laboratory report and not the hypnotic report. The man was declared guilty of manslaughter, but the judge sentenced him only to three months in jail and three months in the alcoholic ward of the State Hospital. Other factors which might have influenced the verdict was the fact that the woman accompanying was not his wife but his mistress, and there was strong community sentiment against him. The case illustrates a situation in which hypnosis helped to resolve a civil suit but did not prevent a criminal conviction involving the same case.

The hypnotic "techniques" for interrogating witnesses or defendants and for efforts to improve memory do not differ from those described in earlier chapters. However, since contaminated memories and inaccurate testimony can have a profound impact, sometimes that of life or death, the forensic examiner using hypnosis must adhere strictly to the safeguards and controls described so as to minimize the sources of bias. Mistakes in this area cannot generally be rectified as they can during therapy. And one must always keep in mind that the validity of hypermnesia itself is currently subject to much criticism and controversy. I do not agree that experimental research has yet proved conclusively that hypnotic memory enhancement should be eliminated in forensic examinations (Watkins,

1989). But I do agree that these studies have placed on the examiner who uses hypnosis to "refresh" memories the burden of proof as to the validity of his findings.

Interrogation of Witnesses

Witnesses may manifest both conscious and unconscious resistance to being hypnotically interviewed. Sometimes this stems from fears about hypnosis itself, in which case the hypnotist will employ all the reassurance and prior explanations possible, such as are described in Chapters 4-7. Real anxiety may also result from a fear of personal harm at disclosing incriminating evidence against the criminal. Witnesses need all the protection possible, from both realistic and unrealistic fears if they are to become hypnotizable and render significant contributions.

The emotional re-living of an assault by a victim may be too traumatic. The subject breaks off the session by emerging suddenly and spontaneously from hypnosis. Or he/she may become so upset that the session must be terminated in the interests of the witnesses' welfare. Special care must be exercised by the examiner in rape cases. Emphasis should be placed on identification of the attacker, not the details of his crime—except in those aspects which will provide the police with valuable leads or enhance the credibility of the witness during possible future testifying in court. Here, especially, does the tact and sensitivity required of professional psychotherapists pay off. That is why fully-qualified mental health professionals should be doing the hypnotizing.

In many cases, however, the chief interrogator is not necessarily the individual who handles the hypnosis. The hypnotist, a psychologist or psychiatrist, induces the hypnotic state and then instructs the subject that the police interrogator wishes to ask some questions. Suggestions can be given that the subject will want to cooperate and will turn to the mental health practitioner in case any disturbance or problem arises. This format should be followed when the hypnotist is prepared to handle the emotional and personal aspects of the induction, but is not skilled in criminal interrogation.

The emotional impact of revivifying a terrifying scheme can be mitigated by changing it from subject to object. This involves a partial dissociation. Instead of instructing the individual to *re-live* the event, or even to *remember* it, the suggestion is given that he will see it happening as if on a movie screen. He himself will not feel the emotions of the moment, but will watch a person on that screen (who looks like himself) experience the event. This technique has also been used in hypnoanalytic therapy when the patient is not ready to re-experience a traumatic event in its full emotional impact. It is similar to "intellectual insight" vs. genuine experiential insight. As a protection to a seriously traumatized individual, the technique is probably warranted. However, most competent practitioners would feel that a full re-living in which no aspects, effective or otherwise, have suppressed is more likely to approximate the truth.

A number of manipulator suggestions have been offered in the interest of gaining more detail. These involve asking the subject to "stop the clock" and have him look at a "still-life" image of the criminal's face or clothing. Sometimes he is asked to "reverse the tape" and play over again the experience. Definitive research has not yet ascertained whether such manipulations create distortions in the memories. Orne (1979) holds that this involves "putting great pressure on the subject to produce something" and thus may impel him more to confabulation if he did not really have adequate perception to support his "memories" in the first place. It would seem that this is a fruitful area for researchers in the field of forensic hypnosis, but for the present considerable caution must be exercised. It is still best to consider hypnotically derived data as hypotheses which should be supported by corroborating evidence from other sources, neither to be accepted as "the truth" nor to be discarded unless proven invalid. Internal consistency may permit greater weight to be given to such evidence, but it should be remembered that thoughts and perceptions once spoken have a way of persisting, even if they are in error. Repetition and self-suggestion can alone be fixating.

Hypnoanalytic Techniques to Induce Hypermnesia

Assuming that one is attempting to elicit memories about a certain past event what steps would be optimal to achieve that aim? First, of course, one secures all possible conscious memories of that situation. Sometimes there is a genuine amnesia because of severe trauma at that time (See Chap 8). In most cases the material is simply forgotten, not repressed or dissociated. After the induction of hypnosis the subject is regressed back to times prior to the event in question, perhaps even to childhood., Regression tends to deepen the hypnosis. Gradually one moves the memory experiences toward the key moment, the day before, that morning, an hour before, a few minutes before, etc. Finally, one tries to describe the situation as vividly as possible as one had learned it from the subject's conscious report.

"It is June 15, 1983. You are waiting in front of the First National Bank. What can you see on the street? What does the entrance to the bank look like?" etc. The aim is to try and reinstate the moment and the"ego state" which was executive at that particular time. Only after you think the subject is actually in that experiential moment do you non-directively question, "What's happening?"

Sometimes it is desirable to switch subject-object by telling him that, "You can see a person standing in front of the bank. He will watch that person who is observing the entrance of the bank. What is happening." If the subject was traumatized by a bank holdup distancing him can sometimes improves the memory. Don't push. If he did not get a good view of the color of the car, and the forensic examiner pushes, he may get a response which came from some movie the subject recently saw of a bank holdup. Occasionally the subject under hypnosis can be reminded that it is easy to make errors. Perhaps he can be asked to "try" different colors on the get-away car and see which one "sticks." In extreme cases Cheek's finger signal method (Rossi and Cheek, 1989) may work better than asking questions to be answered verbally.

The successful finding of lost objects or missing pieces of information through hypnotically-induced hypermnesia has been reported on a number of occasions: the license number of a kidnaper's car, as a consequence of which 26 school children were rescued (Kroger and Douce, 1979), the make and color of a rapist's car which resulted in his apprehension (Lundy, 1987), a piece of lost jewelry (Kluft, 1987a), a lost book (Watkins, 1946). Obviously failure attempts were not re- ported— and I have had my share. But the clear successes argue that hypermnesia has not yet been written off in spite of the negative experimental studies, (Watkins, 1989).

The Simulation of Dissociation

Guilty defendants may attempt to simulate multiple personality or some variant of dissociation in order to get a "psychiatric acquittal." Although most experts in the field do not believe multiple personality can be successfully simulated there are times when the examiner is asked to rule out this possibility. Most commonly the attempt is made to show that the individual is simulating "hypnosis" and hence, since they are closely related, multiple personality also.

Tests for the reality of hypnosis might include the following:

The Double Hallucination Test

A deeply hypnotized individual is asked to hallucinate a person he knows standing in front of him. He is next shown the real person standing behind him, "And then who is this?" "Reals" tend to look back and forth between the two images, the hallucinated person and the real one, and acknowledge seeing both. (Blum and Graef, 1971; Orne, 1979). This is based on the concept of "trance logic" whereby the truly hypnotized person is willing to accept and deal with the inconsistency. Simulators rarely do, and since they have already committed themselves to perceiving the hallucination may even deny seeing the real person. Reals also often report seeing the hallucinated one as blurred or transparent (Sheehan, 1977). Thus the "Hillside Strangler," Kenneth Bianchi, reported seeing his hallucinated attorney as, "The images weren't clear. It was like looking at a strobe light."

The Circle-Touch Test

A circle is drawn on the palm or forearm of a subject. He is hypnotized and given suggestions that there will be no feeling inside the circle. The subject is then given a catch-22 question. "When I touch you outside the circle where you can feel it, you say "Yes." When I touch you inside the circle where you cannot feel it, you say "No." "Reals" were predicted to manifest trance logic by responding "No" when touched inside. Simulators, recognizing the incongruity, were presumed to make no response when touched inside.

However, Eiblmayr (1987), in apparently the only objective, experimental study, found quite the opposite. When permitted to give a "No response" response as well as a "Yes" or "No" highly susceptibles (reals) gave a "No response" response because they didn't feel the touch stimulus at all, since the area had been truly anesthetized. The test differentiated simulators from moderately susceptibles but not from highly susceptibles — and in the opposite direction predicted.

The Source Amnesia Test

Subjects are taught under hypnosis certain obscure facts such as that amethysts, when heated, turned yellow. Good hypnotic subjects, while unable to recall events that transpired under hypnosis, were, on coming out, still able to answer questions about it correctly. However, they did not know the source or confabulated one. This procedure has been found (Evans, 1979); Evans & Thorn, 1966) to differentiate simulators from "reals."

The Ammonia Test for Simulation

Hibbard and Worring (1981) have suggested a procedure as follows: A subject is shown an after-shave lotion bottle which contains ammonia. A casual remark is made that, "I might show you some interesting things that can be done with your sense of smell under hypnosis." A "real" will react pleasantly: a liar will try to cover up. I have used a variant of this technique by asking the hypnotized subject to smell this "beautiful perfume." The deeply hypnotized individual will apparently enjoy the smell. The unhypnotized person will react with immediate avoidance to the ammonia.

There is probably no single test yet which will take the place of long and consistent study to determine the possibilities of lying or simulation. However, Blum & Graef (1971) reported that in a small sample (2 simulators and 4 "reals") they could distinguish the simulators clearly from the reals by the difference score on the *Stroop Color-Word Test* (See Jensen, 1965). This procedure looks promising but needs more confirming research and will not be described here. Blum and Graef did conclude that simulators could not resist being discovered when studied over a period of time.

Confidence and Accuracy of Memory

Hypnotized subjects report their "memories" with much confidence. Perhaps this is because of the focusing and narrowing of attention, a characteristic of hypnosis. Doubts and consideration of alternatives (or views of other ego states not executive at that time) are simply ablated. Accordingly, we should not be surprised that even when witnesses' memories are contaminated and faulty they still express much confidence in them. In fact, research has rather clearly shown (Sheehan, 1988), that the confidence with which a witness defends hypnotically-secured memories bears no relationship to the accuracy of the material. It is important, therefore, that the examiner not allow his subject's confidence to convince him that the recovered memory is true—as unfortunately so often happens in the courtroom.

There is little evidence that hypnosis *per se* distorts memory, but because of its suggestive qualities errors and biases introduced to subjects during or even prior to hypnosis tend to be perpetuated. Distortions of memory can occur out of hypnosis as well as within it and, as Bowers and Hilgard (1988) have pointed out, "considerable care is needed to avoid attributing to hypnosis problems that really belong to the domain of memory *per se.*

There is considerable evidence (Erdelyi, 1988) that hypnosis produces increased memory materials, both accurate and inaccurate. That is why its greatest use may be in producing leads for police investigators. The conflict lies in permitting its use during police investigation and then trying to rule it out when the subject whose hypnotically-elicited leads materially assisted that investigation is not permitted later to testify in court.

While accepting the fact that memories can be created and altered under hypnosis, the extent to which this is done inadvertently and by subtle and indirect cues has not been researched. To assume that this is a continuous and potent source of influence is to believe that the human organism is a helpless pawn when hypnotized, that it has no integrity but is subject to change on the slightest whim of the hypnotist. Research which could truly show under what conditions specifically false memories are created or altered would be of immense help to the discipline of forensic hypnosis. And if experimental studies could provide techniques whereby created memories could be un-done and turned back to relatively realistic memories, then, indeed, would we approach a true science.

Police Artist Sketches Drawn with the Help of Hypnosis

Remembered perceptions elicited under hypnosis may be of value to the composite artist who provides sketches of a possible criminal. The procedure usually is to have the witness consciously supply as many remembered details of the criminal's appearance first. During hypnosis it is important that the artist non-directively question the witness, but that he not be too specific so as to avoid suggesting changes that were not originally the sole idea of the witness. The role of the hypnotist at this time should be to keep the artist from becoming too suggestive in his questioning. Such sessions are often long in duration and it may be necessary to re-hypnotize or deepen several times during them.

Publicity

Since hypnosis is of high interest to the public, practitioners of forensic hypnosis may expect inquiries from newspaper, radio and TV reporters, often with the intention of sensationalizing their procedures or findings. The practitioner should be forewarned of the need for caution when talking to the press, or he may find himself embarrassed by lurid headlines. Often, especially after a case comes to court action, he may be enjoined to confidentiality by a judge's decree. However, reporters for some of the more sensational newspapers or journals are quite skilled in securing reactions to a prominent trial. If, in fact, the guesses of the reporter are substantially correct, the expert witness may be drawn unwittingly into disclosing that which should be confidential. Many news reporters are ethical, sincere and can be trusted, and represent papers or journals who are known for factual reporting. But it should not be forgotten that the job of a reporter is to get a story. When in doubt, the best reaction to an inquiry is simply, "no comment."

The Practitioner of Forensic Hypnosis as an Expert Witness

The rights, obligations and cautions which apply to any expert witness apply to the forensic specialist—as well as a few additional ones. A hypnotherapist who wishes to enter the field of forensic hypnosis would be well advised to understand the pitfalls encountered in this field and to become familiar with court procedure.

Most practitioners would prefer to serve as a "Friend of the Court," hence, be responsible to the judge and to neither of the opposing parties. However, it is more likely that one's services will have been employed by the prosecution or the defense in a criminal action, or by one of the contesting parties in a civil action. Accordingly, one is confronted with a dilemma. Ethically he is required to be as objective as possible, and in court to tell the truth, the whole truth and nothing but the truth. On the other hand, he is being employed by a party which wishes most strongly that the information he can elicit and the evidence he gives support a point of view. Subtle pressures are placed on the expert witness to arrive at the desired conclusions. Since all witnesses are human, this kind of pressure can influence even the most righteous. It is human to see what we want to see. And it is also human to see what our associates and employers want us to see.

Scientific integrity backed by a firm system of ethics is essential in the expert witness. The willingness constantly to question one's own findings, to modify one's point of view in the face of new evidence and the ability to defer judgment may not be always what is wanted by one's employing attorney, but it is a value which we should strive for— especially the expert witness who is inquiring deeply into mental processes and is in a position to influence those processes.

When the facts elicited under hypnosis do not correspond to views of one's employing attorney, these should be resolutely and forcefully shared with that attorney and only with the attorney who has employed one. The information may be of great value to the other side, but the side which has employed the expert witness has the right to that knowledge. It may well be that, after being informed of the expert's findings, the side which employed him will not call him as a witness nor use his reports further. This can cause an economic loss at times, but the witness is rewarded by the knowledge that he has maintained his integrity, that he cannot be bought. In the long run professional integrity will pay off since the expert witness' credibility will be increasingly recognized by attorneys, courts, and juries.

Testifying in Court

A quality product still may not sell if poorly packaged and advertised. The attorney to whom one is responsible is well aware of the fact that many an expert witness has been "shot down" because of poor preparation or an unconvincing appearance on the witness stand. Prior to court appearance, the attorney will coach his expert witness as to what questions he intends to ask and as to what questions may be anticipated from the opposing side during the cross examination. The attorney will want (if he has not requested this before) a fairly complete vita showing degrees, honors, recognitions, publications, membership in scientific societies, listings in who's who publications, past relevant training and experience. He must first qualify his witness as truly an "expert." Expert witnesses are allowed to give opinions not permitted of non-experts. Furthermore, the attorney will endeavor to establish a prestige position for his witness in the eyes of the jury. Following his initial presentation, the judge will usually ask the opposing side if it is willing to accept the credentials of this individual as an "expert" in the field.

Most hypnotic practitioners who are doctoral trained, have taken substantial courses in the field, and are affiliated with one or more of the major scientific hypnosis societies (such as the Society for Clinical and Experimental Hypnosis or the American Society of Clinical Hypnosis) will seldom be challenged as to their expertness. If their credentials are lacking or borderline, they may expect the opposing side to ask searching questions, to seek out weaknesses, and to raise objection—which will be resolved by decision of the judge.

Once expertness in the field of hypnosis has been established, one's attorney will then proceed to ask questions about the examination of the witness, defendants or individuals involved, to present the findings and to render his opinions about these findings. The expert witness should remember that even though he is answering questions from an attorney he is at all times really speaking to the judge and jury. They are the ones who will accept or reject his testimony. They will weigh it against that of others; and they will make the final decision. It is, therefore, wise to address many of one's replies to the jury by looking at them in a firm but friendly manner and stating one's findings in a clear and confident voice.

Following the direct examination by one's attorney, the attorney for the opposing side will begin the cross examination. One should never forget that, if one's previous testimony has been favorable to the side represented by one's employing attorney, the opposition will do all possible to discredit it. That is the nature of the adversary theory of justice. Accordingly, one can expect to have one's experience and training belittled, one's inconsistencies amplified and one's opinions discredited. Sometimes these questions are given with a deferential air or even flattery in the hope that the expert witness will feel pleased and will make statements which can be held against him later. Sometimes the questions are most unflattering and designed to arouse one's anger, so that the witness will lose his composure, become flustered, and appear in a bad light before the jury.

Many years ago, before Ph.D. psychologists were generally accepted as expert witnesses, an opposing attorney asked this writer the following question: "Mr. Watkins, are you licensed to practice medicine in the State of Washington?" The expert witness can expect that the period of cross examination will be an ordeal and recognize that he must maintain the highest degree of alertness if his testimony is to stand up in the eyes of the jury. A general attitude of courteous but firm response and a refusal to become angry usually adds to one's credibility.

If a crucial issue in a case hangs upon hypnotically-derived testimony, the opposing attorney will usually have prepared himself by bringing difficult questions about hypnosis to ask. He may even have his own hypnosis "expert" ready to testify in opposition to you.

Questions such as the following may be expected: "Doctor, can all people be hypnotized?" "How do you know that you actually hypnotized the witness?" "Can people tell lies under hypnosis?" "Can individuals be made to commit crimes under hypnosis?" "What is the scientific evidence that...?" "Are you aware of the findings of Dr. ...?" "In your earlier testimony you stated that...Now you say that...How do you account for the contradiction in your testimony?" "Is it true that under hypnosis people will...? Answer yes or no." "Isn't it true that research shows...?"

Often questions are so framed that one cannot answer a clear "yes" or "no" without doing violence to the truth. A qualified answer is required. If one's own attorney does not raise proper objection so that the question must be re-framed in a more acceptable form, one can appeal to the judge, stating that a qualified answer is required if one is to answer truthfully. The judge is supposed to be fair and objective, and will decide whether a question is or is not properly put.

Summary

The police, courts, attorneys, correctional officers and parole boards will welcome any scientific discipline which can assist in the proper disposal and adjudication of legal problems. Accordingly, clinical practitioners in hypnosis can expect to have requests made for their services. However, while sophistication and skill in clinical hypnotherapy is a prerequisite for qualified practice in forensic hypnosis, this alone is not sufficient. The practitioner should be well versed in the relevant court rulings and decisions made concerning hypnosis, the safeguards and controls in its applications—especially when used to refresh memories, skills in investigative interrogation, court procedures, and effective manners of presentation as an expert witness.

The controversy as to the extent to which anti-social behavior can be hypnotically suggested is still open, but a number of reports indicate that this is possible with some subjects. This is related to the whole question as to just how much influence does the hypnotist have, and to what extent can he/she modify behavior and bias memories.

Any and all of the hypnoanalytic techniques dealt with in previous chapters may be employed in the practice of "forensic" hypnosis. However, their application requires special attention to recommended safeguards and controls to minimize suggestive bias.

The question of the use of memory enhancement through hypnosis is today quite controversial. Experimental studies have questioned its validity and have shown that a subject's confidence in his hypnotically-enhanced memories bears no relation to its correctness, but the research design, validity and freedom from bias in many of those studies have themselves been criticized. Hypnosis has been used to assist police artists in constructing sketches of possible suspects.

Forensic examiners are often asked to assist in arriving at a diagnosis of defendants and to testify as to their perceptions and motivations at the time of an alleged crime. Tests for lying or simulation include the "double hallucination" test, the"circle-touch" test, the "source-amnesia" test and the "ammonia" test.

Forensic hypnosis is a developing field with its possibilities and limitations for assisting the police and the courts still in the process of being determined. It does differ from therapeutic hypnosis in many ways. Its aim is evaluation and diagnosis, not treatment. Yet even here there are significant similarities with therapy. Both seek to understand an individual, and both use that understanding to achieve ways of dealing with that person. In therapeutic hypnosis our goal is change within an individual for his own personal betterment. In forensic hypnosis we employ many of these same "understanding procedures" but in the cause of "justice" and the protection of society. One is for a change designed primarily to benefit the individual, in the other it is for society as a whole. In therapeutic hypnosis the examiner-therapist, after the "understanding," is the primary "change agent." In forensic hypnosis it will be the police and the courts who act upon such "understandings" to achieve socially-desirable goals.

Yet in the final analysis both the forensic examiner and the psychotherapist are concerned with real, live humans, complex organisms who exist though motivation, learning and emotion, conscious and unconscious. As behavioral scientists we must deal with the reality of life and the meanings of that existence as it is manifested within people and between people.

Both forensic and clinical practitioners must accept the limitation that, regardless of objective research findings, regardless of their own knowledges and skills, they will always be confronted with possibilities, but hopefully sometimes with probabilities.. And as humans working with humans we need constantly to remind ourselves that people are not "things" to be manipulated.

It is appropriate, therefore, that in the next and last chapter of this work we consider some fundamental questions related to our own therapeutic selves and to the quality of life which we with our "techniques," forensic, therapeutic, hypnotic or analytic must address if we are to achieve constructive changes in our clients' relations with themselves and with others.

Chapter 11. Forensic Hypnosis

Outline

1. Forensic hypnosis as a new and developing field.

2. Should be practiced by qualified clinicians and scientists trained in legal and court procedures.

3. Stages in the courts' attitudes towards hypnosis.
   a. Complete rejection prior to 1960's.
   b. Partial acceptance with reservations during 1970's.
      (1) Period of over-enthusiasm. Police trained to use hypnosis.
   c. Experimental studies questioning validity of hypermnesia.
      (1) Rejection by California Supreme Court and others.
   d. U.S. Supreme Court permits use by a defendant in own defense.
      (1) Several State courts determine possible acceptance on a case by case basis.

4. Orne publishes minimal safeguards when "enhancing memory" of witnesses.

5. Differences between "laboratory" hypermnesia and "clinical" hypermnesia.

6. Hypnoanalytic techniques to induce hypermnesia.

7. Antisocial behavior controversial. Newer studies report cases.

8. Tests for the simulation of hypnosis.
   a. The double hallucination test.
   b. The circle touch test.
   c. The source amnesia test.
   d. The ammonia test.

9. Sketches of suspects drawn by police artists from descriptions by hypnotized witnesses.

10. Problems of the practitioner of forensic hypnosis.
    a. Publicity.
    b. Testifying in court.
       (1) The direct examination.
       (2) The cross examination.

Chapter 12

Existential Hypnoanalysis and the Therapeutic Self

The new patient slumped into the easy chair.

"What seems to be the trouble, " inquired the therapist?

"Well, nothing I guess," replied the patient slowly.

"Then why are you here?"

"You know Doc, I really don't know. I have everything, a good wife, children, an excellent income, big house, two cars paid for, a cabin at the lake, job security, nothing to worry about, and I'm really happy. Its just—well it's just that I don't seem to get much of a kick out of life. I build things in the shop. My wife and I play tennis at the club. No sexual frustrations. The kids are in college. We're thinking about a round-the-world sailing cruise next year—but there's something missing."

The wheels inside the therapist's head started spinning. Low level depression? Borderline? Maybe an obsessive-compulsive personality? Silently he reviewed the many diagnostic categories found in the DSM III. None of them seemed to fit. Why would an apparently happy and successful person come to a psychotherapist merely because he wasn't getting "a kick" out of life.

The usual suggestions passed through his mind: medical check-up, diet, jogging, more "together" activities, join an organization, meet new people, change work, get a hobby, start a garden, become involved in community activities, church, politics, etc., etc.? None of these seemed to fit either. How come?

Psychotherapists are being increasingly confronted today with patients who don't show the classic anxieties, conversional symptoms and psychosomatic disorders for which treatment strategies have been primarily developed. True, more low-level depressions are being uncovered, while schizoid and borderline characters are diagnosed with greater frequency. But increasing numbers of people today are manifesting a kind of ennui with life, individuals who according to present societal standards "have it made." They don't demonstrate clear-cut "symptoms," such that they can be regarded as "sick." Somehow they are a product of a general cultural malaise, in a society which has everything, one in which most of life's frustrations can be gratified, where there is a pill for every symptom, but a lack of challenge. Our fore-fathers struggled against a hostile nature, starvation, a harsh environment, disease and unfriendly natives to wrest a continent from a wilderness. They were often defeated, but they were never bored.

Today, we are confronted with a cultural deficiency. We have "things," but we lack "souls." With the greatest number of conveniences, labor-saving devices, activities and luxuries of any society that every existed, we have the most number of "bored" people. As therapists, analysts, "human engineers" we have many skills for enhancing perceptions, improving motivations, integrating dissociations and developing understanding through suggestion, reinforcement, interpretation, plus numerous other devices. We are strengthened by our knowledge of unconscious processes and our facilitative techniques of clinical hypnosis. But can we do something about improving the "quality of life." We have the "psychological tweezers" for removing a fly from the soup. Can we also enhance the taste of the soup. Must we only "eliminate the negative," or can we also, as suggested in an old song, "accentuate the positive," and add to the zest for living?

For many people there is a lack of "meaning" in their life's activities. They interact with others, have affairs, listen to TV evangelists, donate to causes and seek therapists. There is no dearth of stimulation. They have developed object representations, and they also have self representations, but somehow the two just don't contact each other significantly enough.

Man has always wrestled with the problem of his own existence. This area has been addressed by existential philosophers, like Kierkegaard (1954), Heidegger (1949), Marcel (1948), Buber (1970), and Tillich (1952). And we can go back to the classical "debate" between Locke (1963), who felt that reality existed in external objects—in "matter," Berkeley (1929), who noted that external reality would not exist unless there was the self of a perceiver—hence mind, and Hume (1963), the skeptic, who used these arguments to "prove" that neither mind nor matter existed, thus bringing philosophy to a nihilism that required the rescue of Kant (1934), who questioned the validity of a "pure reason" that destroys its own self.

The question of what is real, what exists, what has "meaning" became the focus in the mid-20th century of a group of therapists who developed a school of psychological treatment known as "humanistic," that contrasted with the behavioral and psychoanalytic approaches.

Emphasis was put on the role of "the self" in human adjustment and the ability of patients to heal themselves with minimal intervention and control by the therapist. Humanistic-existential approaches to treatment were proposed by Bugental (1967), Satir (1967), Burton (1972), Shostrom (1967) and Jourard (1971). These writers emphasized the encouragement of "authenticity" in the therapist and "spontaneity" in the patient—usually called "a client" to de-emphasize the concept of "illness." They drew inspiration from the writings of John Dewey (1916), who, railing against the wide-spread authoritarianism in schools, advocated a liberal and democratic approach to education which stressed more permissiveness and freedom for students to develop their own interests. The mood was toward less parent-control, less teacher-control, and less therapist-control. Human behavior was to be improved more by the development of inner (self) resources than by the control of outer stimuli—as advocated by the behaviorists. Some psychoanalysts, Perls (1969), Erich Fromm (1973) and Erikson (1964), began turning more attention toward the development rather than the analysis of inner processes. The pendulum was moving from a focus on "interpersonal" relationships toward one on "intra-personal" relationships.

May (1958), attempting some integration between the two, proposed three areas of existence, an *Umwelt*, the external or "around world," (the physical environment) a *Mitwelt*, the world of interpersonal relationships, hence, a "with-world," and an *Eigenwelt*, the "own-world" of self.

From this perspective when we use hypnotic suggestion directed at a patient's external behavior we are intervening in his Umwelt. When we interpret his transference in a hypnoanalytic relationship we are dealing with his Mitwelt. And when we are developing self and object representations to establish ego boundaries we are re-fashioning his Eigenwelt. Each is a kind of reality which can have "meaning" to the patient in the different spheres of his existence.

Existential hypnoanalysis is not some new therapeutic technique which should have a devoted group of disciples, ("I am an Existential Hypnoanalyst.") It is a perspective and a therapeutic goal where the object of our interventions is not merely a "symptom," but rather an approach which aims at enhancing "meaning-in-living" for our bored patients. When Baker (1983), Copeland (1986) and Murray-Jobsis (1984) hypnotically helped their psychotic patients to establish stable ego boundaries, so that self and object representations could meaningfully contact one another, they were practicing existential hypnoanalysis. When Federn (1952) taught his schizophrenics to distinguish between Reality A and Reality B, he, too was practicing existential analysis, although he didn't label it as such.

Once I (Watkins, 1967b) tried to interest behavior therapists in an approach which treated "meaning" as a behavior, a behavior which could be enhanced if its discovery was "reinforced" with therapist praise—as well as by the natural reinforcement that insightful discoveries always receive. It was an attempt to "integrate" two very different therapeutic languages. The paper, although presented internationally, appealed unfortunately to neither humanistic editors nor behavioral editors. It was not published.

The humanistic movement featured such innovators as Rogers (1961), who called our attention to the inherent strengths in the human self, which, when not molested with excessive therapist direction, could through its own resources make significant steps toward new insights and integrations. However, the stereotypes of hypnosis as necessarily being a directive approach tended to alienate Rogerian non-directive or "client-centered" practitioners. I suggested to one devoted disciple of Rogers that he try practicing non-directive therapy under hypnosis. He looked at me in astonishment and replied, "Why, they're the exact opposite. In hypnosis you suggest and direct. We never do that in client-centered therapy."

Once induced, hypnosis is simply an altered state within an intensive relationship setting. There is nothing inherent in hypnosis that requires us to be suggestive and "directive." The ease with which suggestions can be made operative in hypnosis is seductive to the practitioner whose counter-transference needs for controlling others gains encouragement. However, the principles and approaches practiced by non-directive, client-centered therapy can be equally applied under hypnosis if desired. Volney Faw, a professor at Lewis and Clark College practiced Rogerian non-directive therapy with hypnotized clients most successfully•. He utilized the techniques of reflecting feeling ("You feel that your father is hostile toward you"), and the clarification of meanings ("As I understand it, you are telling me that you can't really trust him"), which were advocated by Rogers (1951)—but under hypnosis. His experiences with this approach were apparently not published.

It was from the contributions of this group of philosophers and therapists, and the theories of Paul Federn (1952), plus his own experience with patients, that this writer attempted to apply hypnosis in the implementation of a more humanistic approach to treatment (Watkins, 1967a) and coined the term "Therapeutic Self" (Watkins, 1978).

The Therapeutic Self

Psychotherapy may be studied as science but it is practiced as an art. And in spite of the titles of these two texts, "Hynotherapeutic Techniques" and "Hypnoanalytic Techniques," the techniques are not as important as the "self" of the clinician who practices them. Two equally-trained young resident doctors were rotated on the medical wards of a Veterans Administration Hospital. Wherever Dr. Y was assigned ward morale was excellent and healing took place, be it on the genito-urinary, cardiac or gastro-intestinal wards. However, when, after three months, he was replaced on these same wards by Dr. X. morale dropped. Urinary infections proved more stubborn, complaints of anginal pain were more frequent, and ulcers flared. These two young doctors had both graduated from the University of Oregon Medical School, had equal training, and were ranked comparably among their classmates. Yet Dr. Y had something, which Dr. X lacked, a "therapeutic self."

*Resonance**

What constitutes a therapeutic self? Can we tell who has it, and who not? And how can it be developed in young healing-arts personnel? The theories of Federn (1952) have a contribution to make here. They revolve around the concept of "resonance." Resonance is that

---

• Personal communications and discussions.
* The concept of "resonance" is dealt with in much greater detail in Watkins (1978), Chapter 15

inner experience within a therapist during which he co-feels, (co-enjoys, co-suffers) and co-understands with his patient, though in mini-form. It is a relationship, but not an object relationship. It is a "subject" or self-relationship, one in which he commits himself as a full-fledged ally with his patient. When resonating, the therapist replicates within his own ego as close as he can a facsimile of the other's experiential world—considering the limitations of communication, verbal, postural, etc, and identifies with that replica. When the patient is sad, he, too, is sad. When the patient is successful, he participates in the resulting joy. When treating another he involves himself in a kind of "with-ness." At the moment he is able to experience the patient's world as does the patient. Resonance, therefore, is a temporary identification established for purposes of better understanding the internal motivations, feelings and attitudes of a patient. Resonance describes from an inner, experiential point of view the term "modeling," as employed by behaviorists.

Rogers (1961) has used the term, "accurate empathy." This seems to be very close to "resonance." However, although Rogers defined it as where, "the counselor is perceiving the hates and hopes and fears of the client through immersion in an empathic process," he then delimits empathy by adding, "*without himself* experiencing those hates and hopes and fears." Rogers, apparently, conceived empathy as an "understanding process," but not as a fully "co-experiencing process," as subsumed by the term "resonance." Resonance assumes that we cannot fully understand a process merely by observing it from the outside, as an object. Some understanding is certainly acquired in this way. But a more complete apprehension requires a participation by the therapist (if only in mini form), not merely an outside observing.

Although resonance is relationship it should be clearly distinguished from transference. In transference we impact our object representations by clothing them with the "psychological garments" of our parents or other early, significant figures, and we respond to them as if they were such. In resonance we co-exist with the internalization of the patient as if it is our own self, not as an object. The image of them is now included within our own ego boundaries as part of our self and is sensed in the same way as we experience our own self.

Resonance can be differentiated into "affective resonance," and "cognitive resonance." Resonance as a whole can be objectively rated by individuals listening to taped recordings of therapy sessions. In fact, an objective scoring system for evaluating these phenomena has been developed and submitted to some experimental validation (See Watkins, 1978, Part IV).

Groups of raters, using this scale, scored therapist responses classified as resonant (R), objective (O), and simply facilitative (F). The percentages in each category were determined for published, session recordings of five therapists: Albert Ellis, Carl Rogers, John Cameron, Franz Alexander and John Watkins. However, lest it be assumed that the "best therapists" are those who manifest the greatest amount of resonance another equally important consideration must be taken into account.

If a therapist immerses himself 100% into the patient's feelings and understandings he will not be able to help that one achieve more objectivity in life. There will now be a *folie a deux*, and the two will be sick together. A therapist can understand a patient through both resonance and objectivity, often differently, since these represents two different perspectives, the internal and the external. If the therapist is only "objective" he will not understand the patient's world as does the patient. Hence, his understanding will be incomplete. However, if he lacks objectivity he cannot comprehend the ways in which the patient's perspective differs from external reality and from the expectations of society. He cannot, therefore, hope to move the patient from his neurosis to the reality of an experiential maturity. The therapist must be like a bridge, a therapeutic bridge with one foot in the patient's experiential world, including his pathology, and the other foot in the world of objective reality. A *balance* between resonance and objectivity is optimal. There must not be an over-emphasis on either alone.

Many cognitive, behavior and psychoanalytic therapists emphasize being "objective' when doing therapy. This is in the scientific tradition of adhering to objectivity in the design and execution of experimental research. The practitioner is urged to avoid contaminating the outcome with his own "counter-transference" needs. This increases the problem, however, of initiating in the patient the feeling that he is only a "thing," an object of interest, but not a "person," who evokes "caring" feelings in the therapist. Since patients are accustomed to being treated as "things" by doctors, especially those who are not their "family doctors," they may accept this "object relationship." However, something important is lost therapeutically. As Tillich (1960) most eloquently stated it: "The other person cannot be controlled like a natural object. Every human being is an absolute limit, an unpierceable wall of resistance against any attempts to make him into an object. He who breaks this resistance by external force destroys his own humanity; he never can become a mature person."

"This interdependence of man and man in the process of becoming human is a judgment against a psychotherapeutic method in which the patient is a mere object for the analyst as subject. The inevitable reaction then is that the patient tries in return to make the analyst into an object for himself as subject. This kind of acting and reacting has a depersonalizing effect on both the analyst and the patient."

Even as transference may beget counter-transference, and resonance beget counter-resonance, so does complete "objectivity" beget complete "counter-objectivity." Should the doctor fail to cure, the patient will have no hesitancy in suing him. It may well be that more doctors have been sued for their failure to resonate than because of genuine malpractice. Patients may forgive a "caring," doctor but they deeply resent being treated as objects, as "things."

An equally regrettable trap happens to the therapist who is an over-resonator. In supervising psychology trainees at the Montana State Prison I would often hear their strong feelings of indignation at the "mistreatment" of the inmates by the correctional officers. The poor inmate had been abused by his parents (possibly true), had been "railroaded" into jail by an overly-vindictive prosecuting attorney (less-likely true), and had been sentenced by a judge who wouldn't even listen to him (least-likely true). My trainees not only had learned to resonate well, but their own counter transferences toward their own possibly rejecting parent figures had been stimulated in their resonance with the inmates.

It was necessary to commend them on their ability to resonate but also to say to them, "Whoah! Step back and look at your inmate client from a different point of view, him who is in prison for aggressive acts inflicted on others. Suppose it was your own sister or brother who had been their victims. Would you still feel the same way?" The trainee therapists had to learn to balance their resonating with at least equal objectivity. Otherwise, they could never help their inmate clients rehabilitate and find places back in society. They had learned half the secret of a therapeutic self. Perhaps because of the emphasis on "objectivity" in the experimental side of their graduate studies they had overly reacted against it in the therapeutic side of their training. However, the ability to resonate is extremely important and is not generally studied in the preparation of young psychologists and psychiatrists.

The reason resonance is so effective in therapy is because we all are more prone to "fight" for our own causes than those of others. When we resonate we also "co-suffer" the discomforts of the patient, and, hence, are more impelled to find solutions that will reduce such anxiety—in our own self as well as in the patient. The attorney who resonates with his client adopts the position of the client as his own, and is thus more highly motivated to prepare a strong case. The therapist is more effective when he is an "attorney-for-the-defense" of his patient, protecting him against his pathology, than if he only strives to be 100% "objective."

Sociopaths seem incapable of resonating with others, hence they can victimize people and feel neither anxiety nor remorse—except perhaps concern at the possibility of being caught. Other people are simply "objects," which they manipulate for their own pleasure. Perhaps one of the difficulties in treating them is because of the inability of most therapists to resonate with such characters.

When the therapist listens to the communications of the patient, he is building within himself an increasingly accurate image of that one. He introjects a replica of the other and forms an "object representation." He senses the characteristics of this object and achieves some understanding of it accordingly. However, if he resonates he identifies with this image. He turns it into an "indentofact," and it becomes a self representation. He then co-feels and co-understands the way the patient does. This is additional data, not derived from his original sensing of the object representation—and perhaps not derivable if contacted only as object.

As the therapist moves back and forth from resonance to objectivity he gains greater apprehension of his patient. His interventions become more knowledgeable and effective. Perhaps from his "objective' observation he recognizes that the patient has repressed a murderous rage toward a sister. But from his resonance he realizes that the patient is not ready to accept such an interpretation. It would be too devastating because he, himself, would hurt too much if "we" confronted this problem at this time. The ability to resonate, and to balance it with objectivity gives the analyst a greater therapeutic sensitivity—an internal "third ear" (Reik, 1948).

Federn's theories of ego and object cathexis (discussed in Chapter 9) contribute a rationale to the understanding of resonance. The image of the therapist is first introjected as an object by investing it with "object cathexis" at the time it is internalized. The sensing of this "object" gives the analyst his first knowledge concerning it. Then this object representation is changed into a self representation by removing the object cathexis and investing it with self energy, "ego cathexis." The therapist now experiences the patient as part of his own self and gathers understanding of it from within to add to the knowledge he had received from its sensing as object.

In making a suggestion, interpretation or other intervention the analyst "tests" it on a self-representation to determine whether it is desirable, appropriate, and acceptable before transmitting it to the patient. If his resonance has been correct then his intervention will also be correct and optimal. He and the patient will move (by bits and pieces) toward a resolution of the problem.

Unfortunately, we can never resonate completely. We have our own personal agenda based on our training and life experiences. These may interfere. Resonance will then be only partial. We may have "self-tested" an interpretation and transmitted it to our client, only to find that we were off-base. Out internal G2 ("Intelligence Department") was faulty. We goofed. However, if resonance is still functioning we may notice our mistake and make appropriate correction before great damage has been done.

The more another person is like ourselves, the easier it is to resonate with him or her. Middle-class therapists resonate better with middle-class patients than with those coming from other socio-economic levels, cultures, races or who posses quite different value systems. To resonate with a female patient the male therapist should be experiencing outrage when she is revealing a rape or other sexual abuse. If instead, he is having sexual feelings toward her he is treating her as an object. Male therapists who are afraid of their own "feminine component" (Jung's anima), and fear that it will "take them over," such that they will become homosexual, may not be able to resonate with their female patients. It does not mean they cannot treat such patients, but their "understanding" will of necessity come from their objective sensing—and thus be more limited.

There is another benefit which enhances the effectiveness of the therapist who can resonate. Resonance begats counter-resonance. If I deeply understand my patient, and correctly transmit this under-standing to him, then he will feel understood. My interpretations will have greater credibility and weight. Their timing will be better, and they will be much more effective. The patient senses that a new, constructive force has entered his world. He is encouraged. "We" can do what "I" could never do alone. The motivations for recovery are strengthened and renewed. He accepts more eagerly the therapist's "loan" of self energy. This is why many studies show that the quality of the therapeutic relationship is so much more important than mere "techniques."

The therapist who is willing to commit himself to a resonant, as well as object relationship in the interests of greater therapeutic effectiveness should recognize that it does not come cheaply. He must be willing to resonate, not only with the patient's assets, but also with liabilities. The resonating therapist accepts in to his own self structure the pathology of the patient, even though in mini form. So temporarily, while the patient is getting well, the therapist is getting more "sick." If he undertakes too many therapeutic commitments and resonates too deeply with them he will be destroyed psychologically himself.

A young resident physician once said to me,"Jack, I'm no damned good as a doctor; all my patients are dieing." This conscientious practitioner had been assigned to manage the "terminal tumor ward," a monstrosity to which all the elderly patients with inoperable cancer were assigned. In the guise of "getting experience" this young doctor was being systematically destroyed. If he resonated with his patients he would go down with them; if he didn't, they would be treated as objects—and like so many rejected people, die alone. The solution for such a dilemma is not easy. Perhaps if one can view life as a quality rather than a quantity, then the treating one can be sustained by the recognition that he deserves credit as a good therapist for every minute of pain-free and meaningful existence he can offer his patients. Their therapy then becomes a growth experience for the doctor, not a debilitating trauma.

As the patient recovers, the ego-loan which the doctor has invested into the self-representation of the individual is increasingly payed-back. Though resonance he co-enjoys the therapeutic gains with the patient—and himself grows in strength and maturity as a therapist and a person. When he over-resonates with too many extremely sick individuals, and his ego-economy is on a deficit track, then sooner or later, either he must reduce his therapeutic commitments, lessen his effectiveness—or face "burn-out." The self economy of a therapcutic self, like that of his patients, requires care and nourishment. Vacations, the love of others, plus the rewards of therapeutic success must keep therapists' ego-energy income greater than its out-go, else they will become personal bankrupts. Therapists and analysts need to be very aware of their current energy "balance sheets." Don't try to be a life saver if you are already exhausted from swimming.

Resonance has another effect. The more people get to know one another, the more they resonate with one another, the better their relationship—vice-versa. At the time this chapter is being written

President Reagan and Secretary-General Gorbachev are meeting in Moscow. We can trace the development of their relationship from the early days of name-calling to the present time when they seem to understand one another much better, communicate, and have a genuine friendly relationship. As the two heads of state learn to resonate with one another, fear and suspicion tend to melt—and the future chances of world peace brighten. What we see today might be likened to the psychotherapy of a neurotic (and almost psychotic) world, which if left unchecked make nuclear war and mutual destruction almost inevitable. In their meetings these two world leaders point up the importance of a balance between resonance, the understanding of each other's needs, and objectivity, in which each champions the positions of his own country and does not "give away the store" to the disadvantage of his own people. The balance between "with-ness" (resonance) and the realities of national security (objectivity) demonstrates here the best chance for "treating" at the foreign policy level the major "dissociation" in our world community.

There is a certain mental hygiene necessary as the therapist or analyst practices resonance. If one internalizes a replica of the patient in order to understand him one must temporarily introject his pathology as well as his assets. Otherwise, one's resonant understanding will be incomplete. Yet to do this means "ingesting" that which has been neurotic, immature, pathogenic and maladaptive in the patient's experience and behavior. If it were not so, the patient would not be seeking treatment. To do this will require energy on the part of the therapist because inevitably much of this material will be cognitively dissonant with the therapist's own concepts, values and behaviors. Resonance in therapy, therefore, is energy demanding. The therapist may suffer anxiety or other symptoms if he resonates too strongly, or if his resonance is not mitigated by objectivity and ego strengths. He must now experience within his own self something of what it feels to suffer from a phobia, an obsessive thought, being unable to control compulsive behavior, etc.

We could go on, but it is obvious that if some part of one's self, perhaps almost one half, is to enter into a co-experience with the patient's pathology, an internalized "reality" that has been borrowed from the patient even though only temporarily so, then the therapist is in for some difficult times. He must reconcile the incompatibilities now found in himself and transmit these reconciliations to the patient, bits at a time through "interpretations."

As the therapist reconciles these cognitively dissonant elements within himself the patient, who is co-resonating with him, will receive and integrate the new meanings within his own self. Doctor and patient "heal" together. The therapist experiences these dissonances and maladaptions in mini form permitting his own self to serve as a kind of laboratory experiment wherein the patient's problems are temporarily his own, and where they are both researching for solutions. Furthermore, as the therapist increases his resonance of the patient, the patient will resonate more with the therapist's objectivity. There is a *quid pro quo*, a kind of temporary exchange of egos as the patient increasingly incorporates the values, the coping abilities, and the ego-strengths of the therapist. Of course, those of their therapist should be more mature, more adjusted, more realistic, more in tune with the environmental demands of the culture than those of the patient. If it were not so the two should change places.

Assuming that the therapist's self is more mature and well-adjusted, the patient by counter-resonating with the therapist is erecting within himself a constructive replica of the treating one. Accordingly, he is introjecting a mature and healing object representation. This element can serve as a focus for integrative forces and as a defense against regression to more immature modes of thought and behavior. In fact, this therapist-introject may in time replace destructive object representations built around the much earlier internalization of rejecting or abusing parent figures. The patient now has within himself an object which will "love" him, one which can issue reassurance and constructive suggestions unconsciously to him.

This establishing of an inner therapist object representation can be the beginning of a more benevolent cycle of intra-personal processes which will replace the previous malevolent ones. If the patient invests this introject with ego cathexis, identifies with it and changes it into a self-representation, his attitudes and behaviors will undergo constructive change. As he has been treated by the therapist, so also will he now begin to treat others. And as he interacts with others constructively he is more likely to be rewarded by their actions. It is a matter of new "being." Therapy takes place, not so much because of the impact of the therapist's techniques on the patient, but because of the impact of the doctor's "self."

Theoretically, if the clinician's resonance and his objectivity were both perfect he could not make a wrong interpretation, a false intervention. Through co-feeling and co-understanding he would understand correctly the current position of the patient and just what needs to be said and done. Through his objectivity he would administer those in terms of the reality of society and the environment in which the patient exists. And through his continuous and correct resonance he would know just what could be accepted and integrated by the patient. He would not time the interpretation wrong nor present the patient with more than he was currently prepared to handle.

Unfortunately, therapists are not perfect, either in their resonating abilities, nor in their objectivity. Good therapists will be closer to this ideal than poor ones. But each of us through resonance can probably grasp but a fraction of what is being experienced by the patient—and each of us is subject to the misperceptions, the biases, counter transferences and all the other distortions which accrue to humans. We will make mistakes because psychotherapy is not an exact science; it is an art based upon the best scientific study of which we are capable.

Psychoanalytic theorists have been emphasizing the importance of establishing good "object relationships," hence, interacting realistically with others. But this is not enough. Two people may have clear inner images of the other, but if their relationship is purely an "object" one then they will treat each other as only objects. The optimal interaction would be in the establishing of a "subject-object relationship" in which each individual balances his objectivity with resonance for the other. Through the formation of constructive "subject-object relationships" parents and children would build better families, teachers and pupils would optimize education, labor and management would reach better settlements—and international disagreements could be resolved without war.

But what has hypnosis got to do with all of this? We have defined clinical hypnosis as an altered state of consciousness within an intensive inter-personal relationship. When we are "conscious" we are aware of only a part of the communications which may be emitted by a patient. Accordingly, both our objectivity and our resonance will lack all the data necessary to fully understand the patient. If we are lucky in being gifted with a therapeutic "third ear" (Reik, 1948) then we will be more sensitive therapists than those not so fortunate. Hypnosis does not substitute for a good "third ear," but it can mitigate the deficiency somewhat by eliciting and bringing to our own consciousness data which the patient had previously not presented overtly. Probably a good "third ear" plus hypnosis would be better yet. But the many hypnoanalytic techniques for discovering covert processes in patients are simply an extension of both our "third ears" and the original two. They permit us to sense aspects of our patient which had previously not been brought to our attention and to transmit interventions to the same deeper levels of the patient's personality.

From the other side of the equation hypnosis, by being an intensive inter-personal relationship, facilitates resonance. The release of affect in abreactions plus the allyship with the patient necessary for their safe execution, demands that the therapist resonate. He who neglects to do so, who plows ahead in the release of violent affects without sensing the patient's ability to handle them, risks destructive suicidal, homicidal or psychotic episodes. What is a luxury in ordinary, conscious psychotherapy becomes a necessity during intensive hypnoanalytic therapy. In hypnosis we may be traveling both "deeper" and more rapidly. Dare we be unwilling to co-experience this significant journey with our patient?

Fortunately, there is something about the hypnotic relationship which actively promotes resonance and counter-resonance. "Withness" is more easily achieved. We are impelled to throw our own "self" into the interaction—and are rewarded by the patient's doing likewise. Under hypnosis patients may manifest increased sensitivity to the cues emitted by the hypnotists. Perhaps that is why skeptics and those who research hypnosis with"subjects" do not report observing the phenomena which experienced hypnotherapists find in their "patients." Objectivity alone cannot hope to elicit all that objectivity and resonance together can. Furthermore, subjects who are regarded as experimental "objects" will not reveal the potentialities in their covert processes to hypnotists who do not resonate. Yet resonance itself increases enormously the difficulties in scientific control of experiments. While we might wish otherwise, "experimental selves" do not make the best therapists, even as "therapeutic selves" do not do the best experimental research. Human knowledge advances when approached from both perspectives—and from their communication with one another.

Perhaps a word about the selection and training of "therapeutic selves." Is this an inherent trait, or can it be developed? As in musical talent there are some individuals who seem to be born with it. They exert constructive impact on others even though they have received no graduate training in the healing arts. Others with MD's and PhD's may ply their treatment crafts yet lack highly developed therapeutic selves. Graduate training does not guarantee therapeutic success, although it makes it more probable.

The interaction of person on person is generally more therapeutic than otherwise, and especially so if the treating one is not burdened by excessive immature and neurotic motivations. Talented therapists probably begin with natural abilities which when enhanced by graduate study render them much more effective.

Learning to become a "doctor" in the sense of a healing person can certainly be enhanced if the student has role models: supervisors, training analysts, more experienced colleagues, etc. Not all of these are constructive. I have seen resident doctors who were "chewed out" by their clinical professors, and I have wondered how the future "treaters of men" could be developed from models who were "beaters of men." If we are to have therapeutic selves in the healing arts then our medical and dental schools, graduate departments of psychology, schools of nursing and social work need to be peopled with faculty members who have not merely memorized knowledge and therapeutic "techniques," be they medical, psychological, hypnoanalytic, or whatever. Clinical faculties should be chosen for their impact on the lives and the lives of others, not merely for their scientific expertise. For therapeutic selves beget and develop therapeutic-self structure in others.

Finally, if those of us who hold society's mandate to heal would live up to our full potential then the development of better therapeutic selves along with more scientific and "objective' knowledge should be our constant life goal. And if the ability to interact with others through a balance of resonance and objectivity can be transmitted broadly, then perhaps we will see a world which through its "therapeutic selves" can heal its pathologies of injustice, hatred, crime—and war.

Summary

Many patients today confront a therapist or analyst with a lack of meaning in life rather than the classical neurotic symptoms. They appear to be products of a culture which emphasizes "things" instead of people and meaningful relationships. The "meaning' of life has been much considered by many philosophers over the years. More recently, it has been the "humanistic" branch of psychotherapists who have focused on this problem.

Psychotherapeutic interventions have been focused toward the patient's "Umwelt," or reactions to the exterior world, his "Mitwelt," or inter-personal relations, and his "Eigenwelt," or intra-personal experience within his own self.

The "therapeutic self' is a concept formulated by observing the differential impact of various physicians (who were equally well trained) on their patients. The patients of those who possessed a therapeutic self responded much more favorably to treatment even though all were equally skilled in technical knowledge and therapeutic "techniques."

Resonance is the ability to co-experience (co-suffer and co-enjoy) with another. It involves temporarily internalizing the other, forming first an object representation, and then by investing it with "ego cathexis" changing it into a self representation. It is a partial identification which may be affective, cognitive or both.

When there is a balance of resonance and objectivity therapeutic interventions are maximized, because the therapist or analyst is viewing the patient from two different perspectives simultaneously—as others view the patient, and as he perceives and experiences himself.

Under-resonance leaves the therapist without the sensitive inside understanding of his patient. Over-resonance can result in a folie a deux with the two simply being sick together. Also, since resonance takes energy, too much will personally exhaust the therapist unless he can renew his own store of ego energies from other sources. He must then either reduce his therapeutic commitments, lessen their intensity or face "burn-out." In-come must balance out-go in his own ego economy.

The hypnotic relationship encourages resonance in the therapist and hence, counter-resonance in the patient. The doctor better understands the needs of the patient, can time his interventions better, and the patient is better able to accept such interventions.

The "therapeutic self" of the doctor is not only optimized by a proper balance between resonance and objectivity, but such a balance within parents and teachers can greatly improve their interactions with children. Finally, the same balance could assist diplomats and world leaders in achieving better international relations by helping them to understand the needs of the other without compromising the interests of their own country. If more "therapeutic selves" could be developed in such individuals international conflicts and wars could be better avoided.

The *techniques* of psychotherapy and analysis (hypnotic or non-hypnotic) are our "scientific" heritage of knowledge as healers. But the full use of these for the betterment of our patients, our students, our children and other people in our world rests on a balance between our objectivity and our ability to resonate with these others. Of such, are "therapeutic selves."

Chapter 12. Existential Hypnoanalysis and the Therapeutic Self

Outline

1. Many patients lack "meaning" in their existence rather than suffering from traditional neurotic symptoms.
    a. Due to culture's emphasis on "things" rather than people.

2. Humanistic approaches to psychotherapy.
    a. Existential hypnoanalysis, therapy in the humanistic tradition.

3. Resonance, the ability to co-experience with another.
    a. Temporarily introjecting the other and investing the resulting object representation with ego cathexis, thus changing it to a self-representation.
    b. It may be affective, cognitive or both.

4. The therapeutic self, a balance between resonance and objectivity.
    a. Permits the therapist to understand the patient from two different perspectives: internally and as viewed by others.
    b. Optimize therapeutic interaction.

5. Under-resonance impoverishes therapist's potential.

6. Over-resonance can create a *folie a deux* and may exhaust therapist's personal energies.
    a. Requires renewal of therapist's ego cathexes from external sources.

7. The hypnotic relationship increases resonance in therapist and counter-resonance in patient.
    a. Interventions and interpretations made more effective.

8. Application of therapeutic self concepts and resonance-objectivity balance could assist in many human relationship problems including international diplomacy.

References

Adler, A. *The practice and theory of individual psychology*. Totowa, N.J.: Littlefield, Adams, 1963.

Adler, G. *Studies in analytical psychology*. London: Routledge & Kegan Paul, 1948.

Alexander, F. & French, T.M. *Psychoanalytic Therapy*. New York: Ronald Press, 1946.

Allison, R.B. A new treatment approach for multiple personalities. *Am. J. Clin. Hypn.*, 1974, *17*, 15-32.

Alvarez, W.C. *The neuroses: Diagnosis and management of functional disorders and minor psychoses*. Philadelphia: Saunders, 1951.

American Psychiatric Assoc. *Diagnostic and statistical manual of mental disorders. DSM-III-R*. 3rd. ed. rev., 1987.

Ås, A. The recovery of forgotten language knowledge through hypnotic age regression: A case report. *Am. J. Clin. Hypn.*, 1962, *5*, 21-29.

Baker. E.L. An hypnotherapeutic approach to enhance object relatedness in psychotic patients. *Int. J. Clin. Exp. Hypn.*, 1981, *29*, 136-147.

Baker, E.L. The use of hypnotic techniques with psychotics. *Am. J. Clin. Hypn.,* 1983, *25,* 283-288.

Barber, T.X. Toward a theory of "hypnotic" behavior: The hypnotically induced dream. *J. Nerv. Ment. Disorders,* 1962, *135,* 206-221.

Barber, T.X. The effects of "hypnosis" on learning and recall: A methodological critique. *J. of Clin. Psychol.,* 1965, *21,* 19-25.

Barnett, E.A. *Analytical hypnotherapy: Principles and practice.* Kingston, Ontario: Junica, 1981.

Baskin, W. *Dictionary of santanism.* Secaucus, N.J.: Citadel Press, 1972.

Beahrs, J.O. *Unity and multiplicity: Multilevel consciousness of self in hypnosis, psychiatric disorder and mental health.* New York: Brunner/Mazel, 1982.

Beahrs, J.O. Multiple consciousness, Chap. 5 in *Limits of scientific psychiatry: Role of uncertainty in mental health.* New York: Brunner/Mazel, 1986.

Beck, A. *Cognitive therapy and the emotional disorders.* New York: Internat. Univ. Press, 1976.

Bellak, L. An ego-psychological theory of hypnosis. *Int. J. Clin. & Exp. Hypn.,* 1955, *36,* 375-378

Berkeley, G. *Essay, principles, dialogues,* M.W. Calkins (Ed.), New York: Scribner, 1929.

Berkowitz, L. The case for bottling up rage. *Psychology Today,* 1973, *2,* 24-31.

Berne, E. *Transactional analysis in psychotherapy.* New York: Grove Press, 1961.

Bernheim, H. *Hypnosis and suggestion in psychotherapy.* New Hyde Park, N.Y.: University Books, 1964. (Originally published in 1886 under the title *Suggestive therapeutics.*)

Biddle, W.E. *Hypnosis in the psychoses*. Springfield, Ill., Thomas, 1967.

Blanck, G. & Blanck, R. *Ego psychology: Theory and practice*. New York: Columbia Univ. Press, 1974.

Bliss, E.L. *Multiple personality, allied disorders, and hypnosis*. New York: Oxford Univer. Press, 1986.

Blum, G.S. & Graef, J.R. The detection over time of subjects simulating hypnosis. *Int. J. Clin. & Exp. Hypn.*, 1971, *19*, 211-224.

Boor, M. & Coons, P.M. A comprehensive bibliography of literature pertaining to multiple personality. *Psychological Reports*, 1983, *53*, 295-310.

Bower, G.H. Mood and memory. *Am. Psychologist*, 1981, *36*, 129-148.

Bower, G.H., Monteiro, K.P. & Gilligan, S.G. Emotional mood as a context of learning and recall. *J. of Verbal Learn. & Verbal Behav.*, 1978, *17*, 573-585.

Bowers, K.S. & Hilgard, E.R. Some complexities in understanding memory. In H.M. Pettinati (Ed.), *Hypnosis and memory*. New York: Guilford Press, 1988, pp. 3-18.

Bowers, M.K. Theoretical considerations in the use of hypnosis in the treatment of schizophrenia. *Int. J. Clin. & Exp. Hypn.*, 1961, *9*, 39-46.

Braun, B.G. (Ed.), *The Psychiatric Clinics of North America: Vol. 7. Symposium on multiple personality*. Philadelphia: Saunders, 1984.

Braun, B.G. (Ed.), *Treatment of multiple personality disorder*. Washington, D.C.: Am. Psychiatric Assoc. Press, 1986.

Brenman, M. & Gill, M.M. *Hypnotherapy*. New York: Internat. Univ. Press, 1947.

Brown, D.P. & Fromm, E. *Hypnotherapy and hypnoanalysis*. Hillsdale, N.J.: Lawrence Erlbaum, 1986.

Brown, D.P. & Fromm, E. *Hypnosis and behavioral medicine.* Hillsdale, N.J.:Lawrence Erlbaum, 1987.

Brown, W. The revival of emotional memories and its therapeutic value. *Brit. J. of Med. Psychol.*, 1920, *1*, 16-19.

Buber, M. *I and thou.* New York:Scribner, 1970.

Buck, J.N. The H-T-P technique: A qualitative and quantitative scoring manual. *J. of Clin. Psychol.*, 1948, Monograph Suppl. No. 5.

Bugental, J.F.T. *The search for authenticity: An existential analytic approach to psychotherapy.* New York: Holt, Rinehart & Winston, 1967.

Burton, A. *Interpersonal psychotherapy.* Englewood Cliffs, N.J.: Prentice-Hall, 1972.

Cautella, J.R. & Bennett, A.K. Covert conditioning. In R.J. Corsini (Ed.), *Handbook of innovative psychotherapies.* New York: Wiley, 1981.

Cheek, D.B. Ideomotor questioning for investigation of subconscious "pain" and target organ vulnerability. *Am. J. Clin. Hypn.*, 1962, *5*, 30-41.

Cheek, D.B. & LeCron, L.M. *Clinical hypnotherapy.* New York: Grune & Stratton, 1968.

Christopher, M. *Mediums, mystics and the occult.* New York: Crowell, 1975.

Comstock, C. The therapeutic utilization of abreactive experiences in the treatment of multiple personality disorder. (Presented at the 3rd. Internat. Conference on Multiple Personalities and Dissociative States, Chicago, Ill.: Sept 20, 1986.)

Conn, J.H. Cultural and clinical aspects of suggestion. *Int. J. Clin. & Exp. Hypn.*, 1959, *7*, 175-185.

Conn, J.H. Is hypnosis really dangerous? *Int. J. Clin. & Exp. Hypn.*, 1972, *20*, 61-67.

Cooper, L.M. & London, P. Reactivation of memory by hypnosis and suggestion. *Int. J. Clin. & Exp. Hypn.*, 1973, *21*, 312-323.

Copeland, D.R. The application of object relations theory to the hypnotherapy of developmental arrests: The borderline patient. *Int. J. Clin. & Exp. Hypn.*, 1986, *34*, 157-168.

Coué E. *Self-mastery through conscious autosuggestion*. New York: American Library Service. 1922.

Crawford, H.J. Hypnotizability, day dreaming styles, imagery, vividness, and absorption: A multidimensional study. *J. of Personality & Social Psychol.*, 1982, *42*, 915-926.

Déjerine, J. & Glauckler, E. *The psychoneuroses and their treatment by psychotherapy*. Philadelphia, Lippincott, 1913.

Dement, W.C. & Kleitman, N. Cycle variations in EEG during sleep and their relation to eye movements, body motility and dreaming. *Electroencephalography & Clinical Neurophysiology*, 1957, *9*, 673-690.

Dement, W.C. & Kleitman, N. Your eyes watch the dream action. In R.L. Woods & H.B. Greenhouse (Eds.), *The new world of dreams*. New York: Macmillan, 1974, pp. 292-293.

Dewey, J. *Democracy and education*. New York: Macmillan, 1916.

Dhanens, T.P. & Lundy, R.M. Hypnotic and waking suggestions and recall. *Int. J. Clin. & Exp. Hypn.*, 1975, *23*, 68-79.

Diamond, M.J. It takes two to tango: Some thoughts on the neglected importance of the hypnotist in an interactive hypnotherapeutic relationship. *Am. J. Clin. Hypn.*, 1984, *27*, 3-13.

Dubois, P. *The psychic treatment of nervous disorders*. New York: Funk and Wagnals, 1909.

Eiblmayr, K. Trance logic and the circle-touch test. *Australian J. of Clin. & Exp. Hypn.*, 1987, *15*, 133-145.

Ellenberger, H.F. *The discovery of the unconscious*. New York: Basic Books, 1970.

Erdelyi, M.H. Hypermnesia: The effect of hypnosis, fantasy and concentration. In H.M. Pettinati (Ed.), *Hypnosis and memory*. New York: Guilford, 1988, pp. 95-127.

Erickson, M.H. An experimental investigation of the possible anti-social uses of hypnosis. *Psychiatry*. 1939, *2*, 391-414.

Erickson, M.H. Deep hypnosis and its induction. In L.M. LeCron (Ed.), *Experimental hypnosis*. New York: Macmillan, 1952, pp. 70-112. (also Citadel Press, 1968).

Erickson, M.H. *Advanced techniques of hypnosis and therapy* New York: Grune & Stratton, 1967, (edited by Jay Haley).

Erickson M.H. and Kubie, L.S. The successful treatment of a case of acute hysterical depression by return under hypnosis to a critical phase of childhood. *Psychoanalytic Quarterly,* 1941, *10*, 539-609.

Erikson, E.H. *Insight and responsibility*. New York: Norton, 1964.

Evans, F.J. Contextual forgetting: Posthypnotic source amnesia. *J. Abn. Psychol.*, 1979, *88*, 556-563.

Evans, F.J. & Thorn, W.A.F. Two types of posthypnotic amnesia: Recall amnesia and source amnesia. *Int. J. Clin. & Exp. Hypn.*, 1966, *14*, 162-179.

Federn, P. *Ego psychology and the psychoses*. (E. Weiss, Ed.), New York: Basic Books, 1952.

Federn, P. Narcissism in the structure of the ego. (Read before the Tenth International Psychoanalytic Congress, Sept. 1, 1927). In *Ego psychology and the psychoses*. by Paul Federn, E. Weiss, Ed., New York: Basic Books, 1952a, pp. 38-59.

Fenichel, O. *The psychoanalytic theory of neurosis.* New York: Norton, 1945.

Fisher, C. Subliminal and supraliminal stimulation before the dream. In R.L. Woods & H.G. Greenhouse (Eds.), *The new world of dreams.* New York: Macmillan, 1974, pp. 377-388.

Foulkes, D. Theories of dream formation and recent studies of sleep consciousness. In C.T. Tart (Ed.), A*ltered states of consciousness.* New York: Wiley, pp. 117-131.

Franks, C. *Behavior therapy: Appraisal and status.* New York: McGraw-Hill, 1969.

French T.M. & Fromm, E. *Dream interpretation: A new approach.* New York: Basic Books, 1964. (Republished Internat. Univ. Press, 1986).

Freud, A. *The ego and the mechanisms of defense.* New York: Internat. Univ. Press, 1946.

Freud, S. Further recommendations in the technique of psycho-analysis. Observations on transference love. *Collected papers. Vol. II.* London:Hogarth press and The Institute of Psycho-Analysis, 1924. pp. 377-391.

Freud, S. On narcissism: An introduction. In *Collected papers, Vol. IV.*, London: Hogarth Press and the Institute of Psycho-Analysis, 1933, pp. 30-59.

Freud, S. A general introduction to psycho-analysis. New York: Liveright, 1935.

Freud, S. On the history of the psychoanalytic movement. *Collected papers. Vol. I.* London: Hogarth Press and the The Institute of Psycho-Analysis, 1953a, pp. 287-359.

Freud, S. The interpretation of dreams. In J. Strachey (Ed. and Trans.). *The standard edition of the complete psychological works of Sigmund Freud, Vols. 4 & 5.* London: Hogarth Press. 1953b.

Freud, S. A case of paranoia (dementia paranoides). In *Collected papers, Vol. III*. London: Hogarth Press and the Institute of Psycho-analysis, 1953c, pp. 390-416.

Freud, S. & Breuer, J. On the psychical mechanism of hysterical phenomena. In Freud S. *Collected papers, Vol. I*. London: Hogarth Press and the Institute of Psycho-Analysis, 1953, pp. 24-41.

Fromm, Erich. *The forgotten language*. New York: Rinehart, 1951.

Fromm, Erich. *The anatomy of human destructiveness*. New York: Holt, Rinehart & Winston, 1973.

Fromm, Erika. Transference and counter-transference in hypnosis. *Int. J. Clin. & Exp. Hypn.*, 1968, *16*, 77-84.

Fromm, Erika & Kahn, S. *Self hypnosis: The Chicago paradigm*. New York: Guilford, 1990.

Gill, M.M. & Brenman, M. *Hypnosis and related states*. New York: Int. Univ. Press, 1959.

Gill, M.M. & Menninger, K. Techniques of hypnoanalysis, a case report. In M.M. Gill & M. Brenman (Eds.). *Hypnotherapy: A survey of the literature*. New York: Internat. Univ. Press, 1947, pp. 151-174.

Glover, E. *The technique of psychoanalysis*. New York: Internat. Univ. Press, 1955.

Greenberg, J. *I never promised you a rose garden*. New York: Signet, 1964.

Greenberg, J. R. & Mitchell, S.A. *Object relations in psychoanalytic theory*. Cambridge, Mass.: Harvard Univ. Press, 1983.

Grinker, R.R. & Spiegel, J.P. *War neuroses*. Philadelphia: Blakiston, 1945.

Grof, S. *Realms of the human unconscious: Observations from LSD research*. New York: Viking Press, 1975.

Grof, S. *LSD psychotherapy.* Pomona, Calif.: Hunter House, 1980.

Grof, S. *Beyond the brain: Birth, death and transcendence in psychotherapy.* Albany, N.Y.: State University of New York Press, 1985.

Gruenwald, D. Transference and countertransference in hypnosis. *Int. J. Clin. & Exp. Hypn.*, 1971, *19*, 71-82.

Guntrip, H. *Personality structure and human interaction: The developing synthesis of psychodynamic theory.* New York: Internat. Univ. Press, 1961.

Gutheil, E.A. T*he handbook of dream analysis.* New York: Washington Square Press, 1970. (Originally Liveright, 1951).

Hadfield, J.A. Treatment by suggestion and hypnoanalysis. In E. Miller (Ed.), *The neuroses of war.* Macmillan, 1940, pp. 128-149.

Hall, C.W. *The meaning of dreams.* New York: Harper & Bros., 1953.

Hartmann, H. Notes on the theory of sublimation. In H. Hartmann, *Essays on ego psychology.* New York: Internat. Univ. Press, 1955, p.240.

Hartmann, H. *Ego psychology and the problem of adaptation.* New York: Internat. Univ. Press, 1958.

Heidgger, M. Existence and being. Chicago: Henry Regnery, 1949.

Heisenberg, W. *Physics and philosophy.* New York: Harper, 1958.

Hibbard, W.W. & Worring, R.S. *Forensic hypnosis: The practical application of hypnosis in criminal investigation.* Springfield, Ill.: Thomas, 1981.

Hilgard, E.R. *Hypnotic susceptibility.* New York: Harcourt, Brace & World, 1965.

Hilgard, E.R. *Divided consciousness: Multiple controls in human thought and action.* New York: Wiley, 1977. (Rev. ed. 1986).

Hilgard, E.R. & Loftus, E.F. Effective interrogation of the eyewitness. *Int. J. Clin. & Exp. Hypn.*, 1979, *27*, 342-357.

Hilgard, E.R. & Nowlis, D.P. The contents of hypnotic dreams and night dreams: An exercise in method. In E. Fromm & R. Shor (Eds.), *Hypnosis: Research developments and perspectives.* New York: Aldine, 1972, pp. 510-524.

Hilgard, J.R. Imaginative and sensory-affective involvements in everyday life and in hypnosis. In E. Fromm & R. Shor (Eds.), *Hypnosis: Developments, research and new perspectives.* New York: Aldine, 1979, pp. 482-517.

Hochberg, J.E. *Perception.* (2nd. ed.), Englewood Cliffs, N.J.: Prentice-Hall, 1978.

Hume, D. *The philosophy of David Hume.* (V.C. Chappel, Ed.), New York: Modern Library, 1963.

Huse, B. Does the hypnotic trance favor the recall of faint memories? *J. Exper. Psychol.*, 1930, *13*, 519-529.

Jacobson, E. *The self and the object world.* New York: Internat. Univ. Press, 1964.

Janet, P. *The major symptoms of hysteria.* New York: Macmillan, 1907.

Janov, A. *Primal scream: A revolutionary cure for neurosis.* New York: Putnam, 1970.

Jensen, A.R. Scoring the Stroop test. *Acta Psychologica,* 1965, *24*, 398-408.

Jourard, S. *The transparent self.* New York: Van Nostrand Reinhold, 1971.

Jung, C.G. *Psychology of the unconscious.* New York: Moffat, Yard, 1916.

Jung, C.G. *Psychological types.* Princeton, N.J.: Princeton Univ. Press, 1976/1921.

Jung, C.G. Memories, dreams, reflections. In *Collected works.* New York: Pantheon, 1958, XXVII, pp. 115-117.

Jung, C.G. Chap. II. The eros theory. In *Two essays on analytical psychology.* New York: Pantheon, 1966.

Kant, E. *Critique of pure reason.* New York: Dutton, 1934.

Keet, C.D. Two verbal techniques in a miniature counseling situation. *Psychol. Monographs,* 1948, 148, *62,* no. 294.

Kernberg, O.F. Early ego integration and object relations. *Annals of the New York Academy of Sciences,* 1972, *193,* 233-247.

Kernberg, O.F. *Object relations theory and clinical psychoanalysis.* New York: Jason Aronson, 1976.

Kierkegaard, S. F*ear and trembling and the sickness unto death.* Garden City, N.Y.: Doubleday Anchor, 1954.

Kleinhauz, M., Horowitz, I., & Tobin, Y. The use of hypnosis in police investigation: A preliminary comunication. *J. of Forensic Science Society,* 1977, *17,* No. 2 and 3: 77-80.

Klemperer, E. Past ego states emerging in hypnoanalysis. *J. Clin. & Exp. Hypn.,* 1965, *13,* 132-143.

Klemperer, E. *Past ego states emerging in hypnoanalysis.* Springfield, Ill.: Thomas 1968.

Kline, M.V. *Freud and hypnosis.* New York: Julian Press and The Institute for Research in Hypnosis. 1958.

Kline, M.V. Imagery, affect and perception in hypnotherapy. In M.V. Kline (Ed.), *Psychodynamics and hypnosis: New contributions to the practice and theory of hypnotherapy.* Springfield, Ill.: Thomas, 1967, pp. 41-70.

Kline, M.V. Sensory hypnoanalysis. *Int. J. Clin. & Exp. Hypn.,* 1968, *16,* 85-100.

Kline, P. *Fact and Fantasy in Freudian theory.* London: Methuen, 1972, pp. 208-226.

Kline, V. Ford Motor Co. Inc., 523 F 2d. 1067 (9th Cir. 1975). pp. 75, 78, 94, 95.

Kluft, R.P. Clinical corner. *Internat. Soc. for the Study of Multiple Personality & Dissociation Newsletter*, 1986, *4*, 4-5.

Kluft, R.P. On the use of hypnosis to find lost objects: A case report of a tandem hypnotic technique. *Am. J. Clin. Hypn.*, 1987, *29*, 242-248.

Kluft, R.P. On treating the older patient with multiple personality disorder: "Race against time" or "Make haste slowly." *Am. J. Clin. Hypn.*, 1988, *30*, 257-266.

Kluft, R.P., Frankel, F., Spiegel, D. & Orne, M.T. *Resolved: Multiple personality disorder is a true psychiatric disease entity.* (tape cassette). Mineola, N.Y.: American Audio Assoc., 1988.

Kohut, H. *The analysis of the self.* New York: Internat. Univ. Press, 1971.

Kohut, H. *The restoration of the self.* New York: Internat. Univ. Press, 1977.

Kohut, H. *The search for the self, Vols. 1 & 2.* New York: Internat. Univ. Press, 1978.

Kolb, L.C. Recovery of memory and repressed fantasy in combat-induced post-traumatic stress disorder of Vietnam veterans. In H.M. Pettinati (Ed.), *Hypnosis and memory.* 1988, pp. 265-274.

Kramer, E. *Art therapy with children.* New York: Schocken Books, 1971.

Kris, E. Ego psychology and interpretation in psychoanalytic therapy. *Psychoanalytic Quarterly,* 1951, *20*, 15-31.

Kris, E. The recovery of childhood memories in psychoanalysis. *The psychoanalytic study of the child.* New York: Internat. Univ. Press, 1956, 11, 54-88.

Kroger, W.S. & Douce, R.G. Hypnosis in criminal investigation. *Int. J. Clin. & Exp. Hypn.*, 1979, 27, 358-374.

Kroger, W.S. & Fezler, W.D. *Hypnosis and behavior modification: Imagery and conditioning.* Philadelphia: Lippincott, 1976.

Kubovy, M. & Pomerantz, J.R. *Perceptual organization.* Hillsdale, N.J.: Erlbaum, 1981.

Lambert, G.W. Studies in the automatic writing of Mrs. Verall: X. Concluding reflections. *J. of the Soc. for Psychical Research,* 1971, pp. 271-222.

Laurence, J. & Perry, C. *Hypnosis, will, and memory.* New York: Guilford Press, 1988.

Lavoie, G. & Sabourin, M. Hypnosis and schizophrenia: A review of experimental and clinical studies. In G.D. Burrows & L. Dennerstein (Eds.), *Handbook of hypnosis and psychosomatic medicine.* Amsterdam: Elsevier/North Holland Biomedical Press, 1980.

Lazar, B.S. & Dempster, C.R. Operator variables in successful hypnotherapy. *Int. J. Clin. Exp. Hypn.*, 1984, 33, 28-40.

Levick, M. Art therapy. In R.J. Corsini (Ed.), *Handbook of innovative psychotherapies.* New York: Wiley, 1981.

Levine, M. *Psychotherapy in medical practice.* New York: Macmillan, 1942.

Levy, J. Psychobiological implications of bilateral asymmetry. In *Hemisphere function in the human brain.* S.J. Diamond & J.G. Beaumont (Eds.), New York: Wiley, 1974.

Liebeault, A. *Du summeil et des états analogues considérés surtout au point de vue de l'action moral sur le physique.* Paris: Masson, 1866. (Also Vienna: Deuticke 1892).

Lindner, R.M. *Rebel without a cause.* London: Research Books, 1944.

Locke, J. *The works of John Locke.* Aalen, Germany: Scientia Verlag, 1963.

Loftus, E.F. *Eyewitness testimony.* Cambridge, Mass.: Harvard Univ. Press, 1979.

Lowen, A. *Bioenergetics,* New York: Coward, 1975.

Lowenstein, R.M. The problem of interpretation. *The Psychoanalytic Quarterly,* 1951, *20,* 1-14.

Lundy, R.M. How can we account for reports of hypnotic hypermnesia? Presented, at the 38th annual meeting of the Soc. for Clin. & Exp. Hypnosis, Los Angeles, Oct. 29, 1987.

Machover, K. *Personality projections in the drawing of the human figure.* Springfield, Ill.: Thomas, 1948.

Mahler, M.S. On the first three subphases of the separation-individuation process. *Int. J. Psychoanalysis,* 1972, *53,* 333-338.

Mahler, M.S. Symbiosis and individuation: The psychological birth of the human infant. In *The selected papers of Margaret S. Mahler. Vol. 2.* New York: Jason Aronson, 1974.

Mahler, M.S. *On human symbiosis and the vicissitudes of individuation.* New York: Internat. Univ. Press, 1978.

Mahoney, M.F. *The meaning in dreams and dreaming.* Secaucus, N.J.: Citadel Press, 1976.

Mahoney, M.J. Personal science: A cognitive learning theory. In A. Ellis & R. Grieger (Eds.), *Handbook of psychotherapy and behavioral change: An empirical analysis.* New York: Springer, 1977.

Marcel, G. *The philosophy of existence.* London: Harvill, 1948.

May, R. (Ed.), *Existence: A new dimension in psychiatry and psychology.* New York: Basic Books, 1958.

Means, J.R. et al. Dream interpretation. *Psychotherapy,* Fall 1986, *23,* 448-452.

Meares, A. *Hypnography: A study of the therapeutic use of hypnotic painting.* Springfield, Ill.: Thomas, 1957.

Meares, A. *Shapes of sanity.* Springfield, Ill. Thomas, 1960.

Meares, A. *A system of medical hypnosis.* New York: Julian Press, 1976. (Originally published 1961.)

Meichenbaum, D. *Cognitive behavior modification: An integrative approach.* New York: Plenum, 1977.

Menninger, K. & Holzman, P.S. *Theory of psychoanalytic Technique.* 2d ed., New York: Basic Books, 1973.

Messerschmidt, R. A quantitative investigation of the alleged independent operation of conscious and subconscious processes. *J. Abn. & Soc. Psychol.,* 1927-28, *22,* 325-340.

Moreno, J.L. *Psycho-drama.* New York: Random House, 1946.

Moreno, J.L. & Enneis, J.M. H*ypnodrama and psychodrama. Psychodrama Monographs, No. 27,* New York: Beacon House, 1950.

Moss, C.S. Experimental paradigms for the hypnotic investigation of dream symbolism. *Int. J. Clin. Exp. Hypn.,* 1961, *9,* 105-117.

Moss, C.S. *The hypnotic investigation of dreams.* New York: Wiley, 1967.

Moss, C.S. *Dreams, images, and fantasy: A semantic differential casebook.* Chicago, Ill.: Univ. of Illinois Press, 1970.

Mühl, A. Automatic writing and hypnosis. In L.M. LeCron, (Ed.), *Experimental hypnosis.* New York: Citadel, pp. 426-441, 1952.

Murray, H.A. *Thematic Apperception Test Manual.* Cambridge, Mass.: Harvard Univ. Press, 1943.

Murray-Jobsis, J. Hypnosis with severely disturbed patients. In W.C. Wester & A. H. Smith (Eds.), *Clinical hypnosis: A multidisciplinary approach*. Philadelphia: Lippincott, 1984.

Murray-Jobsis, J. Hypnosis as a function of adaptive regression and of transference: An integrated theoretical model. *Am. J. Clin. Hypn.*, 1988, *30*, 241-247.

Naumburg, M. *Studies of the free art expression of behavior problem children and adolescents as a means of diagnosis and therapy*. New York: Nervous & Mental Disease Publ. Co., 1947.

Naumburg, M. *Schizophrenic art: Its meaning in psychotherapy*. New York: Grune & Stratton, 1950.

Naumburg, M. *Psychoneurotic art: Its function in psychotherapy*. Grune & Stratton, 1953.

Naumburg, M. *Dynamically oriented art therapy: Its principles and practice*. New York: Grune & Stratton, 1966.

Nichols, M.P. & Zax M. *Catharsis in psychotherapy*. New York: Gardner Press, 1977.

Olsen, P. *Emotional Flooding*. New York: Human Sciences Press, 1976.

Orne, M.T. Can a hypnotized subject be compelled to carry out otherwise unacceptable behavior: A discussion. *Int. J. Clin. & Exp. Hypn.*, 1972, *20*, 101-117.

Orne, M.T. Affidavit of Amicus Curiae, Quaglino v. California, U.S. Sup. Ct. No. 77-1288, cert. den. 11/27/78. In E. Margolin (Chm.), *16th annual defending criminal cases: The rapidly changing practice of criminal law. Vol. 2*. New York: Practicing Law Institute, 1978, pp. 831-857.

Orne, M.T. The use and misuse of hypnosis in court. *Int. J. Clin. & Exp. Hypn.*, 1979, *27*, 311-341.

Orne, M.T., Dinges, D.F. & Orne, E.C. *The forensic use of hypnosis*. Washington, D.C.: Nat. Inst. of Justice, 1984.

Orne, M.T., Dinges, D.F. & Orne, E.C. On the differential diagnosis of multiple personality in the forensic context. *Int. J. Clin & Exp. Hypn.*, 1984a, *32*,118-169.

Orne, M.T., Whitehouse, W.G., Dinges, D.F. & Orne, E.C. Reconstructing memory through hypnosis: Forensic and clinical implications. In H.M. Pettinati, (Ed.), *Hypnosis and memory*. New York: Guilford Press, 1988. pp. 21-63.

Osgood, C.E. Semantic differential technique in the comparative study of cultures. *Am. Anthropology,* 1964, *66*, 171-199.

People V. Collingan, 154 Cal. Rptr. 391, 91 Cal. App. 3d 846 (1979).

People v. Eubanks, 1897, 117 Cal. 652, 49 p 1049, pp. 57, 63.

People v. Leyra, 1951, 304 N.Y. 468, 108 N.E., 2d, 673.

People v. Shirley, 641 P.2d 775 (Cal. 1982), cert. denied, 408 U.S. (1982).

People v. Worthington, 105 Cal. 166, 38 P. 689 (1894). Pg. 130.

Perls, F.S. *Gestalt therapy verbatim.* Lafayette, Calif.: Real People Press, 1969.

Pettinati, H.M. Measuring hypnotizability in psychotic patients. *Int. J. Clin. & Exp. Hypn.*, 1982, *30*, 345-353.

Pettinati, H.M. (Ed.), *Hypnosis and memory*. New York: Guilford,1988.

Prince, M. *The dissociation of a personality.* New York: Longmans-Green, 1906.

Putnam, F.W. *Diagnosis and treatment of multiple personality disorder.* New York: Guilford, 1989.

Raginsky, B. The sensory use of plasticine in hypnoanalysis (sensory hypnoplasty). *Int. J. Clin. & Exp. Hypn.*, 1961, *9*, 233-247.

Raginsky, B. Sensory hypnoplasty with case illustrations. *Int. J. Clin. & Exp. Hypn.* 1962. *10*, 205-219.

Raginsky, B. Hypnosis in internal medicine and general practice. In Schneck, J.M. (Ed.), *Hypnosis in modern medicine.* Springfield, Ill.: Thomas, 1963, pp. 29-99.

Raginsky, B. Rapid regression to the oral and anal levels through sensory hypnoplasty. *Int. J. Clin. & Exp. Hypn.*, 1967, *15*, 19-30.

Råmonth, S.M. Dissociation and self-awareness in directed daydreaming. *Scandinavian J. of Psychol.*, 1985a, *26*, 259-276.

Råmonth, S.M. *Multilevel consciousness in meditation, hypnosis, and directed daydreaming.* Upsalla, Sweden: Univ. of UMEA, 1985b.

Rank, O. *Art and artist, creative urge and personality development.* New York: Knopf, 1932.

Rank, O. *The trauma of birth.* New York: Brunner, 1952.

Rapaport, D. The theory of ego autonomy: A generalization. *Bull. Menninger Clin.*, 1958, *22*, 13-35.

Regardie, F. Experimentally induced dreams as psychotherapeutic aids. *Am. J. Psychotherapy*, 1950, *4,* 643-650.

Reich, W. *Character analysis.* New York: Orgone Inst. Press, 1949.

Reik, T. *Listening with the third ear.* New York: Farrar, 1948.

Reik, T. *The search within.* New York: Grove Press, 1956.

Reik, T. *Of love and lust.* New York: Farrar, Strauss & Cudahy, 1957.

Reiser, M. *Handbook of investigative hypnosis.* Los Angeles: Lehi, 1980.

Relinger, H. Hypnotic hypermnesia: A critical review. *Am. J. Clin. Hypn.*, 1984, *26*, 212-225.

Renee (Pseudonym). *Autobiography of a schizophrenic girl.* (with analytic interpretations by Marguerite Sechehaye) New York: Grune & Stratton, 1951.

Rock V. Arkansas. 107 S. Ct. 2704 (1987).

Rogers, C. *Client-centered therapy.* Boston: Houghton-Mifflin, 1951.

Rogers, C. *On becoming a person: A client's view of psychotherapy.* Boston: Houghton-Mifflin, 1961.

Rolf, I. *Rolfing.* Santa Monica, Calif.: Dennis Landman, 1978.

Romero v. Colorado, 1988, *Colorado Lawyer, 17,* 136-147 (Colorado Supreme Court, Nov. 9, 1987).

Rorschach, H. *Psychodiagnostics.* New York: Grune & Stratton, 1949.

Rose, S. Intense feeling therapy. In P. Olsen (Ed.), *Emotional flooding.* New York: Human Sciences Press, 1976, pp. 80-95.

Ross, C.A. *Multiple personality disorder: Diagnosis, clinical features and treatment.* New York: Wiley, 1989.

Rossi, E.L. *Dreams and the growth of personality.* New York: Pergammon Press, 1972.

Rossi, E.L. & Cheek, D.B. *Mind-body therapy: Methods of ideodynamic healing in hypnosis.* New York: Norton 1988.

Rycroft, C.S. *The innocence of dreams.* New York: Pantheon, 1979.

Sacerdote, P. *Induced dreams.* New York: Vantage Press, 1967.

Sanders, S. The Perceptual Alteration Scale: A scale measuring dissociation. *Am. J. Clin. Hypn.,* 1986, *29,* 95-102.

Satir, V. *Conjoint family therapy.* Palo Alto, Calif.: Science & Behavior Books, 1967.

Scagnelli, J. A case of hypnotherapy with an acute schizophrenic. *Am. J. Clin. Hypn.,* 1974, *17,* 60-63.

Scagnelli, J. Hypnotherapy with schizophrenic and borderline patients: A summary of therapy with eight patients. *Am. J. Clin. Hypn.,* 1976, *19,* 33-38.

Scagnelli, J. Hypnotic dream therapy with a borderline schizophrenic: A case study. *Am. J. Clin. Hypn.*, 1977, *20*, 136-145.

Scagnelli, J. Hypnotherapy with psychotic and borderline patients: The use of trance by patient and therapist. *Am. J. Clin. Hypn.*, 1980, *22*, 164-169.

Scagnelli-Jobsis, J. Hypnosis with psychotic patients: A review of the literature and presentation of a theoretical framework. *Am. J. Clin. Hypn.*, 1982, *25*, 33-45.

Scagnelli-Jobsis, J. Hypnosis with psychotic patients: Response to Speigel. *Am. J. Clin. Hypn.*, 1983, *25*, 295-298.

Schilder, P. & Kauders, O. A textbook of hypnosis. In P. Schilder (Ed.). *The nature of hypnosis*. New York: Internat. Univer. Press, 1926.

Scheflin, A.W. and Shapiro, J.L. *Trance on trial*. New York, Guilford, 1989.

Schneck, J.M. *Studies in scientific hypnosis*. Baltimore: Williams and Wilkins, 1954.

Schneck, J.M. *Principles and practice of hypnoanalysis*. Springfield, Ill.: Thomas, 1965.

Schneck, J.M. Observations on the hypnotic nightmare. *Am. J. Clin. Hypn.*, 1974, *16*, 240-245.

Schneidman, E.S. *Make a Picture Story Test (MAPS)*. New York: Psychological Corp., 1947.

Schreiber, F.R. *Sybil*. New York: Warner Paperback Library, 1974.

Schwing, G. *A way to the soul of the mentally ill*. New York: Internat. Univ. Press, 1954.

Sechehaye, M. *Symbolic realization*. Monograph Series on Schizophrenia, No. 2., Internat. Univ. Press, 1951.

Sechehaye, M. *A new psychotherapy in schizophrenia.* New York: Grune & Stratton, 1956.

Shakow, D. & Rosenzweig, S. The use of the tautophone (verbal summator) as an auditory apperceptive test for the study of personality. *Character and Personality,* 1949, *8,* 216-226.

Shaw, H.L. Hypnosis and drama: A note on a novel use of self-hypnosis. *Int. J. Clin. & Exp. Hypn.,* 1978, *26,* 154-157.

Sheehan, P.W. Incongruity in trance behavior: A defining property of hypnosis? *Annals of the N.Y. Acad. of Sciences,* 1977, *296,* 194-207.

Sheehan, P.W. Confidence, memory and hypnosis. In H.M. Pettinati (Ed.), *Memory and hypnosis.* New York: Guilford Press, 1988, pp. 95-127.

Sherman, S.E. *Very deep hypnosis: An experiential and electroencephalographic investigation.* (Unpublished doctoral dissertation. Stanford Univ., 1971.

Shevrin, H. & Luborsky, L. Subconscious stimulation before the dream. In R.L. Woods & H.B. Greenhouse (Eds.), *The new world of dreams.* New York: Macmillan, 1974, pp. 371-377.

Shor, R.E. A phenomenological method for the measurement of variables important to an understanding of the nature of hypnosis. In E. Fromm & R. Shor (Eds.), *Hypnosis: Developments in research and new perspectives.* New York: Aldine, 1979.

Shostrom, E. *Man the manipulator.* Nashville, Tenn.: Abingdon Press, 1967.

Skinner, B.F. The verbal summator and a method for the study of latent speech. *J. Psychol.,* 1939, *34,* 33-38.

Smith, A.H. Sources of efficacy in the hypnotic relationship: An object relations approach. In W.C. Wester & A.H. Smith (Eds.), *Clinical hypnosis: A multidisciplinary approach.* Philadelphia: Lippincott, 1984, pp. 85-114.

Soskis, D.A. *Teaching self-hypnosis: An introductory guide for clinicians.* New York: Norton, 1986.

Spanos, N.P. & McPeake, J.D. Everyday imaginative activities on hypnotic susceptibility. *Am. J. Clin. Hypn.*, 1975, *17*, 245-252.

Sperry, R.W. Lateral specialization of cerebral function in the surgically separated hemispheres. In F.J. McGuigan & R.A. Schoonover (Eds.), *The psychophysiology of thinking.* New York: Academic Press, 1973, pp. 209-229.

Spiegel, D. Vietnam grief work using hypnosis. *Am. J. Clin. Hypn.*, 1981, *24*, 33-40.

Spiegel, D. Hypnosis with psychotic patients: Comment on Scagnelli-Jobsis. *Am. J. Clin. Hypn.*, 1983, *25*, 298-294.

Stampfl, T.G. Implosive therapy: The theory, the subhuman analog, the strategy, and the technique. Part I: The theory. In S.G. Armitage (Ed.), *Behavior modification techniques in the treatment of emotional disorders.* Battle Creek, Mich.: V.A. Publication, 1967.

State v. Harris, 214 Or. 224, 405 P. 2d. 492 (1965). Pg. 69.

State v. Hurd, 86 N.J. 525, 432 A 2d. 86 (1981). pp. 55, 85, 86, 87, 97.

State v. Iwakiri, 682 P. 2d 571 at 577-578 (Idaho 1984).

State v. White, J-3665 (Cir. Ct., Branch 10, Milwaukee Co., Wisc., March 27, 1979; unrep).

Stein, C. Trance, transference and countertransference in the resistive patient. *Am. J. Clin. Hypn.*, 1970, *12*, 213-221.

Stekel, W. *Sadism & masochism, (Vols 1 & 2).* New York: Liveright, 1939a.

Stekel, W. *Impotence in the male, (Vols. 1 & 2)* New York: Liveright, 1939b

Stekel, W. *Sexual aberrations, (Vols. 1 & 2).* New York: Liveright, 1940.

Stekel, W. *Frigidity in women. (Vols. 1 & 2).* New York: Liveright, 1943a.

Stekel, W. *Peculiarities of behavior. (Vols. 1 & 2).* New York: Liveright, 1943b.

Stekel, W. *The interpretation of dreams. (Vols. 1 & 2)* New York: Liveright, 1943c.

Stekel, W. *Compulsion and doubt. (Vols. 1 & 2).* New York: Liveright, 1949.

Stern, M.M. Art therapy. In G. Bychowski & J.L. Despert (Eds.), *Specialized techniques in psychotherapy.* New York: Grune & Stratton, 1952.

Stillerman, B. The management in analytic hypnotherapy of the psychodynamic reaction to the induction of hypnosis. *J. of Clin. & Exp. Hypn.* 1957, *5,* 3-11.

Tart, C.T. A comparison of suggested dreams occurring in hypnosis and sleep. *Int. J. Clin. Exp. Hypn.*, 1964, *12,* 263-289.

Tart, C.T. The hypnotic dream: Methodological problems and a review of the literature. *Psychol. Bull.*, 1965, *63,* 87-99.

Teasdale, J.D. & Fogarty, F.J. Differential effects of induced mood on retrieval of pleasant and unpleasant events from episodic memory. *J. of Abn. Psychol.*, 1979, *88,* 248-257.

Thigpen, C.H. & Cleckley, H.M. *Three faces of Eve.* New York: McGraw-Hill, 1957.

Thorne, F.C. *Principles of personality counseling.* Brandon, Vermont: J. of Clin. Psychol., 1950.

Tillich, P. *The courage to be.* New Haven: Yale Univ. Press. 1952.

Tillich, P. Existentialism, psychotherapy and the nature of man. *Pastoral Psychol.*, 1960, *11*, 10-18.

Trussell, M.A. The diagnostic value of the verbal summator. *J. Abn. Soc. Psychol.*, 1939, *34*, 533-538.

Udolf, R. *Forensic hypnosis: Psychological and legal aspects.* Lexington, Mass.: D.C. Heath, 1983.

Ullman, M. & Zimmerman, N. *Working with dreams.* New York: Delacorte/Eleanor Friede, 1979.

Vogel, G., Foulkes, D. & Trosman, H. Ego functions and dreaming during sleep onset. In C.T. Tart (Ed.), *Altered states of consciousness.* New York: Wiley, 1969, pp. 75-91.

Wadeson, H. *Art Psychotherapy.* New York: Wiley, 1980.

Wadeson, H. Art therapy. In L.E. Abt & I.R. Stuart (Eds.), *The newer therapies: A source book.* New York: Van Nostrand Reinhold, 1982.

Walker, P.C. The hypnotic dream: A reconceptualiztion. *Am. J. Clin. Hypn.*, 1984, *16*, 246-255.

Watkins, H.H. Ego-state therapy. Chap. 22 in J.G. Watkins (Ed.), *The therapeutic self.* New York: Human Sciences Press, 1978. (See also: Chapters 5, 9, 10, 12, 14, & 23.)

Watkins, H.H. The silent abreaction. *Int. J. Clin. Exp. Hypn.*, 1980, *28*, 101-113.

Watkins, J.G. The hypnoanalytic location of a lost object. *J. of Clin. Psychol.*, 1946, *2*, 390-394.

Watkins, J.G. *Hypnotherapy of war neuroses.* New York: Ronald Press, 1949.

Watkins, J.G. Poison-pen therapy, *Am. J. Psychotherapy.* 1949a, *3*, 410-418.

Watkins, J.G. Projective hypnoanalysis. Chap. 19 in L.M. LeCron (Ed.), *Experimental hypnosis.* New York: Macmillan, 1952, pp. 442-462.

Watkins, J.G. Trance and transference. *J. Clin. & Exp. Hypn.*, 1954, 2, 284-290.

Watkins, J.G. *General psychotherapy: An outline and study guide.* (with an Introduction by Lewis M. Wolberg), Springfield, Ill.:, Thomas, 1960.

Watkins, J.G. El puente afectivo: Una tecnica hipnoanalitica. (Translated by Marcelo Lerner). *Acta Hypnologica Latinoamericana.*, 1961, 2, 323-329.

Watkins, J.G. Transference aspects of the hypnotic relationship. In M.V. Kline (Ed.), *Clinical correlations of experimental hypnosis.* Springfield, Ill.: Thomas, 1963.

Watkins, J.G. Symposium on posthypnotic amnesia: Discussion. *Int. J. of Clin. & Exp. Hypn.*, 1966, *XIV*, 139-149

Watkins, J.G. Hypnosis and consciousness from the viewpoint of existentialism. Chap. III in M.V. Kline (Ed.), *Psychodynamics and hypnosis.* Springfield, Ill., Thomas, 1967a. pp. 15-31.

Watkins, J.G. Operant approaches to existential therapy. (Unpublished address. Presented at the Internat. Congress for Psychosomatic Medicine and Hypnosis, Kyoto, Japan, July 12th), 1967b..)

Watkins, J.G. The affect bridge: A hypnonalytic technique. *Int. J. Clin. & Exp. Hypn.*, 1971, *19*, 21-27.

Watkins, J.G. Ego states and the problem of responsibility: A psychological analysis of the Patty Hearst case. *J. of Psychiat. & Law, Winter*, 1976, pp. 471-489.

Watkins, J.G. *The therapeutic self.* New York: Human Sciences Press, 1978.

Watkins, J.G. The Bianchi (L.A."Hillside Strangler") case: Sociopath or multiple personality? *Int. J. Clin. & Exp. Hypn.*, 1984, *32*, 67-111.

Watkins, J.G. *Clinical hypnosis: Vol. 1. Hypnotherapeutic technique.* New York: Irvington, 1987.

Watkins, J.G. Hypnotic hypermnesia and forensic hypnosis: a cross-examination. *Am. J. Clin. Hypn.*, 1989, *32*, 71-83.

Watkins, J.G. & Johnson, R.J. *We, the divided self.* New York: Irvington, 1982.

Watkins, J.G. & Watkins, H.H. *Abreactive technique.* (audio tape). New York: Psychotherapy Tape Library, 1978.

Watkins, J.G. & Watkins, H.H. The theory and practice of ego-state therapy. In H. Grayson (Ed.), *Short term approaches to psychotherapy.* New York: Human Sciences Press, 1979, pp. 176-220.

Watkins, J.G. & Watkins, H.H. Ego states and hidden observers. *J. of Altered States of Consciousness,* 1979-1980, *5,* 3-18.

Watkins, J.G. & Watkins, H.H. *I. Ego states and hidden observers. II. Ego-state therapy: The woman in black and the lady in white.* (Audio tape and transcript), New York: Jeffrey Norton, 1980.

Watkins, J.G. & Watkins, H.H. Ego-state therapy. In R.J. Corsini, (Ed.), *Handbook of innovative psychotherapies.* New York: Wiley, 1981, pp. 252-270.

Watkins, J.G. & Watkins, H.H. Ego-state therapy. In L.E. Abt & I.R. Stuart (Eds.), *The newer therapies: A source book.* New York: Van Nostrand Reinhold, 1982, pp. 137-155.

Watkins, J.G. & Watkins, H.H. Hazards to the therapist in treating multiple personality disorders. *Psychiatric Clinics of North America.* 1984, *7*, 111-119.

Watkins, J.G. & Watkins, H.H. Hypnosis, multiple personality and ego states as altered states of consciousness. In B.W. Wolman & M. Ullman (Eds.), *Handbook of states of consciousness*. New York: Van Nostrand Reinhold, 1986.

Watkins, J.G. & Watkins, H.H. The management of malevolent ego states. *Dissociation*, 1988, *1*, 67-72.

Watkins, J.G. & Watkins, H.H. Ego-state transferences in the treatment of dissociative reactions. In M.L. Fass & D. Brown (Eds.), *Creative mastery in hypnosis and hypnoanalysis: A festschrift for Erika Fromm*. Hillsdale, N.J. Lawrence Erlbaum, 1990, pp. 255-261.

Weiss, E. *The structure and dynamics of the human mind*. New York: Grune & Stratton, 1960.

West, L.J. Psychopathology produced by sleep deprivation. In S.S. Kety, E.V. Evarts & H.L. Williams (Eds.), *Sleep and altered states of consciousness*. Baltimore: Williams & Wilkins, 1967.

Wilbur, C.B. Multiple personality disorder and transference. *Dissociation.*, 1988, *1*, 73-76.

Winicott, D.W. *The maturational processes and the facilitating environment*. New York: Internat. Univ. Press, 1965.

Wolberg, L.R. *Hypnoanalysis*. New York: Grune & Stratton, 1945.

Wolberg, L.R. *Medical hypnosis: Vol. I. Principles of hypnotherapy: Vol. II. Practice of hypnotherapy*. New York: Grune & Stratton, 1948.

Wolman, M.M. (Ed.). *Handbook of dreams: Research, theories and applications*. New York: Van Nostrand Reinhold, 1979.

Woods, R.L. *The world of dreams*. New York: Random House, 1947.

Woods, R.L. & Greenhouse, H.B. *The new world of dreams*. New York: Macmillan, 1974.

Wright, M.E. (With Beatrice A. Wright). *Clinical practice of hypnotherapy*. New York: Guilford Press, 1987.

Subject Index

handwriting, 45, 80, 91, 123, 127-
130, 133-139, 153, 156-158, 185
hallucinated, 158-160
rage (anger), 72, 172, 186
techniques, 114, 175
Dissociation, 64, 155-187, 198, 231, 232,
233, 234
treatment of, 160-186
amnesia, 161-170
multiple personality, 170-185
Don Juan, 14, 28
Doodle, 89-97, 98, 130
Double hallucination test, 267, 274
Drama (socio) spontaneous, 123
Draw-a-Person test, 79
Drawings, 7, 9, 97
Dream (s), 16, 78, 79, 101-120, 125, 152,
209
analysis (interpretation), xi, 4, 8, 86,
106, 111, 153, 231, 241, 248
under hypnosis, 114-117
intuitive approach to, 107, 110,
111, 119
steps in, 107-111
day dreams, 21
first, 110
drive theory (model) of, ix, 191
hypnotic and normal (sleep), 16, 104,
117, 119, 132
inducing, 113, 118
physiological basis of, 104-105, 120
psychoanalytic theory of, 105-106
like psychosis, 16
research in, 106
resolution after insight, 149, 159
transference, 237
work, 105
drive theory of, ix,
hypnotic and normal (sleep), 16, 104
interpretation, xi, 4
like psychosis, 16
psychoanalytic theory of, 105-106
research, 106
steps in, 107-111
work, 105
Drug addiction, vii
DSM IIIR, (Diagnostic and Statistical
Manual), 170
Ego(s), 158, 168, 190
body ego,
boundary, 178, 195, 197, 198, 245,
245, 246, 248, 280, 282
by-passing of x, 3, 6, 11
cathexis (energy), 194, 195, 226, 247,
246, 293, 294
defenses, ix, 10

economy, 287
egotize (egotization), 10, 11, 54
factory, 6, 7
in hypnosis, 60, 118, 234
integration, 242
overwhelmed, 15
participation, 5-7
protection, 27
psychology, ix, 10
self representation, 74, 106, 190-192,
195, 201, 202, 226, 234, 238, 244,
246, 247, 249, 252
state, 25, 123, 124, 175, 176, 186,
196, 197, 224, 260
activation of, 203
characteristics of, 200, 226
child, 208, 210
conflicts, 205
covert, 203
destructive, 204
executive, 197, 282
origin of, 226
parental, 205, 206
therapy (therapist), 160, 189-
226, 201-202
as group and family therapy,
204-205
hypnosis in, 203-204, 226
of therapist, 8, 72, 289
strength, (strengthening), 52, 55, 65,
67, 74, 249
Eigenwelt, 279, 292
Elderly, treatment of, 73
Emotion (emotional)
catharsis, 75
corrective experience, 64
discharge of, 51
release of, 53, 57, 71, 72
re-living 53
Empathy (See also Resonance), 249
accurate, 282
Estrangement, 246
Experience (experiential), 37, 38, 57
co-experience, 74
corrective emotional, 75, 90
organize, 42
Expert witness, 270-271
Eye movements, rapid (REM), 104, 119
Existential
analysis, 280
hypnoanalysis, xii, 37, 246, 277-281,
294
philosophers, 278
Fantasy, 16, 31, 258
erotic, 19, 21
induction, 29

Hypermnesia)
    as regression (See also Regression), 14, 261
    relationship, 14, 19, 20, 29, 232, 235, 259, 279, 294
    self-hypnosis, 60, 118, 234, 249
    simulation of, 261
    stage hypnosis, 254
    state, 9, 13, 14, 20, 27, 232, 242
    susceptibility (suggestibility), 22
    termination of, 26, 27, 29
    theories of, 231
        re-evaluation by psychoanalysts, 4
    training in, 291, 292
        advanced
    visualization, 248
Hypnotist,
    influence, 3
Hypnotizability (See also, Susceptibility), 22, 102, 243
Hysteria (hysterical), ix, 49
    conversion, 161, 202, 278
    tremor
Id, ix, 16, 245
Ideomotor,
    finger signal, 45-46, 47
Identification, 195, 197, 226, 282, 293
    with therapist, 8, 195
Indetofact, 195, 226, 234, 285
Imagination, 102
Image (Imagery), 77, 78, 79, 119, 229
Impressionism, 78
In-and-out technique, 35-36, 46
Indeterminancy, Principle of, 101
Induction, Hypnotic (see Hypnotic induction)
Insanity defense, 261
Insight, 78, 82, 88, 102, 153, 280
    achieving, 4, 11
    cognitive, 53
    effective, 10
    experiential, 180, 215
    intellectual, 2, 10, 150, 265
    in hypnoanalytic therapy, 1
    resolution of neurotic dreams, 149, 159
    true (genuine) 2, 9, 11, 39, 78, 85, 243, 265
    unconscious (covert) 97, 99
Insomnia 205, 224
Integration, x, 73, 173, 177, 182-183, 185, 280
    vs. fusion, 175, 181, 187
Internal self helper (ISH), 173
International, 290, 293, 294

Interpretation, 53, 57, 73, 74, 75, 84, 88, 204, 243
    of induction, 20, 182
    intellectual, 237
    of transference, 227, 233
Interview,
    case history, 34, 43, 47
Introjection, 195, 196, 197, 201, 213, 215, 226, 229, 231, 134, 288, 289, 294
    of analyst, 244, 285
    of drama, 229
Jung (Jungian), 86, 115, 119, 153
    Verbal Association Test, 161
Labor-management conflict, 290
Levitation, arm, (see Hand levitation, Hypnotic induction, also Susceptibility tests).
Libido (See also Cathexis)
    ego, 194
    narcissistic, 194
    object, 194
Life space, comceptions of, 42
Lost object, locating, 266
Madonnas, 79
Make-a-Picutre-Story Test (MAPS), 122
Malpractice, 255
Manslaughter, 263
Meaning, 17, 47, 57, 88
    as behavior, 280
    experiential, 9
    of hypnosis, 5, 28, 29, 31
    of interpersonal interaction 13
    in life, xiii, 278, 287, 292
    psychodynamic, 84
    symbolic, 84, 91
Memory (memories), 38, 42, 60, 229, 230, 248, 253, 254, 265
    accuracy, 268
    birth, 43
    contaminations of, 255, 258, 261, 268
    distortions in, 264, 265
    enhancement (refreshing), 255, 256, 273, 274
    frozen, 65
    pseudo, 46
    recovery of, x, 63
    reconstructrion of, 258
    review of literature, 259
    screen, x
    self-serving 259
    veridical, 9, 46
Metaphor, 78
Minnesota Multiphasic Personality Inventory, 56
Mitwelt, 279, 292

Smoking, 202
Society for Clinical and Experimental Hypnosis (SCEH), 272
Sociopath, 285
Socratic qu3ewstioning, 167
Sodium amytal, 51, 56, 57, 161
Sodium pentothal, 51, 57
Somatic bridge, 62
Souls, lack of, 278
Sports,
   psycholocy, vii
   hypnosis (See Hypnosis)
Springfield rifle, 4,
Stage hypnosis, 254
State (See Ego, state and Hypnotic state)
Stress, 162, 175, 185
Stroop Color Word Test, 268
Stuttering, viii,
Study habits, viii, 202
Subject-object, 189, 225, 234, 266
   relationship, 290
   technique, 77, 196
Subliminal, 105
Suggestibility tests (see Hypnotic suscep-
   tibility, and Hypnotizability)
Suicide, 68, 72, 172, 174, 175, 176, 184, 186, 249
Supreme Court
   California, 258
   Colorado, 259
   Idaho, 259
   New Jersey, 257
   U.S., 255, 259
Surgery, vii
Symbiotic relationship, 245
Symbol (symbolic) 85, 104
   communication, 97, 146, 153
   conventional, 86
   individual, 86
   non-verbal, 89
   para-logic, 109
   penis, 109
   representational, 86
   sexual, 86
   of the unconscious, 145
Symbolic Realization, 89
Tautophone, 133, 153
Teachers, 290
Tests of lhypnotic susceptibility (See Hyp-
   notic susceptibility)
Tests, psychological, 56, 122
Thematic Apperception Test (TAT), 104, 122, 124-126, 153
Theories of hypnosis (See Hypnosis, theo-
   ries of)
Therapeutic self, xii, 185, 277, 281-293

Therapy, (therapist)
   art, 79
   behavior, viii, 33, 283
   bridge, 283
   client-centered, 2, 32, 280
   cognitive, viii, 1, 102, 283
   doodle, 89-97
   existential, 279
   genuine change in, 8,
   hazzards (dangers) to, 172, 184, 187, 240
   goal of, 230
   gestalt, 24
   humanistic, 53, 279
   LSD, 79
   poison-pen, 67-68, 75, 76, 180
   psychoanalytic (See psychoanalysis)
   release, 49
   reconstructive, viii, 1
   self, 289, 291, 292, 293
   self control of, 71
   stress on, 185
   suggestive, 10
Third ear, 22, 33, 89, 109, 195, 290
Training in hypnosis (see Hypnosis, training in)
Trance, hypnotic (see also Hypnosis)
   deep (depth of), 3, 7, 10, 18, 32, 56, 103, 104, 236
   entering, 14, 19
   induction (See also Hypnotic induction), 18
   interviewing under, 33, 45
   intermediate, 3, 7
   optimal, 8, 11
   plenary, 3, 29, 112
   somnambulistic, 112
Trance logic, 267
Transactional analysis, 24, 202
Transference, 15, 17, 21-22, 74, 122, 150, 156, 227-252
   activation of, 10
   analysis of, xi, 4, 231, 238
   counter-transference, 9, 232, 233, 235, 236, 237, 240, 246, 252, 280, 283, 284
   corrective experience within, 64
   dream, 237
   headache, 229
   in hypnoanalysis, 239
   in hypnosis, 241-243
   interpretation, x, 182, 227, 234, 236, 238, 249
   love, 230, 240
   managing (manipulating), 234, 239, 241

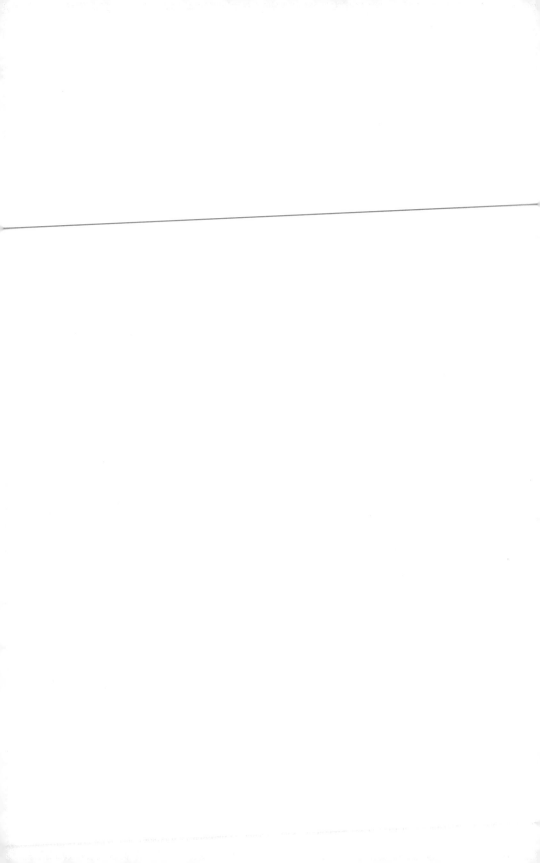

Index of Names

Abt, L.E., 318, 320
Adler, A., 106, 192, 295
Adler, G., 115, 295
Alexander, F., 64, 90, 283, 295
Allison, R.B., 173, 295
Alvarez, W.C., viii, 295
American Psychiatric Association, 170, 174, 295
Armitage, S.G., 316
Ås, A., 378, 295
Baker, E.L., 106, 243, 244, 247, 280, 295, 296
Barber, T.X., 16, 38, 104, 296
Barnett, E.A., 296
Baskin, W., 260, 296
Beahrs, J.O., 171, 244, 296
Beaumont, J.G., 307
Beck, A., viii, 102, 296
Bellak, L., 14, 296
Bennett, A.K., ix, 123, 298
Berkeley, G., 279, 296
Berkowitz, L., 53, 296
Berne, E., 202, 296
Bernheim, H., 254, 296
Biddle, W.E., 244, 297
Blanck, G., 3, 196, 297
Blanck, R., 3, 196, 297
Bliss, E.L., 171, 297
Blum, G.S., 267, 268, 297
Boor, M. 171, 297
Bower, G.H., 63, 64, 297
Bowers, K.S., 258, 269
Bowers, J.K., 245, 250, 297
Braun, B.G., 171, 297

Brenman, M., viii, xi, 14, 15, 111, 123, 232, 233, 234, 297, 302
Breuer, J., xi, 49, 238, 302
Brown, D.P., 52, 68, 69, 248, 297, 298, 321
Brown, W., 51, 298
Buber, M., 278, 298
Buck, J.M., 79, 298
Bugental, J.F.T., 279, 298
Burrows, G.D., 307
Burton, A., 279, 298
Bychowski, G., 317
Calkins, M.W., 296
Cameron, J., 283
Cautela, J.R., ix, 123, 298
Chappel, V.C., 304
Cheek, D.B., 43, 45, 46, 91, 159, 203, 266, 298, 313
Christopher, M., 160, 298
Cleckley, H.M., 170, 317
Comstock, C., 73, 182, 298
Conn, J.H., 6, 254, 298, 299
Coons, P.M., 171, 296
Cooper, L.M., 38, 299
Copeland, D.R., 14, 245, 280, 299
Corsini, R.J., 307, 320
Coué, E., viii, 299
Crawford, H.J., 102, 299
Debussy, C., 78
Degas, E., 78
Déjerine, J., viii, 299
Dement, W.C., 104, 299
Dempster, C.R., 235, 307
Dennerstein, L., 307
Despert, J.L., 317

333

The Wisdom of Milton H. Erickson
Volume 1, Hypnosis & Hypnotherapy

Ronald A. Havens, Editor

The psychiatrist Milton Erickson was a master hypnotist, capable of inducing trances by the most unexpected means—even a mere handshake. Erickson also published numerous books, articles, transcripts, and audiotapes. Erickson's books have sold more than 250,000 copies. *The Wisdom of Milton H. Erickson I: Hypnosis and Hypnotherapy* is the first work to provide a unified survey of the philosophy behind Erickson's techniques.

The material in this volume has been selected from the psychiatrist's lectures, seminars, articles, and books and is carefully organized to offer a clear account of how Erickson conceived of hypnosis, particularly its access to the unconscious and its role in the process of psychotherapy. The reader discovers what hypnosis actually does, explores general considerations on inducing the state, learns specific techniques, and most importantly, comes to understand the contribution that hypnosis can make in the healing or therapeutic process. *The Wisdom of Milton H. Erickson I: Hypnosis and Hypnotherapy* is a valuable guide to the work of one of psychiatry's most original and innovative minds.

...a heroic effort to bring clarity to a hard-to-grasp theory...(This book) is a major reference for students and scholars who want to know what Erickson said and when and where he said it.

Contemporary Psychology

ISBN 0-8290-2413-1 (Paper)
298 pages
$14.95

IRVINGTON PUBLISHERS, INC.
740 Broadway, New York, NY 10003

MC/Visa orders may be telephoned to (603) 669-5933.

The Wisdom of Milton H. Erickson
Volume 2, Human Behavior & Psychotherapy

Ronald A. Havens, Editor

Milton H. Erickson was one of the most creative, dynamic, and effective hypnotherapists and psychotherapists of the twentieth century. Erickson's books have sold more than 250,000 copies. He used unconventional techniques with remarkable success. An indication of the respect Erickson gained from his peers are the words inscribed on his 1976 Benjamin Franklin Gold Medal, the highest award that the International Society of Clinical and Experimental Hypnosis can bestow: "To Milton H. Erickson, M.D.—innovator, outstanding clinician, and distinguished investigator whose ideas have not only helped create the modern view of hypnosis but have profoundly influenced the practice of all psychotherapy throughout the world."

Although he wrote hundreds of papers, articles, and books in his lifetime, Erickson himself never put his techniques and methods into a clear and centralized body of work. *The Wisdom of Milton H. Erickson, II: Human Behavior and Psychotherapy* is an effort to do just that. Along with its companion volume, *The Wisdom of Milton H. Erickson I: Hypnosis and Hypnotherapy*, this book is a collection of Erickson's methods and lessons, including his feelings on the uses of objective observation, the uniqueness of the conscious mind, the realities and abilities of the unconscious mind, the creation and use of a therapeutic environment, and many other aspects of the life and work of this remarkable thinker and teacher.

...a heroic effort to bring clarity to a hard-to-grasp theory...(This book) is a major reference for students and scholars who want to know what Erickson said and when and where he said it.

Contemporary Psychology

ISBN 0-8290-2414-X (Paper)
258 pages
$14.95

IRVINGTON PUBLISHERS, INC.
740 Broadway, New York, NY 10003

MC/Visa orders may be telephoned to (603) 669-5933.